Treatment of Neurodevelopmental Disorders

TREATMENT OF NEURODEVELOPMENTAL DISORDERS

Targeting Neurobiological Mechanisms

Edited by

Randi Jenssen Hagerman, MD

Distinguished Professor of Pediatrics
Endowed Chair in Fragile X Research
Medical Director of the MIND Institute
Sacramento, California

and

Robert L. Hendren, DO

Professor and Vice Chair
Director, Child and Adolescent Psychiatry
University of California, San Francisco
San Francisco, California

OXFORD
UNIVERSITY PRESS

OXFORD
UNIVERSITY PRESS

Oxford University Press is a department of the University of
Oxford. It furthers the University's objective of excellence in research,
scholarship, and education by publishing worldwide.

Oxford   New York
Auckland   Cape Town   Dar es Salaam   Hong Kong   Karachi
Kuala Lumpur   Madrid   Melbourne   Mexico City   Nairobi
New Delhi   Shanghai   Taipei   Toronto

With offices in
Argentina   Austria   Brazil   Chile   Czech Republic   France   Greece
Guatemala   Hungary   Italy   Japan   Poland   Portugal   Singapore
South Korea   Switzerland   Thailand   Turkey   Ukraine   Vietnam

Oxford is a registered trademark of Oxford University Press
in the UK and certain other countries.

Published in the United States of America by
Oxford University Press
198 Madison Avenue, New York, NY 10016

Library of Congress Cataloging-in-Publication Data
Treatment of neurodevelopmental disorders: targeting neurobiological mechanisms / edited by Randi
Jenssen Hagerman and Robert L. Hendren.
     p. ; cm.
Includes bibliographical references.
ISBN 978-0-19-993780-6 (alk. paper)
I. Hagerman, Randi Jenssen, 1949– editor of compilation.   II. Hendren, Robert L., 1949– editor of
compilation.
[DNLM: 1. Nervous System Diseases—pathology.   2. Nervous System Diseases—
therapy.   3. Child.   4. Developmental Disabilities—therapy.   5. Mental Disorders—
pathology.   6. Mental Disorders—therapy. WS 340]
RJ486.6
618.92'80475—dc23
2013045533

9 8 7 6 5 4 3 2 1
Printed in the United States of America
on acid-free paper

CONTENTS

FOREWORD

The science of psychiatry, especially child psychiatry, is in a period of radical change. After decades of focusing exclusively on the psychological and behavioral aspects of development, research in this field now incorporates genomics, neuroimaging, cognitive science, and a range of more distant disciplines. Increasingly behavioral disorders are being addressed as neurodevelopmental disorders, with symptoms best understood in the context of the trajectory of brain development.

This approach is only now becoming feasible as we are getting the tools to study human brain development. The recent results of these studies are stunning. The patterns of gene expression in the developing brain are profoundly different from the expression profiles of the adult brain, with as many as 80% of genes processed differently during fetal brain development. (http://www.brainspan.org) Indeed, the profile of gene expression in the human fetal brain is so different from the postnatal brain, one might consider the fetal brain a different organ altogether. But even the rules for post-natal brain development are extraordinary. In contrast to other organ systems, the brain develops, in part, through the exuberant over-production of cells and connections, followed by a several year sculpting of pathways by massive elimination of much of the neural architecture along with myelination of select fibers for rapid transmission of information. We now know the human brain continues to develop into the third decade, with cortical maturation usually not completed until age 25.

What does this mean for researchers, clinicians, and concerned family members? This prolonged period of brain development provides a critical template for understanding the emergence of behavioral and cognitive symptoms. Why do the symptoms of autism emerge at 18 months while the psychosis of schizophrenia emerges at 18 years? Why are boys more likely to be affected by some neurodevelopmental disorders, such as autism and ADHD? Why do adults with mood disorders often have a history of anxiety disorders in childhood? Developmental neuroscience can begin to address these issues by defining the age-specific changes in brain development, specifically changes in circuits, as a basis for the emergence of symptoms and vulnerabilities.

In truth, this extraordinary period for developmental neuroscience has not been fully translated to alter our diagnosis or treatment of neurodevelopmental disorders. Part of the problem is that we do not know enough. We know that our symptom-based diagnoses are highly heterogeneous, but biomarkers or cognitive tests have yet to provide greater specificity except for those rare Mendelian disorders linked to a single gene. Even for those syndromes where we have identified the genetic basis, bridging from a genetic mutation to a treatment target remains a work in progress. And although we know that refining diagnosis is often a critical step to developing more precise treatments, we are just at the beginning of the long process to graduate our nosology beyond symptom-based diagnosis.

Although we don't know enough, this book demonstrates that the state of our knowledge has advanced considerably and that already, the science of neurodevelopmental disorders can inform the diagnosis and treatment of infants and children. Insights from research on rare syndromes, such as Rett syndrome and Fragile X syndrome, are proving to be useful for our understanding of many aspects of idiopathic autism. And new information from longitudinal neuroimaging studies suggests that we can begin to reframe some attentional disorders as delays in cortical maturation. This volume provides an accessible overview of the state of the art and demonstrates how today's knowledge can improve today's practice.

Clinicians and family members need to appreciate that the tools are improving rapidly and that much of what passes for knowledge today may look overly simplistic or entirely wrong as we get more information. Two recent discoveries remind us we are still at the beginning of a long, surprising journey. Recent studies have revealed genomic variation that is found only in specific brain cells, variation that would not have been suspected from sequencing the DNA in blood. And epigenetics, one way by which nurture alters nature, appears to follow different rules in the brain compared to other organ systems. These new, surprising insights reflect the nature of science – knowledge is iterative and often counterintuitive.

This book represents a milestone in this fascinating journey to understand neurodevelopmental disorders. The next phase will likely be influenced heavily by new technologies. Mapping the changing connections across brain development, the "developmental connectome", will almost certainly give us new insights about neurodevelopmental disorders. Biomarkers for early detection should enable preemptive interventions.

New sensors to monitor the fetal and postnatal environment may finally shed light on causes, enabling prevention. And new intervention technologies from social prosthetics to electroceuticals to targeted cognitive training may offer a rich new range of options for helping children at risk.

But beyond the technologies, the next phase for understanding neurodevelopmental disorders will need to create a new relationship between researchers, clinicians, and families. In the past, translating research to practice has been a major barrier, with estimates of 17 years for many scientific discoveries to be adopted into practice. In the future, progress may be accelerated by moving practice into research; ensuring that clinicians and families partner with researchers in the quest to understand neurodevelopmental disorders. This partnership has already proven effective for cystic fibrosis and childhood cancers.

Now is the time for providers and families who have the greatest stake in progress to become part of the research enterprise for neurodevelopmental disorders. This volume, by translating recent research for a broad audience, provides a roadmap for many such opportunities. Its success will be measured, in part, by how this translation improves current practice. But its promise is also that clinicians and families can become part of the scientific process. By creating registries, supporting research, and even developing clinical trials, they can drive the engine of scientific progress, ensuring the most rapid development of diagnostic biomarkers, preventive interventions, and ultimately cures. For families challenged by a neurodevelopmental disorder, there is no time to waste.

Thomas R. Insel, MD,
National Institute of Mental Health,
Bethesda, MD

PREFACE

This is an extraordinarily exciting time in neuroscience research and treatment. The advances in molecular biology and animal models of most neurodevelopmental disorders have led to the development of targeted treatments that in many cases can reverse the neurobiological abnormalities in animal models. These advances are now being translated into the treatment of patients with neurodevelopmental disorders. This book describes the highlights of these advances for several disorders. Although significant progress has been made, particularly for single gene disorders, the details for how to utilize this knowledge of shared neurodevelopmental mechanisms has not been summarized in one place for the practicing clinician. This book will fill that gap by providing the theoretical underpinnings of the neurodevelopmental model and then describe the disorders where this model can be used to guide evaluation and treatment. This book will stimulate further research in targeted treatments, explain their implications and applications in clinical practice, and demonstrate a new understanding of how neurodevelopmental disorders can be treated.

To illustrate how the advances in targeted treatments are based on a neurobiological understanding of the molecular pathology, thirteen chapters on neurodevelopmental disorders (ND) including single gene disorders, such as fragile X syndrome, tuberous sclerosis, Rett syndrome, Rasopathies (RAS) pathway disorders, Angelman syndrome and phenylketonuria (PKU), and complex genetic disorders, including Down syndrome, schizophrenia, attention-deficit hyperactivity disorder, depression, and autism spectrum disorders, are included in this book. In the single gene disorders, researchers have been more successful in identifying the underlying molecular etiology and targeting treatment than with complex genetic disorders, but the five chapters covering these complex genetic disorders demonstrate how far we have come. Each chapter will describe the relevant research underlying the molecular dysregulation and explore the treatments that have the potential to reverse these problems. For each of these disorders, the evaluation and treatment requires a multimodality approach, including a comprehensive biomedical assessment useful in planning targeted treatments ranging from pharmacological agents and nutritional supplements to cognitive, behavioral, and psychotherapeutic interventions.

We hope that reading this book will make it possible for the pediatrician, geneticist, neurologist, child and adolescent psychiatrist, interested primary care practitioner, educator, and allied therapists to make a neurodevelopmental formulation for each person being evaluated and to better guide the interventions they and the family choose to implement.

Randi Jenssen Hagerman, MD
Distinguished Professor of Pediatrics
Endowed Chair in Fragile X Research
Medical Director of the MIND Institute
University of California Davis Medical Center
Sacramento, California

Robert L. Hendren, DO
Professor and Vice Chair
Director, Child and Adolescent Psychiatry
University of California, San Francisco
San Francisco, California

CONTRIBUTORS

Ruhel Boparai, MD
Department of Psychiatry
University of Kentucky
Kentucky

Khyati Brahmbhatt, MD
Department of Psychiatry and Behavioral Sciences and MIND Institute
University of California Davis School of Medicine
Sacramento, California

Nicole Bush, PhD
Department of Psychiatry
University of California, San Francisco (UCSF) School of Medicine
San Francisco, California

Petrus J. de Vries, MBChB, MRCPsych, PhD
Division of Child and Adolescent Psychiatry
University of Cape Town
Rondebosch
Cape Town, South Africa

Maria Diez-Juan, MS
MIND Institute
University of California at Davis Medical Center
Sacramento, California
Sant Joan de Déu Hospital
Barcelona Spain

Coleman Garrett
Department of Psychiatry
San Francisco VA Medical Center
San Francisco, California

Andre Goldani
Universidade Federal do Rio Grande do Sul
Porto Alegre, Brazil

Randi Jenssen Hagerman, MD
Distinguished Professor of Pediatrics and
Medical Director of the MIND Institute
University of California Davis Medical Center
Sacramento, California

Steven Hamilton, MD, PhD
Department of Psychiatry
University of California, San Francisco (UCSF) School of Medicine
San Francisco, California
Kaiser Permanente Medical Center
San Francisco, California

Jay J. Han, MD
Department of Physical Medicine and Rehabilitation
University of California, Davis Medical Center
Sacramento, California

Emma B. Hare
MIND Institute and Department of Pediatrics
University of California Davis Medical Center
Sacramento, California

Robert L. Hendren, DO
Department of Psychiatry
University of California, San Francisco
UCSF Benioff Children's Hospital
San Francisco, California

Walter E. Kaufmann, MD, PhD
Department of Neurology
Boston Children's Hospital and Harvard Medical School
Boston, Massachusetts

Mary Jacena Leigh, MD
Department of Pediatrics and MIND Institute
University of California Davis Medical Center
Sacramento, California

Daniel Lindqvist, MD, PhD
Department of Psychiatry
University of California, San Francisco (UCSF) School of Medicine
San Francisco, California; and
Department of Psychiatry
Lund University
Lund, Sweden

Bethany M. Lipa, MD
Shriners Hospitals for Children
Philadelphia, Pennsylvania

Reymundo Lozano, MD
MIND Institute and Department of Pediatrics
University of California Davis Medical Center
Sacramento, California

R. Scott Mackin, PhD
Department of Psychiatry
University of California, San Francisco (UCSF) School of Medicine
San Francisco, California

Synthia H. Mellon, PhD
Department of OB-GYN and Reproductive Endocrinology
University of California, San Francisco (UCSF) School of Medicine
San Francisco, California

William C. Mobley, MD, PhD
Department of Neurosciences
University of California, San Diego
La Jolla, California

Billur Moghaddam, MD
Kaiser Permanente Medical Center
Department of Pediatrics, Genetics Division
Sacramento, California

Que T. Nguyen, DO
Department of Physical Medicine and Rehabilitation
University of California, Davis Medical Center
Sacramento, California

Jan Nolta, PhD
Department of Regenerative Medicine
University of California Davis Medical Center
Sacramento, California

Lindsey Partington
Department of Pediatrics and the MIND Institute
University of California Davis Medical Center
Sacramento, California

David Patterson, PhD
Department of Biological Sciences
University of Denver
Denver, Colorado

Katherine A. Rauen, MD, PhD
Department of Pediatrics and the MIND Institute
University of California Davis Medical Center
Sacramento, California

Blake J. Rawdin, MD, PhD
Department of Psychiatry
University of California, San Francisco (UCSF) School of Medicine
San Francisco, California

Victor I. Reus, MD
Department of Psychiatry
University of California, San Francisco (UCSF) School of Medicine
San Francisco, California

Aarti Ruparelia, PhD
Department of Neurosciences
University of California, San Diego
La Jolla, California

Kyle J. Rutledge, PhD
Human Development Graduate Group
University of California, Davis; and
Department of Psychiatry and Behavioral Sciences and MIND Institute
University of California Davis School of Medicine
Sacramento, California

Danielle A. Schlosser, PhD
Department of Psychiatry
University of California, San Francisco (UCSF) School of Medicine
San Francisco, California

Julie B. Schweitzer, PhD
Department of Psychiatry and Behavioral Sciences and MIND Institute
University of California Davis School of Medicine
Sacramento, California

Daniel C. Tarquinio, MS-CL, DO
Department of Neurology
Boston Children's Hospital and Harvard Medical School
Boston, Massachusetts

William E. Tidyman, PhD
Department of Pediatrics
University of California Davis Medical Center
Sacramento, California

Sophia Vinogradov, MD
San Francisco Veterans Administration Medical Center; and
Department of Psychiatry
University of California, San Francisco (UCSF) School of Medicine
San Francisco, California

Edwin Weeber, PhD
Neurobiology of Memory and Learning Laboratory
University of South Florida
Tampa, Florida

Owen M. Wolkowitz, MD
Department of Psychiatry
University of California, San Francisco (UCSF) School of Medicine
San Francisco, California

Treatment of Neurodevelopmental Disorders

CHAPTER 1

Overview of Neurodevelopmental Processes and the Assessment of Patients with Neurodevelopmental Disorders

ROBERT L. HENDREN, ANDRE GOLDANI,
AND RANDI JENSSEN HAGERMAN

INTRODUCTION

We have come a long way in understanding the neurodevelopmental underpinnings of childhood developmental and mental disorders. Yet this knowledge is not regularly woven into our clinical practice as we develop our case formulation leading to the treatment plan. A clinical formulation is a theoretically based explanation or conceptualization of the information obtained from a clinical assessment. It offers a hypothesis about the cause and nature of the presenting problems and is used to develop the treatment plan. This formulation might be behavioral, psychodynamic, familial, cultural, or biomedical. The neurodevelopmental formulation describes the underlying neurodevelopmental processes, from the genetic core to the surface symptoms, and attempts to explain the ongoing process underlying brain/body development in a way that lends itself to biomedical and penetrating psychosocial interventions. These interventions can improve environmental interactions, enhance developmental progression, reverse neurobiological dysfunction, prevent kindling and sensitization (changes in neural substrates from repetition, which increases vulnerability to repeated episodes and may be transmitted genetically), protect through high-risk periods, and promote or create healthy neurodevelopment.

The chapters in this book elucidate a number of pathways, including gamma-aminobutyric acid (GABA) (inhibitory) and glutamate (stimulatory), that show commonalities across several neurodevelopmental disorders so that one targeted treatment may be useful for another disorder if the same pathways are dysfunctional. For instance, a $GABA_A$ agonist is likely to be helpful in fragile X syndrome (Chapter 9) and autism (Chapter 2), but an inverse agonist (antagonist) is likely to be helpful in Down syndrome (Chapter 11). With the advent of whole-exome sequencing (WES) and whole-genome sequencing (WGS), small single nucleotide mutations that are deleterious or copy number variants (CNVs), including duplications and deletions, have been found in up to 50% of individuals with autism spectrum disorder (ASD), with or without intellectual disability (ID) (Jiang et al., 2013; Noh et al., 2013). The identification of these specific mutations allows an understanding of the pathways that are impacted so that some of the targeted treatments that are discussed in this book may be helpful for new mutations, thereby allowing "person-specific treatments." We have also begun to realize that many disorders, including the complex disorders of ASD, depression, schizophrenia, attention-deficit hyperactivity disorders (ADHD), and single gene disorders, may be modified by additional mutations that influence multiple pathways and may add intellectual disability, epilepsy, or other problems to the basic phenotype (Jiang et al., 2013).

DISCUSSION OF KEY ELEMENTS IN NEURODEVELOPMENT

Neurodevelopment is a dynamic and ongoing process beginning shortly after conception and transpiring rapidly in early childhood, continuing throughout adolescence, and slowing in early adulthood before deteriorating in aging. This process is guided by genetic and epigenetic processes whereby genes interact with the environment to form the neurodevelopmental underpinnings of who we are. The following subsections describe basic elements of this process, and these concepts will be used in each chapter throughout the book.

Synaptogenesis refers to the formation of synapses between neurons occurring when the axons and dendrites grow. Synaptogenesis continues throughout life but occurs most rapidly from early in gestation through the first two years of life. During critical periods of growth, neuronal *pruning* occurs, whereby neurons, axons, and synapses compete for neural growth factors in the gray matter, reducing the overall number of neurons and creating more efficient synaptic configurations. The number of neurons increases until adolescence and decreases thereafter, although neurogenesis continues to occur even in aging. Gray matter peaks in the frontal lobes at 12.1 years in males and 11 years in females; in the temporal lobes at 16.5 years in males and 16.7 years in females; and in the parietal/occipital areas there is a linear increase throughout adolescence (Giedd, 2008). Pruning is influenced by environmental factors such as hormones, toxins, and learning.

Myelination is another important process that occurs during neurodevelopment. Myelin is an outgrowth of the oligodendrocyte that forms a layer or sheath and serves as "electrical insulation," typically around only the axon of a neuron. The production of myelin begins in the fourteenth week of fetal development, occurs quickly, and continues through adolescence to young adulthood. Myelin and glial cells are receiving increasing attention in psychiatric disorders such as ASD, schizophrenia, and depression (see Chapters 2, 3, and 4). "Demyelination" refers to the loss of the myelin sheath and is well known to occur in neurodegenerative autoimmune diseases such as multiple sclerosis, the fragile X-associated tremor ataxia syndrome (FXTAS), Guillain-Barré syndrome, and in inherited demyelinating diseases such as leukodystrophy. Demyelination has been suggested to occur in autism as a result of neuroinflammation (see Chapter 2).

Epigenetics is the study of how the environment can influence gene expression and even pass it along through generations without altering the DNA structure. It is a promising field in neurodevelopmental disorders because it elucidates the causal link between environmental factors and the developing disorder. The most studied epigenetic process consists of alterations of the chromatin structure. The two most important mechanisms known to alter chromatin are DNA methylation and histone modification. These alterations can either silence or activate the expression of the genes; they also are potentially reversible and preventable (Boks et al., 2012; Gapp et al., 2012; Kofink et al., 2013). Therefore, elucidating this complex and dynamic process could yield new targets in the treatment of neurodevelopmental disorders. There are many neurodevelopmental disorders associated with methylation changes or epigenetic dysregulation, including Angelman syndrome (Chapter 10), fragile X syndrome (Chapter 9), Rett syndrome (Chapter 6), and Rubinstein-Taybi syndrome (Arrowsmith et al., 2012; LaSalle, 2011). However, how epigenetic dysregulation leads to a clinically significant cognitive or developmental disorder and which environmental factors influence this is a growing area of research (Cortessis et al., 2012; El-Sayed et al., 2013). For instance, the use of topoisomerase inhibitors, including topotecans, have the potential to reverse the silent paternal allele of Ube3a in neurons to compensate for the loss of maternal UBE3a in

Angelman syndrome (Powell et al., 2013; Chapter 10). The use of valproic acid can up-regulate expression of the *FMR1* gene to a minor degree both in normal patients and in those with a mosaic fragile X mutation (Chapter 9). Furthermore, there are other biomedical areas, like oncology, where epigenetic treatment is already becoming a reality for patients—such as the histone deacetylase inhibitors in the treatment of cutaneous T cell lymphoma (Arrowsmith et al., 2012). While epigenetic processes can be used to elucidate the mechanisms of disordered development, as we understand them better, they become treatment targets allowing us to bolster healthy processes and increase the body's resilience.

DNA methylation, a core component of epigenetic processes, is a process in which a methyl group is added to a specific part of the DNA and generally silences expression of the gene if the "promotor" (control region of the DNA that initiates transcription of the gene) is methylated, as in the full mutation of fragile X syndrome (Chapter 9). In mammals it usually takes place at the regions where there are densely clustered cytosine-guanine dinucleotides (CpG), known as CpG islands (CGIs). The CGIs are often located in the promoter regions of genes. This whole process leads to silencing by either of two mechanisms: creation of negative DNA charges that prevents chromatin opening, or recruitment of transcriptional repressors (Gapp et al., 2012; Kofink et al., 2013). Like much of the rest of the study of epigenetics, its relevance to neurodevelopment is still primarily preclinical. However, abnormal methylation provides important direction as to possible etiologies of neurodevelopmental disorders, with implications regarding GABAergic neurons and brain-derived neurotrophic factor (BDNF) expression in schizophrenia, mood disorders (Grayson & Thomas, 2013; Ikegame et al., 2013), fragile X syndrome (Heulens et al., 2011), and premutation disorders (Hagerman & Hagerman, 2013). Also, it seems that some psychoactive drugs, including valproate, can alter DNA methylation (Boks et al., 2012).

GENE–ENVIRONMENT INTERACTION AND ENDOPHENOTYPE

Changes in epigenetic marks, such as DNA methylation and histone acetylation, are associated with a broad range of disease traits, including cancer, asthma, metabolic disorders, and various reproductive conditions. It seems plausible that changes in epigenetic state may be induced by environmental exposures such as malnutrition, tobacco smoke, air pollutants, metals, organic chemicals, other sources of oxidative stress, and the microbiome, particularly if the exposure occurs during critical periods of development.

Thus, epigenetic changes could represent an important pathway by which environmental factors influence disease risk, both within individuals and across generations.

This process of gene–environment interaction and the resulting endophenotype might be viewed schematically as a model in which the layers of the earth represent the expression of the genotype through various layers to the phenotype, the "*terroir* model" of neurodevelopment (Figure 1.1). The surface of the earth represents the personal expression and symptoms we see (phenotype), and the core of the earth represents the genes of that person (genotype). In between is the complex and interactive layering of developmental processes that represent the endophenotype. Interventions targeting the surface at Level 4 might include behavioral interventions, such as applied behavior analysis and the provision of external structure. Levels 3 to 4 can be targeted with occupational therapy, physical therapy, speech and language therapy, and cognitive behavioral therapy. Level 3–targeted interventions include pharmacotherapies, while interventions targeting Level 2 might be a biomedical approach, such as methylation through methylcobalamin or folinic acid; a nutraceutical approach, such as omega 3 fatty acids, or high-dose micronutrients, or antioxidants targeting oxidative stress, inflammation, or immune function. A Level 1 intervention could be one that results in gene modification. None of these interventions targets solely one level. For instance, a behavioral approach

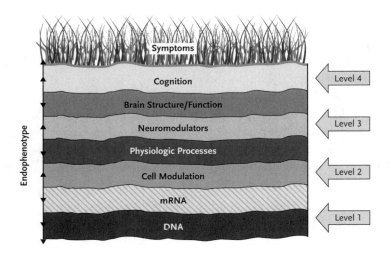

Figure 1.1:
Translating from "*Terroir*" Model
Terroir is a French word that refers to characteristics in the earth and climate that interact with the plant's genetics to impart a unique quality to a product of the plant, such as wine.

might target a symptom seen at Level 1, but the intervention process may "resculpt" neurons. An example is evidenced by the normalization of the electroencephalogram (EEG) in young children with autism who benefit from the Early Start Denver Model of behavioral intervention (Dawson, 2013; see Chapter 2). These level-based interventions will be discussed further in the following paragraph on epigenetic processes, and in each of the chapters.

EPIGENETIC PROCESSES

Immune Etiology of Neurodevelopmental Disorders

Models to explain the immune etiology of neurodevelopmental disorders include direct cause–effect relationships with the immune system and the brain having a common route to shared dysfunction; and the associated but independent adverse responses of the developing brain, the immune system, the endocrine system, and the gastrointestinal (GI) tract (Bilbo & Schwarz, 2012). Inflammatory processes can have both beneficial and deleterious consequences, determined by the magnitude and duration of inflammation. Cell components such as microglia, Kupffer cells (hepatic resident macrophages), and alveolar and testicular macrophages serve critical homeoregulatory functions in tissues and organs in the body (Dietert & Dietert, 2008).

Astrocytes and Microglia

Microglia are the resident macrophages of the brain and spinal cord, and thus act as the first and main form of active immune defense in the central nervous system (CNS) (Lawson et al., 1992). Microglia (and astrocytes) are distributed in large non-overlapping regions throughout the brain and spinal cord (Bushong et al., 2002; Kreutzberg, 1995). They are constantly scavenging the CNS for plaques, damaged neurons, and infectious agents (Gehrmann et al., 1995). Microglial dysfunction results in behavioral defects and is also associated with aging disorders, ASD, Down syndrome, and other disorders (Aguzzi et al., 2013; Siew et al., 2013).

Inflammation

Inflammation is a vital process necessary for tissue recovery, repair, and regeneration (Khansari & Sperlagh, 2012); however, it can be harmful if dysfunctional. In the past few years, more evidence has accumulated linking neurodevelopmental disorders and an inflammatory pathogenesis. Although mainly providing correlational data, subsets of patients with major depressive disorder (MDD) have been reported with higher levels of proinflammatory cytokines (see Chapter 4). Also, chronic inflammatory illnesses are associated with higher rates of depression, and patients administered cytokines are at higher risk for MDD (Khansari & Sperlagh, 2012; Krishnadas & Cavanagh, 2012). Furthermore, abnormal levels of cytokines and infection during intrauterine life are associated with other conditions, such as schizophrenia. The cytokines IL-1, IL-6, and tumor necrosis factor-α (TNFα) can be either neurotropic or toxic, depending on their levels (Muller et al., 2013). In addition, in a pathological condition, microglia (the resident macrophage in the CNS) and astrocytes (providing metabolic support to the neuron) can participate in an inflammatory response within the CNS. Genetic disorders, which affect both astrocytes and neurons, may have the most important influence on CNS dysfunction through the astrocytes. Specific gene knock-in models to astrocytes have demonstrated this for several disorders, including Angelman syndrome (Chapter 10), prion disorders, and fragile X premutation disorders (Chapter 9). The inflammatory explanation may also be based on a permeable blood–brain barrier, with peripheral immune cytokines reaching the CNS: influencing neurotransmission, affecting the HPA-axis, and contributing to even more inflammation, or even altering BDNF and adult neurogenesis (Khansari & Sperlagh, 2012).

MicroRNAs

The molecular landscape is also becoming more complex with the discovery of microRNA (miRNAs)—small sequences of approximately 22 nucleotides from non-coding RNA. The miRNAs are regulatory in that they mediate post-transcriptional gene silencing and impact protein expression by inhibiting mRNA translation or promoting RNA decay (Siew et al., 2013). There are over 2000 miRNAs in the CNS, and besides controlling gene expression, they also control cytokine production and are known to be dysregulated in many disorders, including depression, Down syndrome (Siew et al., 2013), fragile X syndrome (Bagni et al., 2012; Edbauer et al., 2010), *FMR1* premutation involvement (Sellier et al., 2013), ASD, and most likely all neurodevelopmental disorders. Dysregulation of miRNAs leads to many overlapping problems among neurodevelopmental disorders. For example, in Down syndrome, overexpression of miR-155 and miR-802 represses MeCP2 (Siew et al., 2013), the protein that is missing in Rett syndrome and is important for repression of protein expression at different times in development (Chapter 6). miR-155 is overexpressed in both Alzheimer disease and Down syndrome, and this in turn represses complement factor H (CFH), which is an essential repressor of immune function. CFH repression is an important factor leading to more inflammation in both Down syndrome and Alzheimer disease (Siew et al., 2013).

There is still much to learn about this field, more specifically whether inflammation or miRNA dysregulation precipitates, perpetuates, or is a consequence of neurodevelopmental disorders (Khansari & Sperlagh, 2012). But whatever role inflammation may have, it can be clinically significant, ranging from an etiological formulation to a biomarker of disease progression and thus to a treatment option. Therapies based on small interfering RNA (siRNA) and locked nucleic acid (LNAs) hold promise for changing miRNA dysregulation and subsequent inflammation and thereby treating neurodevelopmental disorders (Chapter 14).

Oxidative Stress

Oxidative stress occurs with the intracellular imbalance between pro-oxidative stress and the antioxidant defense mechanisms (ADOS). The former represents the reactive oxygen species (ROS) that are formed during cellular aerobic metabolism. To neutralize them, the ADOS comprise an arsenal that ranges from enzymatic (e.g., superoxide dismutase, catalase, glutathione peroxidase) to nonenzymatic components (e.g., glutathione, methionine) (Frustaci et al., 2012). Therefore, when there is an excess of ROS and/or a lack of ADOS, the intracellular environment is vulnerable to oxidative stress—that is, tissue-damaging effects like peroxidation, DNA and protein damage, and even cell death (de Diego-Otero et al., 2009; Stohs, 1995). Although still an incipient field of study, oxidative stress has already been strongly associated with disorders like bipolar disorder, depression, schizophrenia, Alzheimer disease, fragile X syndrome, fragile X premutation involvement, Down syndrome, and ASD, and most likely, all neurodevelopmental disorders (de Diego-Otero et al., 2009; Hagerman & Hagerman, 2013; Hansen & Obrietan, 2013; Zhang & Yao, 2013). Polymorphisms in oxidative pathway genes, altered antioxidant levels, and enzymatic activity have been associated with severity of symptoms and the psychiatric phase of the disease in neurodevelopmental disorders (Zhang & Yao, 2013). Therefore, an aspect of treatment for neurodevelopmental disorders that has been neglected for most disorders is the use of antioxidants.

Mitochondrial Dysfunction

Like epigenetics, mitochondrial dysfunction is a currently a growing field of neurodevelopmental interest with still much to elucidate. Considered the "power generator" of the cell (Marazziti et al., 2012), this rod-shaped organelle plays a major role in several other key functions of the neuron cell (e.g., amino-acid, lipid, and steroid metabolism; modulation of calcium levels; and production of free radicals; Manji et al., 2012). These functions have a direct influence in generating neurotransmission, plasticity, and cellular resilience to stress (Manji et al., 2012). However, there is still much to learn, given that biomedical evidence that links mitochondrial dysfunction and neurodevelopmental disorders is mainly statistical correlations. More specifically, recent reviews have gathered articles that range from schizophrenia, mood disorders, fragile X syndrome, fragile X premutation disorders, ASD, ADHD, and Alzheimer disease, but in many cases lack a clear disease-provoking mechanism (Marazziti et al., 2012). An exception to this is our understanding of RNA toxicity seen in fragile X premutation cells, where the level of *FMR1*-mRNA is increased over normal levels (Tassone et al., 2000), leading to sequestration of critical proteins for neuronal cell functioning, such as Sam 68, an important splicing protein, and DROSHA and DGCR8, two proteins critical for miRNA maturation (Sellier et al., 2013). This sequestration leads to a significant drop of several miRNA levels (Sellier et al., 2013) and significant dysregulation of frataxin and subsequent mitochondrial deficits (Napoli et al., 2011; Ross-Inta et al., 2010). It is likely that most of the premutation problems seen, including developmental delays and ASD (Kaplan et al., 2012) in some; and chronic fatigue (Summers et al., in press), migraine headaches (Au et al., 2013), restless legs syndrome (Summers et al., in press), depression, anxiety, and even FXTAS (Napoli et al., 2011) in others; are related to these mitochondrial problems (P. Hagerman, 2013; Hagerman & Hagerman, 2013). In idiopathic ASD, there was some degree of mitochondrial dysfunction in all ten randomly selected patients who participated in detailed mitochondrial function studies (Giulivi et al., 2010; Chapter 2). For the other disorders, it is interesting to observe that the mining of this promising field of mitochondrial dysfunction is being carried out with all types of biomedical approaches—such as genetics, proteomics, postmortem studies, and pharmacological and neuroimaging studies (Manji et al., 2012; Marazziti et al., 2012; Park & Park, 2012)—thus exemplifying the need for an integrative approach (the *terroir* model" going from core DNA to surface symptoms, described above) to unveil new ways to address and treat mitochondrial dysfunction in neurodevelopmental and neurodegenerative disorders.

Free Fatty Acid Metabolism

Fatty acids are carboxylic acids with a long aliphatic tail, which are important for energy production and storage. They also are essential components of cell membranes (IUPAC-Goldbook, 2012). One well-known type of fatty acid is the omega-3 (which contains a double bond on the 3 carbon starting from its tail, thus the nomenclature). Even though other areas of health care, like cardiology, are extensively studying this compound, there is limited research in the field of neurodevelopment. However, recent studies have associated long-chain omega-3 deficiencies with mental disorders like major depressive disorder, bipolar disorder, anxiety disorder, schizophrenia, ASD, and ADHD (McNamara & Strawn, 2013). Several potential mechanisms of action of omega-3s have already been examined. One is its anti-inflammatory activity. For instance, it competes with omega-6 fatty acids, such as arachidonic acid, which are precursors of inflammatory messengers (Bloch & Hannestad, 2012). Moreover, omega-3 may also have a crucial role in the CNS cell membrane fluidity, influencing the structure and the function of the proteins located in it (Bloch & Hannestad, 2012).

Excitatory/Inhibitory Imbalance

An inhibitory/excitatory (I/E) imbalance is a model for social and cognitive deficits that has been proposed and studied in fragile X disorders, ASD, schizophrenia, and ID (Rubenstein & Merzenich, 2003). It postulates that, in certain key central nervous system areas, there is either an over-excitability, or under-inhibition, or over-inhibition (Down syndrome), which would cause increased "noise" and subsequent altered information signaling. This is caused by structural or functional abnormalities of neurotransmitting systems (Buxbaum & Patrick, 2012). New laboratory techniques, such as optogenetics, a neuromodulation technique that allows one to control the activity of individual neurons on a living tissue, has allowed scientists to probe and link GABAergic and other synapse-related systems to this concept (Yizhar et al., 2011).

Hormonal Effects

Attenuated hypothalamic-pituitary-adrenal (HPA) axis function is associated with the activation of innate immune responses (low-grade inflammation), and enhanced HPA axis function and elevated cortisol levels can be associated with stress in several neurodevelopmental disorders, including fragile X disorders (Hessl et al., 2006), depression (Brouwer et al., 2006), and ASD (Schupp et al., 2013).

Microbiome

The "microbiome" has recently gained a special attention in the medical field due to the recognition of the huge amounts of bacteria living in the human gut and their influence on health and development (Foster & McVey Neufeld, 2013; Mulle et al., 2013). The effects of the microbiome go beyond just participating in the breakdown of polysaccharides. It has documented relevance in the immune system and in pathologies such as inflammatory bowel disease, obesity, and heart disease. In neurodevelopmental disorders, the gut-brain axis is still a growing field, but several links have been found. It has a role in mechanisms such as HPA axis programing, reactivity, and activation of stress circuits through gut vagal innervation in early-life mouse models. Also, some evidence points to the interaction of the microbiome's diversity and probiotic supplementation with levels of BDNF, with GABA receptors' expression, and with serotonin turnover in key brain areas; also with gut permeability, which would allow translocation of pathogens in the bloodstream. Recent clinical trials using probiotics and other dietary interventions are appearing in the literature, and although modest in benefit, they seem promising as a treatment addition for depression, autism, and other neurodevelopmental disorders.

Other Epigenetic Pathways

Several other possible epigenetic pathways have been studied that lead to neurodevelopmental dysfunction. For example, membrane signal transduction pathway, neurotrophin production, neurogenesis and synaptogenesis, neuronal resilience to physiological stressors, and neurodevelopmental perturbations in serotonin and dopamine neurotransmission have been described (McNamara & Strawn, 2013), and more such pathways are likely to be recognized as epigenetic research progresses.

BIOMARKERS

A "biomarker" generally refers to a measured characteristic, which may be used as an indicator of some biological state or condition. Biomarkers are often measured and evaluated to examine normal biological processes, pathogenic processes, or pharmacological responses to a therapeutic intervention.

Once a proposed biomarker has been validated, it can be used to diagnose disease risk, to determine the presence of disease in an individual, to tailor treatments for the disease in an individual (choices of drug treatment or administration regimes), and to assess outcomes of treatment. In evaluating potential drug therapies, a biomarker may be used as a surrogate for a natural endpoint such as survival or irreversible morbidity. If a treatment alters the biomarker, which has a direct connection to improved health, the biomarker serves as a surrogate endpoint for evaluating clinical benefit. An example of a magnetic resonance imaging (MRI) biomarker is the recent discovery of excess fluid surrounding the brain in toddlers who are siblings of a patient with ASD (Shen et al., 2013). The presence of this excess fluid is associated with the development of ASD by three years of age. Early intervention with Early Start Denver Model (ESDM) or a biomedical intervention may be indicated for these high-risk patients. In fragile X syndrome, there is upregulation of the mTOR system (Hoeffer et al., 2012) and also elevation of matrix metalloproteinase 9 (MMP9) levels because of the lack of the inhibitory effects of fragile X mental retardation protein (FMRP) (Dziembowska et al., 2013). Treatment with minocycline, a targeted treatment for fragile X syndrome, will lower these levels and may be helpful as an outcome marker (Dziembowska et al., 2013; Leigh et al., 2013) (Chapter 9). The use of event-related potentials (ERPs) that characterize the processing of auditory or visual information through the brain electronically holds great promise for measuring effects of targeted treatments. The use of minocycline as a targeted treatment for fragile X syndrome demonstrated significant improvements in ERP compared to children treated with placebo (Schneider et al., 2013).

TREATMENT TARGETS

Targeted treatments have been utilized both in animal models and in patients with a variety of genetic disorders. Each chapter in this book outlines the neurobiological and phenotypical involvement in animal models and in patients with specific disorders. However, several neurodevelopmental disorders have complex genetic and epigenetic features that led to their phenotype, and for some there are no signal genetic markers for the diagnosis; therefore, the diagnosis is made phenotypically, as in schizophrenia, ADHD, and ASD. The research needs new biomarkers. However,

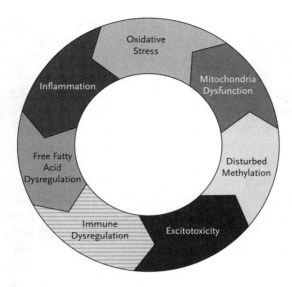

Figure 1.2:
Moving Treatment Targets

these biomarkers may reflect neurobiological changes or epigenetic processes that may be found active only during particular periods of time (Figure 1.2) and do not define the disorder, only the process that led to it. Therefore, treatment research should recruit subjects for trials based on the state of their previously validated endophenotypical biomarkers (Hendren et al., 2009) to find out if an intervention is targeting an active biomedical process in the subject at that time. For instance, identifying an inflammatory process through a biomarker such as a cytokine abnormality could be entry criteria for a study of an anti-inflammatory agent proposed to benefit a neurodevelopmental disorder. Other biomarkers of the active epigenetic process might be such measures as glutathione (GSH) metabolites, glutamate and g-aminobutyric acid, MRI changes, genomic arrays, and others based on the current gene-by-environment interactions altering the epigenetic process (Bent & Hendren, 2010), and these are discussed further in studies presented throughout this book.

CHALLENGES OF BIOMEDICAL EPIGENETIC RESEARCH

Many challenges exist for designing and carrying out clinical trials to demonstrate the efficacy of biomedical or nutraceutical treatments. Since the effect size is often small, sample sizes must be large. Complex genetic neurodevelopmental disorders are heterogeneous spectrum disorders, so sample selection may be over- or under-inclusive. Trial duration is often long, creating resistance and ethical dilemmas in holding other treatments constant. Biomarkers to serve as inclusion criteria related to treatment targets are poorly determined. Blinding may be difficult due to the nature and complexity of the treatment. Formulations may be variable in their potency and safety. Many traditional Institutional Review Boards (IRBs) may also be reluctant to try these mostly unproven treatments. Furthermore, some of the treatments are not eligible for patents, making them less appealing to industry or investor sponsorship.

Biomedical treatments include both conventional treatments, such as psychopharmacological agents, and less studied and less medically accepted treatments, such as nutraceuticals, as well as other types of treatments, including devices like transcranial magnetic stimulation.

Traditionally, research in psychiatry has been guided by *Diagnostic and Statistical Manual of Mental Disorders* (DSM) symptom–based diagnoses and selection criteria for clinical trials were based on these symptom clusters. Biomarkers have not yet been reliable or valid markers of a known etiological process; and, in past trials, results may have varied widely due to the heterogeneity of the DSM disorders. Recently, progress in biomarker research has led to the commitment by the National Institute of Mental Health (NIMH) to the Research Domain Criteria project (RDoC) as a basis for future NIMH funding for biomarker-based research (Cuthbert & Insel, 2013; Insel et al., 2010). The fundamental goal of RDoC is to define basic dimensions of functioning to be studied across multiple units of analysis, from genes to neural circuits to behaviors, cutting across disorders as traditionally defined. The intention is to translate rapid progress in basic neurobiological and behavioral research to an improved integrative understanding of psychopathology and the development of new and/or optimally matched treatments for mental disorders.

CLINICAL NEURODEVELOPMENTAL ASSESSMENT

Clinical neurodevelopmental assessment is evolving in its depth and complexity. Standards such as neuropsychological testing, neuroimaging, and biomedical labs are being expanded to include measures of gene expression, microarray, oxidative stress, mitochondrial function, immune/inflammatory processes, hormones, toxins, and allergens. However, many of these markers are only searched for in research laboratories. In the medical workup that is sanctioned for ID or ASD in the general clinic, chromosome testing has been the norm, but it is replaced now by chromosomal microarray (CMA) testing, which has a higher yield of abnormalities (15% to 20%; Miller et al., 2010) than does high-resolution chromosome testing (3%). However, if an individual demonstrates an obvious phenotype for a chromosome deletion syndrome such as velocardiofacial syndrome (22q11.2 deletion syndrome), the fluorescence in situ hybridization (FISH) testing can be ordered for a specific region. If nothing is seen, then a CMA can be ordered next. Overall, for ASD and ID, the CMA is the best first-tier test to do. Fragile X DNA testing, also a first-tier test, should be ordered for those who have ID or ASD, no matter what the physical phenotype demonstrates, because many with the full mutation or premutation involvement will not have the typical features of loose connective tissue described in Chapter 9. Approximately 2% to 3% of all patients with ID and 1% to 6% of those with ASD will have a fragile X mutation. The full mutation is associated with ASD, and also the premutation can cause ASD, particularly in boys who have seizures (Chonchaiya et al., 2012).

More recent data have shown that whole-exome sequencing and whole-genome sequencing have a yield of up to 50% in patients with ASD (Jiang et al., 2013), and these techniques will take over diagnostic testing because of their ability to find single nucleotide changes or mutations. It is important to remember that FISH testing or microarray testing will not pick up single nucleotide variations/mutations (SNV). The drawback of WES and WGS is that they are expensive, on the order of $8,000 for a trio (i.e., parents and the proband), and often insurance will not cover this unless it is carefully justified by the physician. However, the price will decrease as it is demonstrating more utility and there is competition across laboratories. Many laboratories offer a set of genes that will be sequenced for ASD or seizures or X-linked ID, and this may be more cost-effective and focused on the main clinical symptoms. One lesson that is emerging, particularly in the autism field, is that there can be two or more interactive mutations that can have an additive effect in a patient (Jiang et al., 2013). This has also been demonstrated by Noh et al. (2013), who have identified an ASD network of 187 genes that have a significantly interconnected interaction, and deletions or duplications of SNVs in this network that have a high risk for leading to ASD. They have found many patients who have two or more mutations in this network leading to a higher likelihood for ASD. This network is particularly important for synapse formation, structure, or maintenance; vesicle transport, calcium transport; and cell junction organization (Noh et al., 2013). In assessing CNVs in those with the fragile X premutation who have ASD or seizures, there is a high rate of second genetic mutations associated with autism (Lozano et al., 2014).

There is a variety of additional studies to detect other mutations associated with ID or ASD, and they include organic and amino acids of blood and urine. Specific gene-sequencing where clinically indicated, such as *MeCP2* in a patient with a Rett phenotype or *PTEN* in a patient with autism and a large head, can be done at a much lower expense than WES or WGS. MR spectroscopy (MRS) can be utilized to look for mutations that impact creatine transport into the CNS, including L-arginine:glycine amidotransferase (AGAT), guanidinoacetate N-methyltransferase (GAMT) deficiency, and the X-linked creatine transporter deficiency (CRT; SLC6A8). Although dietary manipulation can help the first two disorders, it is not efficacious for CRT deficiency. Recently a new, targeted treatment for CRT deficiency has been reported, specifically cyclocreatine, which will bypass the creatine transporter and move right into the mitochondria of the CNS and improve mitochondrial function (Kurosawa et al., 2012). Cyclocreatine treatment has led to profound improvements in cognitive abilities, spatial learning, and memory deficits in the mouse model for CRT deficiency. Studies are now being initiated in humans with CRT deficiency.

Thirteen disorders for which remarkable progress has been made to transform our practice of medicine are included in this book. As a bookend to this introductory chapter, this volume concludes with a chapter that is focused on what changes can be made now in our clinics to move us closer to reversing the cognitive and behavioral deficits in children and adults with neurodevelopmental disorders.

DISCLOSURES

Dr. Hendren has received research grants from Forest Pharmaceuticals, Inc., Curemark, BioMarin Pharmaceutical, Roche, Shire, Autism Speaks, the Vitamin D Council, and NIMH, and is on advisory boards for BioMarin, Forest, Coronado, BioZeus, and Janssen.

Andre Goldani has nothing to disclose.

Dr. Hagerman has received funding from Novartis, Roche, Seaside Therapeutics, Curemark and Forest for treatment trials in fragile X syndrome and autism. She has also consulted with Genentech and Novartis regarding treatment trials for fragile X syndrome.

REFERENCES

Aguzzi, A., Barres, B. A., & Bennett, M. L. (2013). Microglia: Scapegoat, saboteur, or something else? *Science, 339*(6116), 156–161.

Arrowsmith, C. H., Bountra, C., Fish, P. V., Lee, K., & Schapira, M. (2012). Epigenetic protein families: A new frontier for drug discovery. *Nature Reviews. Drug Discovery*, *11*(5), 384–400.

Au, J., Akins, R., Berkowitz-Sutherland, L., Tang, H. T., Chen, Y., Boyd, A., et al. (2013). Prevalence and risk of migraine headaches in adult fragile X premutation carriers. *Clinical Genetics*, *84*(6), 546–551.

Bagni, C., Tassone, F., Neri, G., & Hagerman, R. (2012). Fragile X syndrome: Causes, diagnosis, mechanisms, and therapeutics. *Journal of Clinical Investigation*, *122*(12), 4314–4322.

Bent, S., & Hendren, R. L. (2010). Improving the prediction of response to therapy in autism. *Neurotherapeutics*, *7*(3), 232–240.

Bilbo, S. D., & Schwarz, J. M. (2012). The immune system and developmental programming of brain and behavior. *Frontiers in Neuroendocrinology*, *33*(3), 267–286.

Bloch, M. H., & Hannestad, J. (2012). Omega-3 fatty acids for the treatment of depression: Systematic review and meta-analysis. *Molecular Psychiatry*, *17*(12), 1272–1282.

Boks, M. P., de Jong, N. M., Kas, M. J., Vinkers, C. H., Fernandes, C., Kahn, R. S., et al. (2012). Current status and future prospects for epigenetic psychopharmacology. *Epigenetics*, *7*(1), 20–28.

Brouwer, J. P., Appelhof, B. C., van Rossum, E. F., Koper, J. W., Fliers, E., Huyser, J., et al. (2006). Prediction of treatment response by HPA-axis and glucocorticoid receptor polymorphisms in major depression. *Psychoneuroendocrinology*, *31*(10), 1154–1163.

Bushong, E. A., Martone, M. E., Jones, Y. Z., & Ellisman, M. H. (2002). Protoplasmic astrocytes in CA1 stratum radiatum occupy separate anatomical domains. *Journal of Neuroscience22*(1), 183–192.

Buxbaum, J. D., & Hof, P. R. *The Neuroscience of Autism Spectrum Disorders*. UK: Oxford, 2012. Print.

Chonchaiya, W., Au, J., Schneider, A., Hessl, D., Harris, S. W., Laird, M., et al. (2012). Increased prevalence of seizures in boys who were probands with the *FMR1* premutation and co-morbid autism spectrum disorder. *Human Genetics*, *131*(4), 581–589.

Cortessis, V. K., Thomas, D. C., Levine, A. J., Breton, C. V., Mack, T. M., Siegmund, K. D., et al. (2012). Environmental epigenetics: Prospects for studying epigenetic mediation of exposure-response relationships. *Human Genetics*, *131*(10), 1565–1589.

Cuthbert, B. N., & Insel, T. R. (2013). Toward the future of psychiatric diagnosis: The seven pillars of RDoC. *BMC Medicine*, *11*, 126.

Dawson, G. (2013). Early intensive behavioral intervention appears beneficial for young children with autism spectrum disorders. *Journal of Pediatrics*, *162*(5), 1080–1081.

de Diego-Otero, Y., Romero-Zerbo, Y., el Bekay, R., Decara, J., Sanchez, L., Rodriguez-de Fonseca, F., et al. (2009). Alpha-tocopherol protects against oxidative stress in the fragile X knockout mouse: An experimental therapeutic approach for the *Fmr1* deficiency. *Neuropsychopharmacology*, *34*(4), 1011–1026.

Dietert, R. R., & Dietert, J. M. (2008). Potential for early-life immune insult, including developmental immunotoxicity in autism and autism spectrum disorders: Focus on critical windows of immune vulnerability. *Journal of Toxicology and Environmental Health. Part B, Critical Reviews*, *11*(8), 660–680.

Dziembowska, M., Pretto, D. I., Janusz, A., Kaczmarek, L., Leigh, M. J., Gabriel, N., et al. (2013). High MMP-9 activity levels in fragile X syndrome are lowered by minocycline. *American Journal of Medical Genetics.Part A, 161A*(8), 1897–1903.

Edbauer, D., Neilson, J. R., Foster, K. A., Wang, C. F., Seeburg, D. P., Batterton, M. N., et al. (2010). Regulation of synaptic structure and function by FMRP-associated microRNAs miR-125b and miR-132. *Neuron, 65*(3), 373–384.

El-Sayed, A. M., Koenen, K. C., & Galea, S. (2013). Putting the "epi" into epigenetics research in psychiatry. *Journal of Epidemiology and Community Health, 67*(7), 610–616.

Foster, J. A., & McVey Neufeld, K. A. (2013). Gut-brain axis: How the microbiome influences anxiety and depression. *Trends in Neurosciences, 36*(5), 305–312.

Frustaci, A., Neri, M., Cesario, A., Adams, J. B., Domenici, E., Dalla Bernardina, B., et al. (2012). Oxidative stress-related biomarkers in autism: Systematic review and meta-analyses. *Free Radical Biology & Medicine, 52*(10), 2128–2141.

Gapp, K., Woldemichael, B. T., Bohacek, J., & Mansuy, I. M. (2012). Epigenetic regulation in neurodevelopment and neurodegenerative diseases. *Neuroscience.* Advance online publication. doi: 10.1016/j.neuroscience.2012.11.040

Gehrmann, J., Matsumoto, Y., & Kreutzberg, G. W. (1995). Microglia: Intrinsic immuneffector cell of the brain. *Brain Research. Brain Research Reviews, 20*(3), 269–287.

Giedd, J. N. (2008). The teen brain: Insights from neuroimaging. *Journal of Adolescent Health, 42*(4), 335–343.

Giulivi, C., Zhang, Y. F., Omanska-Klusek, A., Ross-Inta, C., Wong, S., Hertz-Picciotto, I., et al. (2010). Mitochondrial dysfunction in autism. *Journal of the American Medical Association, 304*(21), 2389–2396.

Grayson, L., & Thomas, A. (2013). A systematic review comparing clinical features in early age at onset and late age at onset late-life depression. *Journal of Affective Disorders, 150*(2), 161–170.

Hagerman, P. (2013). Fragile X-associated tremor/ataxia syndrome (FXTAS): pathology and mechanisms. *Acta Neuropathologica, 126*(1), 1–19.

Hagerman, R., & Hagerman, P. (2013). Advances in clinical and molecular understanding of the *FMR1* premutation and fragile X-associated tremor/ataxia syndrome. *Lancet Neurology, 12*(8), 786–798.

Hansen, K. F., & Obrietan, K. (2013). MicroRNA as therapeutic targets for treatment of depression. *Neuropsychiatric Disease and Treatment, 9,* 1011–1021.

Hendren, R. L., Bertoglio, K., Ashwood, P., & Sharp, F. (2009). Mechanistic biomarkers for autism treatment. *Medical Hypotheses, 73*(6), 950–954.

Hessl, D., Glaser, B., Dyer-Friedman, J., & Reiss, A. L. (2006). Social behavior and cortisol reactivity in children with fragile X syndrome. *Journal of Child Psychology and Psychiatry, and Allied Disciplines, 47*(6), 602–610.

Heulens, I., Braat, S., & Kooy, R. F. (2011). Metabonomics adds a new dimension to fragile X syndrome. *Genome Medicine, 3*(12), 80.

Hoeffer, C. A., Sanchez, E., Hagerman, R. J., Mu, Y., Nguyen, D. V., Wong, H., et al. (2012). Altered mTOR signaling and enhanced *CYFIP2* expression levels in subjects with fragile X syndrome. *Genes, Brain, and Behavior, 11*(3), 332–341. PMID:22268788 PMCID:PMC23319643.

Ikegame, T., Bundo, M., Murata, Y., Kasai, K., Kato, T., & Iwamoto, K. (2013). DNA methylation of the BDNF gene and its relevance to psychiatric disorders. *Journal of human genetics, 58*(7), 434–438.

Insel, T., Cuthbert, B., Garvey, M., Heinssen, R., Pine, D. S., Quinn, K., et al. (2010). Research domain criteria (RDoC): Toward a new classification framework for research on mental disorders. *American Journal of Psychiatry, 167*(7), 748–751.

IUPAC-Goldbook. (2012). Fatty acids. Retrieved March 5, 2014, from http://goldbook. iupac.org/F02330.html.

Jiang, Y. H., Yuen, R. K., Jin, X., Wang, M., Chen, N., Wu, X., et al. (2013). Detection of clinically relevant genetic variants in autism spectrum disorder by whole-genome sequencing. *American Journal of Human Genetics, 93*(2), 249–263.

Kaplan, E. S., Cao, Z., Hulsizer, S., Tassone, F., Berman, R. F., Hagerman, P. J., et al. (2012). Early mitochondrial abnormalities in hippocampal neurons cultured from *Fmr1* pre-mutation mouse model. *Journal of Neurochemistry, 123*(4), 613–621.

Khansari, P. S., & Sperlagh, B. (2012). Inflammation in neurological and psychiatric diseases. *Inflammopharmacology, 20*(3), 103–107.

Kofink, D., Boks, M. P., Timmers, H. T., & Kas, M. J. (2013). Epigenetic dynamics in psychiatric disorders: Environmental programming of neurodevelopmental processes. *Neuroscience and Biobehavioral Reviews, 37*(5), 831–845.

Kreutzberg, G. W. (1995). Microglia, the first line of defence in brain pathologies. *Arzneimittel-Forschung, 45*(3A), 357–360.

Krishnadas, R., & Cavanagh, J. (2012). Depression: An inflammatory illness? *Journal of Neurology, Neurosurgery, and Psychiatry, 83*(5), 495–502.

Kurosawa, Y., Degrauw, T. J., Lindquist, D. M., Blanco, V. M., Pyne-Geithman, G. J., Daikoku, T., et al. (2012). Cyclocreatine treatment improves cognition in mice with creatine transporter deficiency. *Journal of Clinical Investigation, 122*(8), 2837–2846.

LaSalle, J. M. (2011). A genomic point-of-view on environmental factors influencing the human brain methylome. *Epigenetics, 6*(7), 862–869.

Lawson, L. J., Perry, V. H., & Gordon, S. (1992). Turnover of resident microglia in the normal adult mouse brain. *Neuroscience, 48*(2), 405–415.

Leigh, M. J., Nguyen, D. V., Mu, Y., Winarni, T. I., Schneider, A., Chechi, T., et al. (2013). A randomized double-blind, placebo-controlled trial of minocycline in children and adolescents with fragile X syndrome. *Journal of Developmental and Behavioral Pediatrics, 34*(3), 147–155.

Lozano, R. H., RJ, Duyzen, M., Budirovic, D., Lozano, C., Rothfuss, M., Eichler, E., et al. (2014). Are genomic studies necessary in autism and neurological disorders of fragile X premutation carriers?

Manji, H., Kato, T., Di Prospero, N. A., Ness, S., Beal, M. F., Krams, M., et al. (2012). Impaired mitochondrial function in psychiatric disorders. *Nature Reviews. Neuroscience, 13*(5), 293–307.

Marazziti, D., Baroni, S., Picchetti, M., Landi, P., Silvestri, S., Vatteroni, E., et al. (2012). Psychiatric disorders and mitochondrial dysfunctions. *European Review for Medical and Pharmacological Sciences, 16*(2), 270–275.

McNamara, R. K., & Strawn, J. R. (2013). Role of long-chain omega-3 fatty acids in psychiatric practice. *PharmaNutrition, 1*(2), 41–49.

Miller, D. T., Adam, M. P., Aradhya, S., Biesecker, L. G., Brothman, A. R., Carter, N. P., et al. (2010). Consensus statement: Chromosomal microarray is a first-tier clinical diagnostic test for individuals with developmental disabilities or congenital anomalies. *American Journal of Human Genetics, 86*(5), 749–764.

Mulle, J. G., Sharp, W. G., & Cubells, J. F. (2013). The gut microbiome: A new frontier in autism research. *Current Psychiatry Reports, 15*(2), 337.

Muller, N., Myint, A. M., Krause, D., Weidinger, E., & Schwarz, M. J. (2013). Anti-inflammatory treatment in schizophrenia. *Progress in Neuro-Psychopharmacology and Biological Psychiatry, 42*, 146–153.

Napoli, E., Ross-Inta, C., Wong, S., Omanska-Klusek, A., Barrow, C., Iwahashi, C., et al. (2011). Altered zinc transport disrupts mitochondrial protein processing/import in fragile X-associated tremor/ataxia syndrome. *Human Molecular Genetics, 20*(15), 3079–3092.

Noh, H. J., Ponting, C. P., Boulding, H. C., Meader, S., Betancur, C., Buxbaum, J. D., et al. (2013). Network topologies and convergent aetiologies arising from deletions and duplications observed in individuals with autism. *PLoS Genetics, 9*(6), e1003523.

Park, C., & Park, S. K. (2012). Molecular links between mitochondrial dysfunctions and schizophrenia. *Molecules and Cells, 33*(2), 105–110.

Powell, W. T., Coulson, R. L., Gonzales, M. L., Crary, F. K., Wong, S. S., Adams, S., et al. (2013). R-loop formation at Snord116 mediates topotecan inhibition of Ube3a-antisense and allele-specific chromatin decondensation. *Proceedings of the National Academy of Sciences of the United States of America, 110*(34), 13938–13943.

Ross-Inta, C., Omanska-Klusek, A., Wong, S., Barrow, C., Garcia-Arocena, D., Iwahashi, C., et al. (2010). Evidence of mitochondrial dysfunction in fragile X-associated tremor/ataxia syndrome. *Biochemical Journal, 429*(3), 545–552.

Rubenstein, J. L., & Merzenich, M. M. (2003). Model of autism: increased ratio of excitation/inhibition in key neural systems. *Genes, Brain, and Behavior, 2*(5), 255–267.

Schneider, A., Leigh, M. J., Adams, P., Nanakul, R., Chechi, T., Olichney, J., et al. (2013). Electrocortical changes associated with minocycline treatment in fragile X syndrome. *Journal of Psychopharmacology (Oxford, England), 27*(10), 956–963.

Schupp, C. W., Simon, D., & Corbett, B. A. (2013). Cortisol responsivity differences in children with autism spectrum disorders during free and cooperative play. *Journal of Autism and Developmental Disorders, 43*(10), 2405–2417.

Sellier, C., Freyermuth, F., Tabet, R., Tran, T., He, F., Ruffenach, F., et al. (2013). Sequestration of DROSHA and DGCR8 by expanded CGG RNA repeats alters microRNA processing in fragile X-associated tremor/ataxia syndrome. *Cell Reports, 3*(3), 869–880.

Shen, M. D., Nordahl, C. W., Young, G. S., Wootton-Gorges, S. L., Lee, A., Liston, S. E., et al. (2013). Early brain enlargement and elevated extra-axial fluid in infants who develop autism spectrum disorder. *Brain : A Journal of Neurology, 136*(Pt 9), 2825–2835.

Siew, W. H., Tan, K. L., Babaei, M. A., Cheah, P. S., & Ling, K. H. (2013). MicroRNAs and intellectual disability (ID) in Down syndrome, X-linked ID, and fragile X syndrome. *Frontiers in Cellular Neuroscience, 7*, 41.

Stohs, S. J. (1995). The role of free radicals in toxicity and disease. *Journal of Basic and Clinical Physiology and Pharmacology, 6*(3–4), 205–228.

Summers, S., Cogswell, J., Goodrich, J., Mu, Y., Nguyen, D., Brass, S., et al. (in press). Fatigue and body mass index in the fragile X premutation carrier.

Summers, S., Cogswell, J., Goodrich, J., Mu, Y., Nguyen, D., Brass, S., et al. (2013). Prevalence of restless legs syndrome and sleep quality in carriers of the fragile X premutation. *Clinical Genetics*, doi: 10.1111/cge.12249.

Tassone, F., Hagerman, R. J., Chamberlain, W. D., & Hagerman, P. J. (2000). Transcription of the *FMR1* gene in individuals with fragile X syndrome. *American Journal of Medical Genetics, 97*(3), 195–203. PMID:11449488.

Yizhar, O., Fenno, L. E., Prigge, M., Schneider, F., Davidson, T. J., O'Shea, D. J., et al. (2011). Neocortical excitation/inhibition balance in information processing and social dysfunction. *Nature, 477*(7363), 171–178.

Zhang, X. Y., & Yao, J. K. (2013). Oxidative stress and therapeutic implications in psychiatric disorders. *Progress in Neuro-Psychopharmacology and Biological Psychiatry, 46,* 197–199.

CHAPTER 2

Autism: Neurobiological Mechanisms and Targeted Treatments

ROBERT L. HENDREN AND RANDI JENSSEN HAGERMAN

INTRODUCTION

Autism can be reliably diagnosed by or before age three, but the diagnosis is usually not made until age two when there is a lack of development of functional language (National Institute of Health [NIH], 2005). The ratio of boys to girls is variably reported between three to five boys to one girl. There is no effective means of prevention and no fully effective treatment. Early intervention is effective and improves prognosis (Autism Speaks, 2013).

The prevalence of autism 25 or more years ago was 1/10,000; 10 years ago it was 1/500–1/1,000, and currently is reliably reported at 1/88 but maybe as frequent as 1/50 or 2% of the male population (Blumberg et al., 2013). With a ratio of 5:1 boys:girls, this prevalence figure for boys becomes 1 in 54. There has been a 78% increase between 2002 and 2008 and a greater than 600% increase in prevalence over the past two decades (Doherty, 2013). Possible explanations for the apparent increase with varying degrees of support include diagnostic expansion and substitution, better reporting, increased recognition, increasing acceptability, moving to a location because they reportedly have better services and may be more likely to count autism cases, environmental toxins, infectious and immune vulnerability, and epigenetics (Rutter, 2005).

CLINICAL FEATURES

The DSM IV developed the classification category of pervasive developmental disorders (PDD), which contained autism and related disorders, but illnesses in this larger category have been increasingly referred to as autism spectrum disorders (ASD). Included in the PDD category was autistic disorder, including high-functioning autism; Asperger's disorder; PDD NOS ("not otherwise specified"); Rett's syndrome; and childhood disintegrative disorder as described by the *Diagnostic and Statistical Manual of Mental Disorders* (4th ed., text rev., *DSM-IV-TR*; American Psychiatric Association, 2000). In the DSM-IV, there are three major symptom domains in PDD. The first is impaired social interaction characterized by a lack of empathy, impaired nonverbal communication, failure to develop relationships, and a lack of reciprocity associated with impaired social skills. This impaired social interaction is not due to a lack of attachment, as children with autism do attach to their primary caregiver (Oppenheim et al., 2009). Children with autism do not engage in attention-sharing behaviors; do not recognize emotional expression, gesture, and nonverbal vocalizations; do not know social (pragmatic) rules of interpersonal communication; and have a deficit in joint attention, theory of mind, and affective reciprocity (Robertson et al., 1999).

The second symptom domain in the DSM-IV refers to restricted, repetitive, stereotyped behaviors. This includes excessive circumscribed preoccupations, inflexible motor mannerisms, preoccupation with parts of the whole, and difficulty with transitions. The third symptom domain refers to language abnormalities, with no significant language delay or cognitive delay in Asperger's syndrome, but it is present in autism. Finally, the symptoms are not due to schizophrenia.

DSM-5 has renamed the overarching PDD category "autism spectrum disorder" (ASD), and the three domains have been condensed to two: 1. social/communication deficits; and 2. fixated interests and repetitive behaviors. Several social/communication criteria were merged and streamlined to clarify diagnostic requirements (APA, 2013). For social/communication deficits, this includes social-emotional reciprocity (e.g., conversation, joint attention), nonverbal communicative behaviors (e.g., eye contact, body language, facial expression, gestures); and developing and maintaining relationships (e.g., imaginative play, making friends).

Restricted, repetitive patterns of behavior, interests, or activities include stereotyped/repetitive speech, motor movements, or use of objects; excessive adherence to routines and rituals or excessive resistance to change; highly restricted, fixated interests, abnormal in intensity or focus; hyper-/hypo-reactivity to sensory input or unusual interest in sensory aspects of the environment. Finally, the symptoms must be present in early childhood (but they may not become fully manifest until social demands exceed the child's limited capacities), and the symptoms together limit and impair everyday functioning. Also, there are three levels of severity—requiring support, substantial support, or very substantial support.

There has been substantial controversy regarding the changes to the diagnostic categories in DSM-5, the detailed discussion of which is beyond the purpose of this chapter. A quick summary of the reasons for the changes is that there are no consistent differences demonstrated in diagnostic practices for autism, Asperger's disorder, and PDD NOS; that there is a lack of evidence for differentiation at present or with time; that delays in language are not unique or universal; and that the diagnosis may change over time. Reasons given for not creating the change include concern about a loss of identity that comes from the Asperger's diagnosis, stigma, and possibly a loss of qualification for services for both Asperger's and PDD-NOS diagnoses. There is also concern about how we compare prevalence and other research studies using the new criteria. Comparative testing and field-testing have not been fully conclusive to date and probably will not be until DSM-5 has been in place for some time. It is unlikely that more severely affected children will lose a diagnosis that qualifies them for services. The new category, "social communication disorder," may cover some of the milder cases but may not qualify the individual for services (Lord & Jones, 2012; Volkmar et al., 2012).

NEUROBIOLOGICAL ABNORMALITIES AND EPIGENETICS

There are now thought to be over 400 genetic mutations that can lead to ASD (Iossifov et al., 2012). Most are rare and have only been described in a handful of patients, such as the Neuroligin mutations (*NLGN3* and *NLGN4*) or the neurexin mutations (*NRXN1*), all of which are synaptic adhesion molecules (Betancur, 2011; Zoghbi & Bear, 2012). These mutations and many others lead to synaptic dysfunction, which is a theme not only in ASD but also in many other neurodevelopmental disorders described in this volume. The study of more common genetic causes of ASD, including fragile X syndrome (*FMR1*), tuberous sclerosis (*TSC1* and 2), 15q11-13 duplication, Angelman syndrome (*UBE3A*), Rett syndrome (*MECP2*), Phelan-McDermid syndrome (*SHANK3*, and also *SHANK2*), Cowden syndrome (*PTEN*), and neurofibromatosis (*NF1*) mutations have led to significant insight regarding how a mutation can lead to "synatopathy" or deficits in synaptic connections and plasticity through a variety of mechanisms (Figure 2.1).

Many of the pathways that are dysfunctional in these disorders are overlapping, leading to new avenues for treatment for more than one disorder. The most dramatic example of this is fragile X syndrome (FXS) leading to a loss of the fragile X protein (FMRP) which regulates the translation of hundreds of other messages from multiple genes associated with autism, including *SHANK3, NRXN1, NLGN3* and *4, PTEN,* and many others (Darnell et al., 2011; Iossifov et al., 2012). Reports of lowered levels of FMRP in the brain of adults with idiopathic autism suggest that many types of autism may dysregulate FMRP, as will other psychiatric disorders such as schizophrenia (Fatemi & Folsom, 2011; Fatemi et al., 2012).

The loss of FMRP upregulates the level of many proteins because of the lack of translational suppression rendered by the presence of FMRP (Osterweil et al., 2010; Qin et al., 2005). There is upregulation of the metabotropic glutamate receptor 5 (mGluR5) pathway leading to upregulation of the serine/threonine kinase mammalian target of rapamycin (Akt-mTOR) pathway, which is also seen in Angelman syndrome, tuberous sclerosis, cardiofaciocutaneous (CFC) syndrome, and neurofibromatosis; however, in Rett syndrome the Akt-mTOR pathway is decreased (Zoghbi & Bear, 2012). In Angelman syndrome, *UBE3A,* which normally directs proteolysis via the proteasome, is not working, so there is upregulation of the levels of *UBE3A* target proteins, one of which is Arc (Zoghbi & Bear, 2012). The over-expression of Arc leads to internalization of α-amino-3-hydroxy-5-methyl-4-isoxazolepropionic acid (AMPA) receptors and impaired synaptic transmission in Angelman syndrome (Greer et al., 2010). Arc is also regulated by FMRP. For disorders such as Angelman syndrome with upregulation of the Akt-mTOR pathway, there may be benefit from an mGluR5 antagonist that is used in FXS (Jacquemont et al., 2011), as described in the chapter on fragile X–associated disorders.

The mutations in TSC1 or 2 that cause tuberous sclerosis release the inhibition of mTOR as described in Chapter 8, and the targeted treatment, rapamycin, downregulates the over-activation or mTOR. Although one would expect that rapamycin would be clinically helpful in FXS, this has been shown not to be the case in the FXS animal model (Osterweil et al., 2010).

EPIGENETICS

In addition to a clear neurodevelopmental genetic vulnerability to autism, an interaction with environmental risks is increasingly appreciated, adding to the complex etiology of ASD (Hallmayer et al., 2011). Documented environmental risk factors include prenatal or early postnatal exposure to viral infections (e.g., rubella), valproic acid, and thalidomide. Many more are proposed without firm etiological evidence, such as the influence of mercury, lead, environmental toxins, vaccines, or lack of vitamin D (Herbert, 2010; Landrigan, 2010). Other associations with autism in the offspring include advanced parental age, particularly of fathers (Durkin et al., 2008;

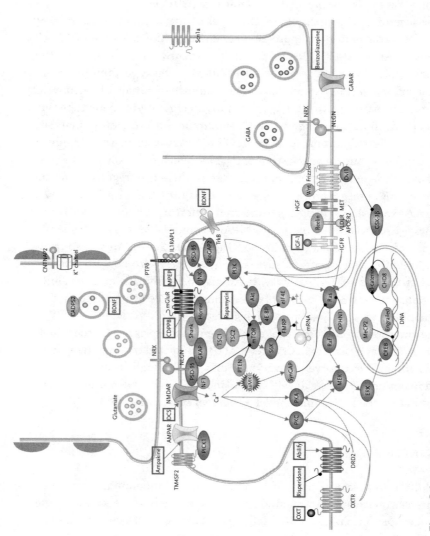

Figure 2.1:

Signaling pathways and possible treatments for ASD

Won, H., Mah, W., & Kim, E. (2013), Autism spectrum disorder causes, mechanisms, and treatments: focus on neuronal synapses. *Frontiers in Molecular Neuroscience*, 6, 19. doi:10.3389/fnmol.2013.00019. eCollection 2013. PubMed PMID: 23935565; PubMed Central PMCID: PMC3733014.

Shelton et al., 2010); maternal metabolic conditions (Krakowiak et al., 2012); and influenza or fever during pregnancy (Zerbo et al., 2013). Many of these suggest an epigenetic influence one or more generations beyond the index change (Frans et al., 2013).

There are many studies associating ASD and environmental pollution. Environmental mercury release from coal-burning plants is associated with special education rates and autism disorder in an ecological study in Texas (Palmer et al., 2006). Children with autism are more likely to be exposed to traffic-related air pollution during gestation and during the first year of life (Volk et al., 2013). Maternal residence near agricultural pesticide applications is associated with ASD in California's central valley (Roberts et al., 2007).

Epigenetic mechanisms by which these gene–environment interactions are detected in biomarkers of underlying neurodevelopmental processes in autism include immune abnormalities/inflammation (Goines & Van de Water, 2010); oxidative stress (James et al., 2009); disturbed methylation (James et al., 2009); mitochondrial dysfunction (Frye & Rossignol, 2011; Giulivi et al., 2010; Manji et al., 2012); free fatty acid metabolism (Bell et al., 2010); an imbalance between excitatory and inhibitory neuromodulators (Rubenstein, 2010); hormonal effects (Harony & Wagner, 2010); and microglia activation (Cunningham, 2013).

The theme of an imbalance of stimulatory systems (glutamate) and inhibitory systems (GABA) is recurrent in the study of many of the causes of ASD. Currently there is a variety of mouse models of autism that have been studied with the use of a GABA agonist or an mGluR5 antagonist, as described below (Silverman et al., 2013; Silverman et al., 2012).

Mitochondrial dysfunction has also been described in patients with idiopathic autism (Giulivi et al., 2010; Napoli et al., 2013) and in known genetic causes of ASD (de Diego-Otero et al., 2009; Frye & Rossignol, 2011). This has implications for treatment, including the use of antioxidants or supplements that could enhance the function of deficient electron-transport enzymes.

Guilivi and colleagues have demonstrated how environmental toxicants can worsen the function of mitochondrial enzymes in patients who may be vulnerable to these effects (Napoli et al., 2013). BDE-49 (2,2',4,5 tetrabromodiphenyl ether) is a flame retardant that is currently in furniture, carpets, and car seats, and previously in baby clothing. It is one of a family of polybrominated diphenyl ethers (PBDEs) that can be absorbed through the skin, and it accumulates in fat and breast milk. At the lowest concentrations, BDE-49 restricts the ability of mitochondria to make ATP by inhibiting two protein complexes (cytochrome C oxidase and adenosine triphosphate [ATP] synthase). BDE-49 increases oxidative stress and disrupts the flow of protons across the inner mitochondrial membrane in neuron cell culture. In neuronal precursor cells, researchers have shown that a reduction of PTEN overactivated the P13Kinase/Akt pathway and caused mitochondrial dysfunction. With inhibition of PTEN, the cytochrome c oxidase activity was reduced by 50%, but with exposure to BDE-49, there was an accumulative 70% reduction in enzymatic activity, leading to a dramatic hit in ATP production that can cause developmental problems, including ASD. A neuron without appropriate ATP levels will not connect well to other neurons, leading to developmental problems, and greater risk for death of the neuron.

DIAGNOSTIC METHODS

Because of the intrinsic heterogeneity of the molecular etiology of autism, it is essential to carry out a detailed genetic workup in anyone who receives the clinical diagnosis of autism or ASD (Miller et al., 2010). It important to rule out the most common genetic forms of autism, including fragile X mutations, either full mutation or premutation, with an FMR1 DNA test, including both PCR and Southern Blot testing. In addition, microarray testing (CGH array) will pick up the deletions and duplications that can be found in a proportion of those with autism, such as a 15q deletion or duplication. The yield of clinically important abnormalities with a CGH array is up to 10%, and it is a part of the workup that is usually covered by medical insurance (Murdoch & State, 2013). Previous experience is important for determining which copy number variant (CNV) is important clinically and which is a normal common variant. If a significant abnormality is found, then parental studies are indicated to see if this is an inherited change or a *de novo* change unique to the child. If it is present in one of the parents who presumably does not have autism or ASD, it is more likely to be a normal variant. Usually the parental genomes are done without further charge, but not always. The CNV studies have also shown that often a second genetic hit may occur, for instance a SHANK2 deletion and CYFIP deletion, and both are important and ASD-related. So the second hit can be a modifier to the primary hit and have an additive effect to the abnormalities that can be seen in neuron cell cultures (Leblond et al., 2012).

More recent research has yielded a higher rate of abnormalities with whole-exome or whole-genome sequencing (Murdoch & State, 2013), both of which are far more expensive than microarrays, and often extensive documentation of need is required by the insurance companies to have this covered, with a cost of approximately $5,000–$8,000 per study or trio (parents and proband). The cost of these studies will decrease over time, and many private diagnostic companies offer whole-exome sequencing.

Several private genetic companies are now offering gene sequencing to find point mutations in genes such as *NRXN1, NLGN3/4, PTEN*, etc., that are known to cause autism if mutated. If a patient has a clinical feature that makes you think about a certain mutation, such as a big head suggesting a *PTEN* mutation, then these studies can often be justified to insurance companies. A number of new genetic mutations have been found through whole-exome sequencing verified by four reports associated with autism including *SNC2A, CHD8, DYRKIA,POG2, GRIN2B*, and *KATNAL2* (Murdoch & State, 2013). These genes are associated with a variety of functions, including sodium or glutamate channel binding, microtubule function, chromatin binding, and kinase activity, all of which can impact synaptic plasticity.

In the future, there may be biomarkers administered to detect a high risk for a diagnosis of autism/ASD. For instance, an immune panel has been developed to test a mother who may be at high risk for immune dysfunction leading to autism in a second child once the first has been identified with autism (Goines & Van de Water, 2010). Another example of biomarkers is the documentation of an increase in the Akt-mTOR pathway, which can be seen in FXS and in other subtypes of ASD (Hoeffer et al., 2012). Another biomarker is elevation of matrix metalloproteinase 9 (MMP9), which is upregulated with a deficit in FMRP, and this suggests that the developmental problems may respond to minocycline, an antibiotic that lowers MMP9, as is seen in FXS and in Angelman syndrome (Dziembowska et al., 2013). A recent neuroimaging study by Shen et al. (2013) of siblings at high risk for autism demonstrated significantly elevated extra-axial fluid at 6 to 24 months in the brains of infants who subsequently developed ASD compared to those who did not develop autism. The babies who developed ASD also had larger cerebral volumes, and both of these features can be considered biomarkers of autism risk (Shen et al., 2013).

RELATED DISORDERS

ASD has many medical and psychiatric comorbidities, confirming the heterogeneity of the category. Regressive autism occurs in 20% to 47% (Werner & Dawson, 2005); gastrointestinal abnormalities in 30% to 70% (Buie et al., 2010); seizure disorder develops in adolescence and young adulthood in 30% (Tharp, Ozonoff, Rogers, & Hendren, 2003); intellectual disability is listed as occurring in up to 70% of those with full-syndrome autism (APA, 2000), but this may decrease with early, effective intervention; and mitochondrial dysfunction is identified in up to 100% (Giulivi et al., 2010), as described above. Higher than expected rates of other medical conditions, such as eczema, allergies, asthma, ear and respiratory infections, and headache, are reported in those with ASD (Kohane et al., 2012).

The high rate of seizures in ASD is particularly important because of the neurochemical changes that occur in the brain during seizures. Bernard et al. (2013) have recently reported that early-life seizures in a rat model disrupt the normal signaling process involving FMRP/S6K/PP2A, a complex that works together to regulate translation of messages important for synaptic plasticity. With seizures, FMRP and the related proteins will pull away from the dendrites and move into the nuclear area of the neuron, which disrupts the function of FMRP regarding synaptic plasticity and enhances metabotropic long-term depression (weakening of the synaptic connections). These rats that have a normal *FMR1* gene subsequently have FMRP dysregulation caused by the seizures, and they develop autistic features in a socialization paradigm (Bernard et al., 2013). This concept helps explain the finding that the frequency of seizures correlate with the severity of autism in individuals with idiopathic autism or genetic disorders associated with autism, including tuberous sclerosis and neurofibromatosis (van Eeghen et al., 2013).

Psychiatric diagnoses to rule out in the differential diagnosis or when considering co-morbidity (APA, 2013) include ADHD, obsessive compulsive disorder, tics and Tourette syndrome, overanxious disorder, bipolar disorder, depressive disorder, and psychotic disorder. Aggression occurs in 53% of children with ASD at some time, is more common when the children are younger; and is often associated with medical co-morbidities (Mazurek et al., 2013).

CURRENT TREATMENTS AND MANAGEMENT

Commonly utilized interventions with evidence for efficacy are behavioral interventions, family support, and speech and language therapy. Commonly utilized, but with less published evidence for their efficacy, are occupational therapy, social skills groups, and cognitive behavioral therapy (CBT). Up to 70% of children with ASD are reported to be using some form of biological treatment (Wong & Smith, 2006), while up to 74% of children recently diagnosed with autism use complementary and alternative medicine (CAM) (Hanson et al., 2007), often with little or no published evidence of benefit.

Behavioral treatments have the strongest evidence for treatment efficacy and include applied behavioral analysis (ABA), whose basic principles consist of reinforcement, extinction, stimulus control, and generalization (Granpeesheh et al., 2009). Therapies under this ABA umbrella include discrete trials training; treatment, education of autistic and related communication-handicapped children (TEACCH) (Vismara & Rogers, 2010); pivotal response training (Koegel et al., 2001); incidental teaching approach: Floor Time is derived from the Developmental, Individual-difference Relationship-based (DIR) model whose premise is communication can be improved by meeting children at their developmental level and building on their strengths. (Greenspan S, 2008); relationship development intervention (RDI) (Vismara & Rogers, 2010); and the Early Start Denver Model (ESDM) (Dawson et al., 2010; Wallace & Rogers, 2010). A recent study of the utilization of ESDM in children with ASD over a two-year period demonstrated dramatic improvements in the EEG brain wave pattern such that they were indistinguishable from normal; such changes did not occur in those with ASD who were treated with community interventions for autism (Dawson, 2013).

Other interventions for specific symptoms associated with autism employ assisted communication; interactive, computer-based, multi-touch screens; tablet-based programs; collaborative story telling (Hourcade, 2013); and following areas of intense interest (e.g., "Horse Boy," Temple Grandin).

Psychotropic medications have variable evidence of benefit for symptoms associated with ASD but not for the core symptoms. Medications for ADHD used to treat symptoms of distractibility, impulsivity, and hyperactivity associated with ASD show modest benefit, but the response rate is lower, and there is greater risk for side effects than with ADHD alone (Handen et al., 2011; Research Units for Pediatric Psychopharmacology (RUPP), 2005).

Selective serotonin reuptake inhibitors (SSRIs) have long been thought to benefit autism-associated aggression, impulsivity, anxiety, social relations, and repetitive behaviors (Hollander et al., 2005; Posey et al., 2006). However, a recent large (n = 149) randomized controlled trial of citalopram for repetitive behaviors in children aged 5 to 17 demonstrated no difference between placebo and active medication, with a 34% placebo response rate (King et al., 2009).

The trials of alpha-2 adrenergic agonists (clonidine, guanfacine) are few, but their use for treatment of overactivity, sensory responses, irritability, and hyperactivity is not uncommon (Handen et al., 2008). Reports of modest benefits for divalproex in ASD have been few, and mostly from the same group (Hollander et al., 2010).

The only medications approved for the treatment of autism are risperidone and aripiprazole, both approved for the treatment of irritability in ASD (Aman et al., 2005; McCracken et al., 2002; Owen et al., 2009). Other medications that have published reports of benefit to symptoms associated with autism include propranolol (Narayanan et al., 2010), amantadine (King et al., 2001), D-cycloserine (Posey et al., 2004), cholinesterase inhibitors (Chez et al., 2004), nicotinic agonists (Deutsch et al., 2010), memantine (Chez et al., 2007; Erickson et al., 2007), naltrexone (Brown & Panksepp, 2009), buspirone (Buchsbaum et al., 2001), divalproex (Hollander et al., 2001), and risperidone plus memantine (Ghaleiha et al., 2013). The use of bumetanide, a diuretic that is a chloride-importer agonist that reduces intracellular chloride levels and reinforces GABAergic activity, was found effective in improving autism symptoms (by CGI and Childhood Autism Rating Scale [CARS]) in a controlled trial of 60 children ages 3 to 11 with ASD, when given for 3 months in a dose of 1 mg/day (Lemonnier et al., 2012).

Neutraceutical/biomedical/CAM treatments are commonly used in the treatment of ASD, but the published evidence for them is scant. CAM treatment has been divided into food sensitivities and gastrointestinal function (gluten-free/casein-free diet, secretin, digestive enzymes, Pepcid, antibiotics); putative immune mechanism or modulators (antifungals, intravenous immunoglobulin [IV Ig], omega-3, vitamin A/cod liver oil); methylation (methylcobalamine, folinic acid); and neurostimulation (transcranial magnetic stimulation). The list of potential biomedical treatments is longer than appropriate for this chapter, but there are recent reviews (Hendren, 2013; Lofthouse et al., 2012).

TARGETED TREATMENTS

Animal Studies

The use of animal models for a variety of neurodevelopmental disorders has been helpful in the development of targeted treatments, because the neurobiological abnormalities can be documented and targeted treatments can be assessed before they are tried in patients with the disorder. Since autism is a heterogeneous disorder, there are several animal models. The laboratory of Jacki Crawley has been a leader in studying these animal models for autism, and recent studies have assessed targeted treatments for the autistic behavior that they demonstrate. Silverman et al. (2011) have initially shown that an mGluR5 antagonist was helpful in decreasing self-grooming behavior in the BTBR (Black and Tan BRachyury) animal model for autism. A more recent study of a long-acting metabotropic glutamate receptor 5 (mGluR5) antagonist, CTEP, developed by Pfizer, in the BTBR mouse model for autism improved several features of the autism phenotype, including self-grooming, marble-burying, nose-to-nose sniffing time, and social interaction time (Silverman et al., 2012). Arbaclofen, a GABA$_B$ agonist developed for FXS, has also been helpful in the animal model for autism. These studies suggest that the targeted treatments for FXS will also be helpful in autism, and clinical trials for some of these medications have been tried in autism.

Targeted Treatments in Patients with ASD

The success of Arbaclofen in a subgroup of patients with FXS who also have autism or significant social deficits (Berry-Kravis et al., 2012) led to the studies of Arbaclofen in patients with ASD without FXS. An initial open-label study carried out by Seaside Therapeutics demonstrated significant changes in all of the primary outcome measures, including the Clinical Global Impression Scale–Improvement (CGI-I), the Aberrant Behavioral Checklist, and the Vineland. This has subsequently led to a double-blind controlled trial of Arbaclofen in children and young adults up to age 25 years with ASD at multiple centers in the United States that was completed in 2012 but was not successful, although not published. Preliminary data suggests that a subgroup of children with autism may respond well, but arbaclofen was not efficacious for the overall group (Veenstra-VanderWeel et al., 2013) and the company has since folded.

Therapeutic strategies targeting the mechanisms of epigenetic expression in ASD include those that target immune function or inflammatory processes, such as melatonin, IV/IG, corticosteroids, vitamin D, hyperbaric oxygen treatment (HBOT), and omega-3 fatty acids. Methylation might be targeted by folic/folinic acid, while oxidative stress might be targeted by N-acetyl cysteine (NAC) and methyl B12. Aberrant functioning of neuro-modulators such as N-methyl-D-aspartate (NMDA) receptor and/or altered glutamate might be targeted by memantine. While reviewing all of these is beyond the scope of this chapter, they are covered elsewhere (Hendren, 2013). We will review a few of the more interesting and promising ones below.

Methyl cobalamine (B12) has been shown to normalize markers of oxidative stress found to be abnormal in children with autism (James et al., 2004). Based on this, a double-blind, placebo, cross-over trial of methyl B12 administered subcutaneously in the buttocks at a dosage of 67.5–75 mcg/kg every three days for six weeks (Wellness Labs) was carried out.

Thirty subjects completed the 12-week, double-blind study (Bertoglio et al., 2010). While no statistically significant mean differences in behavior tests or in glutathione status were found between the active and placebo groups, nine subjects (30%) demonstrated clinically significant improvement on the Clinical Global Impression Scale (CGI) and at least two additional behavioral measures. Responders exhibited significantly increased plasma concentrations of GSH and the ratio of oxidized GSH/reduced GSSG (glutathione disulfide). In a separate study, 48 out of 50 new subjects have been enrolled in an ongoing study that is planning a larger sample size at the University of California, San Francisco, funded by Autism Speaks (Widjaja et al., 2013)

Aberrant functioning of N-methyl-D-aspartate (NMDA) receptor and/or altered glutamate excitotoxicity may play a role in autism; and based on this, Forest Pharmaceuticals conducted a double-blind placebo-controlled multisite study of memantine in autism. Results will soon be reported. There is a case series demonstrating significant improvement in language and socialization in children with autism treated with memantine (Chez et al., 2007).

A high prevalence (75%) of folate receptor-α autoantibodies (FRAs), an autoantibody that prevents folic acid from entering the brain (cerebral folate deficiency), is reported in children with ASD (Frye et al., 2013). Improvement in ASD symptoms with high-dose folinic acid (2 mg/kg/day; max 50 mg; in two divided doses) for 12 weeks of treatment in children with ASD suggests improvement in mitochondrial function, specifically the ability of the mitochondria to be resilient against oxidative stress.

N-acetyl cysteine (NAC) is a glutamatergic modulator and an antioxidant with published studies for several disorders. A 12-week, double-blind, randomized, placebo-controlled study of NAC in children with autistic disorder was reported (Hardan et al., 2012). NAC was initiated at 900 mg daily for four weeks, then 900 mg twice daily for four weeks, and 900 mg three times daily for four weeks. Thirty-three subjects (31 male subjects, 2 female subjects; aged 3.2–10.7 years) were randomized. Oral NAC was well tolerated, with limited side effects. Compared with placebo, NAC resulted in significant improvements on ABC irritability subscale ($F = 6.80$; $p < .001$; $d = .96$).

Melatonin is an endogenous neurohormone that causes drowsiness and sets the body's "sleep clock." Review and meta-analysis of 35 studies (Rossignol, 2009) reported that, of 18 treatment studies, there were five randomized controlled trials (RCTs) ($N = 61$, 2–10 mg/day) where sleep duration (44 min, effect size (ES) = 0.93) was increased, sleep onset latency was decreased (39 min, ES = 1.28), but nighttime awakenings were unchanged. Side effects were minimal to none. Therefore, there is evidence that this intervention can be helpful for some sleep problems. It is easy to obtain over the counter and it is also an antioxidant, so it may helpful for oxidative stress in the neurons.

Preliminary evidence suggests that omega-3 fatty acids, which may reduce inflammatory processes, may reduce hyperactivity in children with autism spectrum disorder. Two small pilot studies found non-significant trends suggesting that omega-3 fatty acids may reduce hyperactivity in children with ASD (Amminger et al., 2007; Bent et al., 2011), and omega-3 fatty acids have been found to have a favorable safety profile (Gillies et al., 2012).

A randomized controlled trial of oral vitamin/mineral micronutrients for three months with 141 children and adults with ASD improved the nutritional and metabolic status of children with autism, including improvements in methylation, glutathione, oxidative stress, sulfation, ATP, nicotinamide adenine dinucleotide (NADH), and nicotinamide adenine dinucleotide phosphate (NADPH) (Adams et al., 2011). The supplement group had significantly greater improvements than did the placebo group on the Parental Global Impression–R average change (p = 0.008), hyperactivity (p = 0.003), and tantruming (p = 0.009) (Adams et al., 2011).

Oxytocin, with reported benefits to trust/socialization, is being studied in several ongoing clinical trials (Andari et al., 2010; Gregory et al., 2009; Guastella et al., 2010).

Future Prospects

The future will lead to the use of mGluR5 antagonists in autism/ASD, and both Roche and Novartis are planning to fund these trials at multiple centers once the benefit in FXS is clarified. It is likely that these trials will begin in 2015, starting with adolescents and adults, and then will be carried out in young children once safety is demonstrated for the adolescents and adults. There will also be further development of $GABA_A$ agonists for ASD, including ganaxolone and perhaps allopregnanolone, once safety is established by the companies and the Food and Drug Administration.

We will see a growth in trials targeting underlying epigenetic processes related to the neurodevelopment of ASD. As suggested in Chapter 1, this will include selecting subjects for trials based on biomarkers rather than symptom-based diagnoses, and using agents that push these patients toward resilience, health, and clinical improvement.

DISCLOSURES

Dr. Hendren has received research grants from Forest Pharmaceuticals, Inc., Curemark, BioMarin, Roche, Autism Speaks, the Vitamin D Council, and the National Institute of Mental Health. He is on advisory boards for BioMarin, Forest, Coronado Bioscience, BioZeus and Janssen, but is on no speakers' bureaus.

Dr. Hagerman has received funding from Seaside Therapeutics, Roche, Novartis, Curemark, and Forest Pharmaceuticals for treatment studies in ASD and fragile X syndrome. Dr. Hagerman also consults with Novartis and Roche/Genentech regarding treatment studies.

REFERENCES

Adams, J. B., Audhya, T., McDonough-Means, S., Rubin, R. A., Quig, D., Geis, E., et al. (2011). Effect of a vitamin/mineral supplement on children and adults with autism. *BMC Pediatrics*, *11*, 111.

Aman, M. G., Arnold, L. E., McDougle, C. J., Vitiello, B., Scahill, L., Davies, M., et al. (2005). Acute and long-term safety and tolerability of risperidone in children with autism. *Journal of Child and Adolescent Psychopharmacology*, *15*(6), 869–884.

Amminger, G. P., Berger, G. E., Schafer, M. R., Klier, C., Friedrich, M. H., & Feucht, M. (2007). Omega-3 fatty acids supplementation in children with autism: A double-blind randomized, placebo-controlled pilot study. *Biological Psychiatry*, *61*(4), 551–553.

Andari, E., Duhamel, J. R., Zalla, T., Herbrecht, E., Leboyer, M., & Sirigu, A. (2010). Promoting social behavior with oxytocin in high-functioning autism spectrum disorders. *Proceedings of the National Academy of Sciences of the United States of America*, *107*(9), 4389–4394.

American Psychiatric Association. (2000). *Diagnostic and statistical manual of mental disorder (4th ed., text rev.)*. Washington, D.C.: Author.

American Psychiatric Association. (2013). *Diagnostic and statistical manual of mental disorders* (5th ed., text rev.) Arlington, VA: American Psychiatric Publishing.

AutismSpeaks. (2013). Facts about Autism. Retrieved June 9, 2013, from www.autismspeaks.org/what-autism/facts-about-autism.

Bell, J. G., Miller, D., MacDonald, D. J., MacKinlay, E. E., Dick, J. R., Cheseldine, S., et al. (2010). The fatty acid compositions of erythrocyte and plasma polar lipids in children with autism, developmental delay or typically developing controls and the effect of fish oil intake. *The British Journal of Nutrition*, *103*(8), 1160–1167.

Bent, S., Bertoglio, K., Ashwood, P., Bostrom, A., & Hendren, R. L. (2011). A pilot randomized controlled trial of omega-3 fatty acids for autism spectrum disorder. *Journal of Autism and Developmental Disorders*, *41*(5), 545–554.

Bernard, P. B., Castano, A. M., O'Leary, H., Simpson, K., Browning, M. D., & Benke, T. A. (2013). Phosphorylation of FMRP and alterations of FMRP complex underlie enhanced mLTD in adult rats triggered by early life seizures. *Neurobiology of Disease*, 59, 1–17.

Berry-Kravis, E. M., Hessl, D., Rathmell, B., Zarevics, P., Cherubini, M., Walton-Bowen, K., et al. (2012). Effects of STX209 (arbaclofen) on neurobehavioral function in children and adults with fragile X syndrome: A randomized, controlled, phase 2 trial. *Science Translational Medicine, 4*(152), 152ra127

Bertoglio, K., Jill James, S., Deprey, L., Brule, N., & Hendren, R. L. (2010). Pilot study of the effect of methyl B12 treatment on behavioral and biomarker measures in children with autism. *Journal of Alternative and Complementary Medicine, 16*(5), 555–560.

Betancur, C. (2011). Etiological heterogeneity in autism spectrum disorders: More than 100 genetic and genomic disorders and still counting. *Brain Research, 1380*, 42–77.

Blumberg, S. J., Bramlett, M. D., Kogan, M. D., Schieve, L. A., Jones, J. R., & Lu, M. C. (2013). *Changes in Prevalence of Parent-reported Autism Spectrum Disorder in School-Aged U.S. Children: 2007 to 2011–2012*. Retrieved from http://www.cdc.gov/nchs/data/nhsr/nhsr065.pdf.

Brown, N., & Panksepp, J. (2009). Low-dose naltrexone for disease prevention and quality of life. *Medical Hypotheses, 72*(3), 333–337.

Buchsbaum, M. S., Hollander, E., Haznedar, M. M., Tang, C., Spiegel-Cohen, J., Wei, T. C., et al. (2001). Effect of fluoxetine on regional cerebral metabolism in autistic spectrum disorders: A pilot study. *The International Journal of Neuropsychopharmacology/Official Scientific Journal of the Collegium Internationale Neuropsychopharmacologicum, 4*(2), 119–125.

Buie, T., Fuchs, G. J., 3rd, Furuta, G. T., Kooros, K., Levy, J., Lewis, J. D., et al. (2010). Recommendations for evaluation and treatment of common gastrointestinal problems in children with ASDs. *Pediatrics, 125*(Suppl 1), S19–S29.

Chez, M. G., Aimonovitch, M., Buchanan, T., Mrazek, S., & Tremb, R. J. (2004). Treating autistic spectrum disorders in children: Utility of the cholinesterase inhibitor rivastigmine tartrate. *Journal of Child Neurology, 19*(3), 165–169. Retrieved from http://www.cdc.gov/ncbddd/autism/data.html.

Chez, M. G., Burton, Q., Dowling, T., Chang, M., Khanna, P., & Kramer, C. (2007). Memantine as adjunctive therapy in children diagnosed with autistic spectrum disorders: An observation of initial clinical response and maintenance tolerability. *Journal of Child Neurology, 22*(5), 574–579.

Cunningham, C. (2013). Microglia and neurodegeneration: The role of systemic inflammation. *Glia, 61*(1), 71–90.

Darnell, J. C., Van Driesche, S. J., Zhang, C., Hung, K. Y., Mele, A., Fraser, C. E., et al. (2011). FMRP stalls ribosomal translocation on mRNAs linked to synaptic function and autism. *Cell, 146*(2), 247–261.

Dawson, G. (2013). Early intensive behavioral intervention appears beneficial for young children with autism spectrum disorders. *The Journal of Pediatrics, 162*(5), 1080–1081.

Dawson, G., Rogers, S., Munson, J., Smith, M., Winter, J., Greenson, J., et al. (2010). Randomized, controlled trial of an intervention for toddlers with autism: The Early Start Denver Model. *Pediatrics, 125*(1), e17–e23.

de Diego-Otero, Y., Romero-Zerbo, Y., el Bekay, R., Decara, J., Sanchez, L., Rodriguez-de Fonseca, F., et al. (2009). Alpha-tocopherol protects against oxidative stress in the fragile X knockout mouse: An experimental therapeutic approach for the Fmr1 deficiency. *Neuropsychopharmacology: Official Publication of the American College of Neuropsychopharmacology, 34*(4), 1011–1026.

Deutsch, S. I., Urbano, M. R., Neumann, S. A., Burket, J. A., & Katz, E. (2010). Cholinergic abnormalities in autism: Is there a rationale for selective nicotinic agonist interventions? *Clinical Neuropharmacology, 33*(3), 114–120.

Doherty, H. L. (2013). Facing autism in New Brunswick: Autism news and opinion. Retrieved March 5, 2014 from http://autisminnb.blogspot.com

Durkin, M. S., Maenner, M. J., Newschaffer, C. J., Lee, L. C., Cunniff, C. M., Daniels, J. L., et al. (2008). Advanced parental age and the risk of autism spectrum disorder. *American Journal of Epidemiology*, *168*(11), 1268–1276.

Dziembowska, M., Pretto, D. I., Janusz, A., Kaczmarek, L., Leigh, M. J., Gabriel, N., et al. (2013). High MMP-9 activity levels in fragile X syndrome are lowered by minocycline. *American Journal of Medical Genetics. Part A*, *161A*(8), 1897–1903.

Dziembowska, M., Pretto, D. I., Janusz, A., Kaczmarek, L., Leigh, M. J., Gabriel, N., et al. (2013). High MMP-9 activity levels in fragile X syndrome are lowered by minocycline. *American Journal of Medical Genetics.Part A*, *161A*(8), 1897–1903.

Erickson, C. A., Posey, D. J., Stigler, K. A., Mullett, J., Katschke, A. R., & McDougle, C. J. (2007). A retrospective study of memantine in children and adolescents with pervasive developmental disorders. *Psychopharmacology*, *191*(1), 141–147.

Fatemi, S. H., Aldinger, K. A., Ashwood, P., Bauman, M. L., Blaha, C. D., Blatt, G. J., et al. (2012). Consensus paper: pathological role of the cerebellum in autism. *Cerebellum*, *11*(3), 777–807.

Fatemi, S. H., & Folsom, T. D. (2011). Dysregulation of fragile X mental retardation protein and metabotropic glutamate receptor 5 in superior frontal cortex of individuals with autism: A postmortem brain study. *Molecular Autism*, *2*, 6.

Frans, E. M., Sandin, S., Reichenberg, A., Langstrom, N., Lichtenstein, P., McGrath, J. J., et al. (2013). Autism risk across generations: a population-based study of advancing grandpaternal and paternal age. *JAMA Psychiatry*, *70*(5), 516–521.

Frye, R. E., & Rossignol, D. A. (2011). Mitochondrial dysfunction can connect the diverse medical symptoms associated with autism spectrum disorders. *Pediatric Research*, *69*(5 Pt 2), 41R–47R.

Frye, R. E., Sequeira, J. M., Quadros, E. V., James, S. J., & Rossignol, D. A. (2013). Cerebral folate receptor autoantibodies in autism spectrum disorder. [Research Support, Non-U.S. Gov't]. *Molecular Psychiatry*, *18*(3), 369–381.

Ghaleiha, A., Asadabadi, M., Mohammadi, M. R., Shahei, M., Tabrizi, M., Hajiaghaee, R., et al. (2013). Memantine as adjunctive treatment to risperidone in children with autistic disorder: A randomized, double-blind, placebo-controlled trial. *The International Journal of Neuropsychopharmacology/Official Scientific Journal of the Collegium Internationale Neuropsychopharmacologicum*, *16*(4), 783–789.

Gillies, D., Sinn, J., Lad, S. S., Leach, M. J., & Ross, M. J. (2012). Polyunsaturated fatty acids (PUFA) for attention deficit hyperactivity disorder (ADHD) in children and adolescents. *Cochrane Database of Systematic Reviews*, *7*, CD007986.

Giulivi, C., Zhang, Y. F., Omanska-Klusek, A., Ross-Inta, C., Wong, S., Hertz-Picciotto, I., et al. (2010). Mitochondrial dysfunction in autism. *JAMA: The Journal of the American Medical Association*, *304*(21), 2389–2396.

Goines, P., & Van de Water, J. (2010). The immune system's role in the biology of autism. *Current Opinion in Neurology*, *23*(2), 111–117.

Granpeesheh, D., Tarbox, J., & Dixon, D. R. (2009). Applied behavior analytic interventions for children with autism: A description and review of treatment research. *Annals of Clinical Psychiatry: Official Journal of the American Academy of Clinical Psychiatrists*, *21*(3), 162–173.

Greenspan S. W. S. (2008). *Engaging Autism: Using the Floortime Approach to Help Children relate, Communication, and Think*. Philadelpha, PA: Da Capo Press.

Greer, P. L., Hanayama, R., Bloodgood, B. L., Mardinly, A. R., Lipton, D. M., Flavell, S. W., et al. (2010). The Angelman Syndrome protein Ube3A regulates synapse development by ubiquitinating arc. *Cell*, *140*(5), 704–716.

Gregory, S. G., Connelly, J. J., Towers, A. J., Johnson, J., Biscocho, D., Markunas, C. A., et al. (2009). Genomic and epigenetic evidence for oxytocin receptor deficiency in autism. *BMC Medicine, 7*, 62.

Guastella, A. J., Einfeld, S. L., Gray, K. M., Rinehart, N. J., Tonge, B. J., Lambert, T. J., et al. (2010). Intranasal oxytocin improves emotion recognition for youth with autism spectrum disorders. *Biological Psychiatry, 67*(7), 692–694.

Hallmayer, J., Cleveland, S., Torres, A., Phillips, J., Cohen, B., Torigoe, T., et al. (2011). Genetic heritability and shared environmental factors among twin pairs with autism. *Archives of General Psychiatry, 68*(11), 1095–1102.

Handen, B. L., Sahl, R., & Hardan, A. Y. (2008). Guanfacine in children with autism and/or intellectual disabilities. *Journal of Developmental And Behavioral Pediatrics: JDBP, 29*(4), 303–308.

Handen, B. L., Taylor, J., & Tumuluru, R. (2011). Psychopharmacological treatment of ADHD symptoms in children with autism spectrum disorder. *International Journal of Adolescent Medicine and Health, 23*(3), 167–173.

Hanson, E., Kalish, L. A., Bunce, E., Curtis, C., McDaniel, S., Ware, J., et al. (2007). Use of complementary and alternative medicine among children diagnosed with autism spectrum disorder. *Journal of Autism and Developmental Disorders, 37*(4), 628–636.

Hardan, A. Y., Fung, L. K., Libove, R. A., Obukhanych, T. V., Nair, S., Herzenberg, L. A., et al. (2012). A randomized controlled pilot trial of oral N-acetylcysteine in children with autism. *Biological Psychiatry, 71*(11), 956–961. PMID:22342106.

Harony, H., & Wagner, S. (2010). The contribution of oxytocin and vasopressin to mammalian social behavior: Potential role in autism spectrum disorder. *Neuro-Signals, 18*(2), 82–97.

Hendren, R. (2013). Autism: Biomedical complementary treatment approaches. *Child and Adolescent Psychiatric Clinics of North America, 22*(3), 443–456.

Herbert, M. R. (2010). Contributions of the environment and environmentally vulnerable physiology to autism spectrum disorders. *Current Opinion in Neurology, 23*(2), 103–110.

Hoeffer, C. A., Sanchez, E., Hagerman, R. J., Mu, Y., Nguyen, D. V., Wong, H., et al. (2012). Altered mTOR signaling and enhanced CYFIP2 expression levels in subjects with fragile X syndrome. *Genes, Brain, and Behavior, 11*(3), 332–341. PMID:22268788 PMCID:PMC23319643.

Hollander, E., Chaplin, W., Soorya, L., Wasserman, S., Novotny, S., Rusoff, J., et al. (2010). Divalproex sodium vs. placebo for the treatment of irritability in children and adolescents with autism spectrum disorders. *Neuropsychopharmacology: Official Publication of the American College of Neuropsychopharmacology, 35*(4), 990–998.

Hollander, E., Dolgoff-Kaspar, R., Cartwright, C., Rawitt, R., & Novotny, S. (2001). An open trial of divalproex sodium in autism spectrum disorders. *The Journal of Clinical Psychiatry, 62*(7), 530–534.

Hollander, E., Phillips, A., Chaplin, W., Zagursky, K., Novotny, S., Wasserman, S., et al. (2005). A placebo controlled crossover trial of liquid fluoxetine on repetitive behaviors in childhood and adolescent autism. *Neuropsychopharmacology: Official Publication of the American College of Neuropsychopharmacology, 30*(3), 582–589.

Hourcade, J. P. (2013). Open autism software. Retrieved March 5, 2014, from http://homepage.divms.uiowa.edu/~hourcade/projects/asd/.

Iossifov, I., Ronemus, M., Levy, D., Wang, Z., Hakker, I., Rosenbaum, J., et al. (2012). De novo gene disruptions in children on the autistic spectrum. *Neuron, 74*(2), 285–299.

Jacquemont, S., Curie, A., des Portes, V., Torrioli, M. G., Berry-Kravis, E., Hagerman, R. J., et al. (2011). Epigenetic modification of the *FMR1* gene in fragile X syndrome is associated with differential response to the mGluR5 antagonist AFQ056. *Science Translational Medicine, 3*(64), 64ra61. PMID:21209411.

James, S. J., Cutler, P., Melnyk, S., Jernigan, S., Janak, L., Gaylor, D. W., et al. (2004). Metabolic biomarkers of increased oxidative stress and impaired methylation capacity in children with autism. *The American Journal of Clinical Nutrition, 80*(6), 1611–1617.

James, S. J., Melnyk, S., Fuchs, G., Reid, T., Jernigan, S., Pavliv, O., et al. (2009). Efficacy of methylcobalamin and folinic acid treatment on glutathione redox status in children with autism. *The American Journal of Clinical Nutrition, 89*(1), 425–430.

King, B. H., Hollander, E., Sikich, L., McCracken, J. T., Scahill, L., Bregman, J. D., et al. (2009). Lack of efficacy of citalopram in children with autism spectrum disorders and high levels of repetitive behavior: Citalopram ineffective in children with autism. *Archives of General Psychiatry, 66*(6), 583–590.

King, B. H., Wright, D. M., Handen, B. L., Sikich, L., Zimmerman, A. W., McMahon, W., et al. (2001). Double-blind, placebo-controlled study of amantadine hydrochloride in the treatment of children with autistic disorder. *Journal of the American Academy of Child and Adolescent Psychiatry, 40*(6), 658–665.

Koegel, R. L., Koegel, L. K., & McNerney, E. K. (2001). Pivotal areas in intervention for autism. *Journal of Clinical Child Psychology, 30*(1), 19–32.

Kohane, I. S., McMurry, A., Weber, G., MacFadden, D., Rappaport, L., Kunkel, L., et al. (2012). The co-morbidity burden of children and young adults with autism spectrum disorders. *PloS One, 7*(4), e33224.

Krakowiak, P., Walker, C. K., Bremer, A. A., Baker, A. S., Ozonoff, S., Hansen, R. L., et al. (2012). Maternal metabolic conditions and risk for autism and other neurodevelopmental disorders. *Pediatrics, 129*(5), e1121–e1128.

Landrigan, P. J. (2010). What causes autism? Exploring the environmental contribution. *Current Opinion in Pediatrics, 22*(2), 219–225.

Leblond, C. S., Heinrich, J., Delorme, R., Proepper, C., Betancur, C., Huguet, G., et al. (2012). Genetic and functional analyses of *SHANK2* mutations suggest a multiple hit model of autism spectrum disorders. [Research Support, Non-U.S. Gov't]. *PLoS Genetics, 8*(2), e1002521.

Lemonnier, E., Degrez, C., Phelep, M., Tyzio, R., Josse, F., Grandgeorge, M., et al. (2012). A randomised controlled trial of bumetanide in the treatment of autism in children. [Randomized Controlled Trial Research Support, Non-U.S. Gov't Video-Audio Media]. *Translational Psychiatry, 2*, e202.

Lofthouse, N., Hendren, R., Hurt, E., Arnold, L. E., & Butter, E. (2012). A review of complementary and alternative treatments for autism spectrum disorders. *Autism Research and Treatment, 2012*, 870391.

Lord, C., & Jones, R. M. (2012). Annual research review: Re-thinking the classification of autism spectrum disorders. *Journal of Child Psychology and Psychiatry, and Allied Disciplines, 53*(5), 490–509.

Manji, H., Kato, T., Di Prospero, N. A., Ness, S., Beal, M. F., Krams, M., et al. (2012). Impaired mitochondrial function in psychiatric disorders. *Nature reviews. Neuroscience, 13*(5), 293–307.

Mazurek, M. O., Vasa, R. A., Kalb, L. G., Kanne, S. M., Rosenberg, D., Keefer, A., et al. (2013). Anxiety, sensory over-responsivity, and gastrointestinal problems in children with autism spectrum disorders. *Journal of Abnormal Child Psychology, 41*(1), 165–176.

McCracken, J. T., McGough, J., Shah, B., Cronin, P., Hong, D., Aman, M. G., et al. (2002). Risperidone in children with autism and serious behavioral problems. *New England Journal of Medicine, 347*(5), 314–321. PMID:12151468.

Miller, D. T., Adam, M. P., Aradhya, S., Biesecker, L. G., Brothman, A. R., Carter, N. P., et al. (2010). Consensus statement: Chromosomal microarray is a first-tier clinical diagnostic test for individuals with developmental disabilities or congenital anomalies. *American Journal of Human Genetics, 86*(5), 749–764.

Murdoch, J. D., & State, M. W. (2013). Recent developments in the genetics of autism spectrum disorders. *Current Opinion in Genetics & Development, 23*(3), 310–315.

Napoli, E., Wong, S., & Giulivi, C. (2013). Evidence of reactive oxygen species-mediated damage to mitochondrial DNA in children with typical autism. *Molecular Autism, 4*(1), 2.

National Institutes of Health. (2005, 11/30/2012). Autism overview. Retrieved March 7, 2014, from http://www.cdc.gov/ncbddd/autism/facts.html.

Narayanan, A., White, C. A., Saklayen, S., Scaduto, M. J., Carpenter, A. L., Abduljalil, A., et al. (2010). Effect of propranolol on functional connectivity in autism spectrum disorder—a pilot study. *Brain Imaging and Behavior, 4*(2), 189–197.

Oppenheim, D., Koren-Karie, N., Dolev, S., & Yirmiya, N. (2009). Maternal insightfulness and resolution of the diagnosis are associated with secure attachment in preschoolers with autism spectrum disorders. *Child Development, 80*(2), 519–527.

Osterweil, E. K., Krueger, D. D., Reinhold, K., & Bear, M. F. (2010). Hypersensitivity to mGluR5 and ERK1/2 leads to excessive protein synthesis in the hippocampus of a mouse model of fragile X syndrome. *The Journal of Neuroscience: The Official Journal of the Society for Neuroscience, 30*(46), 15616–15627.

Owen, R., Sikich, L., Marcus, R. N., Corey-Lisle, P., Manos, G., McQuade, R. D., et al. (2009). Aripiprazole in the treatment of irritability in children and adolescents with autistic disorder. *Pediatrics, 124*(6), 1533–1540.

Palmer, R. F., Blanchard, S., Stein, Z., Mandell, D., & Miller, C. (2006). Environmental mercury release, special education rates, and autism disorder: An ecological study of Texas. *Health & Place, 12*(2), 203–209.

Posey, D. J., Erickson, C. A., Stigler, K. A., & McDougle, C. J. (2006). The use of selective serotonin reuptake inhibitors in autism and related disorders. *Journal of Child and Adolescent Psychopharmacology, 16*(1–2), 181–186.

Posey, D. J., Kem, D. L., Swiezy, N. B., Sweeten, T. L., Wiegand, R. E., & McDougle, C. J. (2004). A pilot study of D-cycloserine in subjects with autistic disorder. *The American Journal of Psychiatry, 161*(11), 2115–2117.

Qin, M., Kang, J., Burlin, T. V., Jiang, C., & Smith, C. B. (2005). Postadolescent changes in regional cerebral protein synthesis: An in vivo study in the FMR1 null mouse. *The Journal of Neuroscience: The Official Journal of the Society for Neuroscience, 25*(20), 5087–5095.

Roberts, E. M., English, P. B., Grether, J. K., Windham, G. C., Somberg, L., & Wolff, C. (2007). Maternal residence near agricultural pesticide applications and autism spectrum disorders among children in the California Central Valley. *Environmental Health Perspectives, 115*(10), 1482–1489.

Robertson, J. M., Tanguay, P. E., L'Ecuyer, S., Sims, A., & Waltrip, C. (1999). Domains of social communication handicap in autism spectrum disorder. *Journal of the American Academy of Child and Adolescent Psychiatry, 38*(6), 738–745.

Rossignol, D. A. (2009). Novel and emerging treatments for autism spectrum disorders: A systematic review. *Annals of Clinical Psychiatry: Official Journal of the American Academy of Clinical Psychiatrists, 21*(4), 213–236.

Rubenstein, J. L. (2010). Three hypotheses for developmental defects that may underlie some forms of autism spectrum disorder. *Current Opinion in Neurology, 23*(2), 118–123.

Research Units on Pediatric Psychopharmacology. (2005). Randomized, controlled, crossover trial of methylphenidate in pervasive developmental disorders with hyperactivity. *Archives of General Psychiatry, 62*(11), 1266–1274.

Rutter, M. (2005). Incidence of autism spectrum disorders: Changes over time and their meaning. *Acta Paediatrica, 94*(1), 2–15.

Shelton, J. F., Tancredi, D. J., & Hertz-Picciotto, I. (2010). Independent and dependent contributions of advanced maternal and paternal ages to autism risk. *Autism Research: Official Journal of the International Society for Autism Research, 3*(1), 30–39.

Shen, M. D., Nordahl, C. W., Young, G. S., Wootton-Gorges, S. L., Lee, A., Liston, S. E., et al. (2013). Early brain enlargement and elevated extra-axial fluid in infants who develop autism spectrum disorder. *Brain: A Journal of Neurology, 136* (Pt 9), 2825–2835

Silverman, J. L., Babineau, B. A., Oliver, C. F., Karras, M. N., & Crawley, J. N. (2013). Influence of stimulant-induced hyperactivity on social approach in the BTBR mouse model of autism. *Neuropharmacology, 68*, 210–222.

Silverman, J. L., Smith, D. G., Rizzo, S. J., Karras, M. N., Turner, S. M., Tolu, S. S., et al. (2012). Negative allosteric modulation of the mGluR5 receptor reduces repetitive behaviors and rescues social deficits in mouse models of autism. *Science Translational Medicine, 4*(131), 131ra151. PMID:22539775.

Tharp, B., Ozonoff, S., Rogers, S., & Hendren, R. L. (Ed.). (2003). *Autism Spectrum Disorders: A Research Review for Practitioners.* Arlington, VA: American Psychiatric Publishing, Inc.

van Eeghen, A. M., Pulsifer, M. B., Merker, V. L., Neumeyer, A. M., van Eeghen, E. E., Thibert, R. L., et al. (2013). Understanding relationships between autism, intelligence, and epilepsy: A cross-disorder approach. *Developmental Medicine and Child Neurology, 55*(2), 146–153.

Veenstra-VanderWeel, J., Hehn, J. S. v., Kuriyama, N., Cherubini, M., Bear, M. F., & Cook, E. H. (2013). *Randomized, controlled, phase 2 trial of STX209 (Arbaclofen) for social function in ASD.* Presentation at International Meeting for Autism Research (IMFAR), May 2, 2013, San Sebastian, Spain.

Vismara, L. A., & Rogers, S. J. (2010). Behavioral treatments in autism spectrum disorder: What do we know? *Annual Review of Clinical Psychology, 6*, 447–468.

Volk, H. E., Lurmann, F., Penfold, B., Hertz-Picciotto, I., & McConnell, R. (2013). Traffic-related air pollution, particulate matter, and autism. *JAMA Psychiatry, 70*(1), 71–77.

Volkmar, F. R., Reichow, B., & McPartland, J. (2012). Classification of autism and related conditions: Progress, challenges, and opportunities. *Dialogues in Clinical Neuroscience, 14*(3), 229–237.

Wallace, K. S., & Rogers, S. J. (2010). Intervening in infancy: Implications for autism spectrum disorders. *Journal of Child Psychology and Psychiatry, and Allied Disciplines, 51*(12), 1300–1320.

Werner, E., & Dawson, G. (2005). Validation of the phenomenon of autistic regression using home videotapes. *Archives of General Psychiatry, 62*(8), 889–895.

Widjaja, F., Choi, J., James, J., & Hendren, R. (2013). Clinical and laboratory results from randomized controlled trial of methylcobalamine injections for children with autism. Paper presented at the Poster at the International Meeting for Autism Research (IMFAR), May 4, 2013, San Sebastian, Spain.

Wong, H. H., & Smith, R. G. (2006). Patterns of complementary and alternative medical therapy use in children diagnosed with autism spectrum disorders. *Journal of Autism and Developmental Disorders, 36*(7), 901–909.

Zerbo, O., Iosif, A. M., Walker, C., Ozonoff, S., Hansen, R. L., & Hertz-Picciotto, I. (2013). Is maternal influenza or fever during pregnancy associated with autism or developmental delays? Results from the CHARGE (CHildhood Autism Risks from Genetics and Environment) study. *Journal of Autism and Developmental Disorders, 43*(1), 25–33.

Zoghbi, H. Y., & Bear, M. F. (2012). Synaptic dysfunction in neurodevelopmental disorders associated with autism and intellectual disabilities. *Cold Spring Harbor Perspectives in Biology, 4*(3), a009886.

CHAPTER 3

Targeted Treatments in Schizophrenia

DANIELLE A. SCHLOSSER, COLEMAN GARRETT,
AND SOPHIA VINOGRADOV

INTRODUCTION

Schizophrenia is a psychiatric illness that is characterized by *psychosis*, a general term that means "loss of touch with reality." Although individuals experiencing psychosis have been observed throughout history and the meaning of their behavior has been understood in various cultural contexts (for example, as a manifestation of supernatural forces), Emil Kraepelin, a German psychiatrist from the nineteenth century, was the first to describe schizophrenia to the medical field (Kraepelin, 1919). His initial description referred to an illness that began at an early age and was characterized by progressive deterioration in cognitive function; he termed it *dementia praecox*, analogous to the late-onset neurodegenerative disorder discovered by his colleague Alois Alzheimer (Kraepelin, 1919). Shortly thereafter, Swiss psychiatrist Eugen Bleuler coined the term *schizophrenia* to describe his clinical observations of symptoms in patients, resulting in a shift of emphasis on the key features of the illness.

The word *schizophrenia* comes from the Greek roots *schizo* (split) and *phrene* (mind), and was used by Bleuler to capture the fragmented thinking seen in individuals with this disorder. Bleuler emphasized not only the thinking disturbances, which he referred to as *positive symptoms*, but also the "fundamental deficits" of experience, which he referred to as *negative symptoms*. The framework for delineating symptoms as *positive* versus *negative* originates from John Hughlings Jackson, a British neurologist who first used the term *negative symptoms* to describe an absence of essential functions due to a loss of higher level neurobiological functions. Conversely, *positive symptoms* were defined as those that result from excitation or the release of lower levels from higher inhibitory control (York & Steinberg, 2006). Thus, even during its inception as a nosological entity, schizophrenia was conceptualized as an illness with strong analogies to neurological disorders—a concept that now, 100 years later, has been confirmed by a wealth of research evidence. At the present time, in fact, we understand schizophrenia to be a neurocognitive disorder, caused by dysfunction in key neural systems in the brain that normally allow us to process sensory information, to create and retrieve memories, and to engage in adaptive planning, abstraction, and problem-solving.

For much of the late twentieth century, the Kraepelian characterization of schizophrenia as a neurodegenerative brain disease, combined with accumulating data indicating a wide range of cognitive deficits in individuals with the illness, led to a stance of therapeutic nihilism. Treatment was seen as palliative only, and the goal was to stabilize the most troublesome of symptoms and to provide enough psychosocial support to permit some kind of community functioning. Indeed, until recently, the typical outcomes have been discouraging. Fewer than 14% of patients sustain an enduring recovery within the first five years of illness, and only another 16% later on (Harrison et al., 2001; Robinson, Woerner, McMeniman, Mendelowitz, & Bilder, 2004). Schizophrenia ranks within the top 10 causes of the global burden of illness, ranking fifth for males and sixth for females in the leading global causes of years lost because of disability (WHO, 2008).

In the past 15 years, however, there has been a radical shift in our understanding of schizophrenia. We now understand it to be not only a neurocognitive disorder, but also a neurodevelopmental disorder: one with antecedents during gestation, and a developmental course that unfolds at first mostly silently, and then with increasing signs and symptoms, until the onset of the first episode of psychosis during adolescence or early adulthood. In addition, we now understand it to be a syndrome rather than a disease per se—that is, a final common clinical phenotype with multiple different etiopathogenic factors contributing to its onset and expression. This new perspective has spurred research that has unequivocally demonstrated that, with early detection and targeted intervention, more specific and personalized treatment approaches can be developed than have been available thus far. More importantly, intact developmental and brain plasticity mechanisms can be harnessed in an adaptive manner in the young schizophrenia patient to promote ongoing psychosocial engagement, healthier neural system functioning, increased resilience to stress, symptom reduction, and functional recovery. In this chapter, we will:

1) Review the core clinical features of the illness, with an emphasis on early detection;
2) Briefly summarize current findings on the etiology and pathophysiology of schizophrenia;
3) Describe ways in which these findings are leading to the development of targeted treatments that focus on the biological bases of schizophrenia, with the ultimate goal of promoting meaningful functional recovery for young individuals.

ESSENTIAL FEATURES OF SCHIZOPHRENIA: EMPHASIS ON EARLY DETECTION

Epidemiological Features of Schizophrenia

Despite the fact that schizophrenia results in a marked reduction in reproductive fitness, it continues to persist in the human population at a global lifetime prevalence of around 0.7%, with moderate variations in prevalence across geographic locales and cultures (Jablensky, 1997; McGrath & Richards, 2009). This suggests that the factors that contribute to schizophrenia are ubiquitous and that some aspects of the vulnerability to psychosis may be advantageous. In a mild and attenuated version, psychotic spectrum traits can be allied with creativity, the ability to pursue a goal in a reward-independent manner, asceticism, and single-minded devotion to a cause, and can appear as an important aspect of spiritual and transcendent experiences.

In its full-blown version, however, schizophrenia is a veritable "cancer of the mind" and is arguably among the most devastating and costly of human illnesses. It strikes adolescents and young adults in their prime, impeding participation in critical social-emotional, educational, and vocational developmental experiences. It robs them of their key human faculties: the ability to perceive and respond adaptively to the environment; the ability to communicate effectively; the ability to plan for the future and engage in task-relevant behavior; and the ability to interact satisfactorily with others. The symptoms of schizophrenia can lead to a pervasive sense of being in mortal danger, and can cause behavior that is bizarre, withdrawn, or violent—engendering incalculable fear and suffering for patients, their family members, and society. In addition to its human toll, schizophrenia costs society more than depression, dementia and other medical illness across most of the lifespan (Bartels, Clark, Peacock, Dums, & Pratt, 2003).

Although men and women experience schizophrenia at similar rates, women tend to experience a later onset (the peak ages of onset are 20–28 years for males and 26–32 years for females) as well as a better course of illness (Riecher-Rössler & Häfner, 2000). On average, 55% of male patients will experience onset before 25 years of age, versus 30% of women (Goldstein, Tsuang, & Faraone, 1989). This may be due to neurodevelopmental differences between males and females, the neuroprotective effects of female hormones, or to the fact that females may experience less exposure to severe psychosocial stressors. Mortality is high, and the average life expectancy of people with schizophrenia is 10 to 15 years less than those without, the result of increased co-occurring physical health problems and a higher suicide rate, which are often inadequately addressed in current treatment settings. Medical comorbidities are a significant public health problem in schizophrenia and include metabolic disorders such as diabetes, dyslipidemia, and hypertension—some of which may be in part secondary to current pharmacological treatment regimens (McEvoy et al., 2005). Psychiatric comorbities are extremely common and include depression, anxiety, and substance abuse. The majority of deaths in schizophrenia are due to cardiovascular disease (Nasrallah & Newcomer, 2004), and about 5%–10% of individuals dying of suicide, usually within the first three years of illness onset (Alaräisänen et al., 2009; Pompili, Lester, Innamorati, Tatarelli, & Girardi, 2008).

Core Clinical Features of Schizophrenia

Patients with schizophrenia demonstrate a number of different psychotic symptoms, and these symptoms wax and wane over the course of the illness. Researchers classify these psychotic symptoms into three major groupings—positive, negative, and disorganized—and it appears that each grouping may be associated with specific forms of dysfunction in brain circuitry. Schizophrenia is highly heterogeneous in its clinical presentation, and any given patient may exhibit just a few, or several, or most of the symptoms described below. In addition to these three symptom groups, schizophrenia is characterized by cognitive dysfunction and psychosocial impairment; thus, the core clinical features of schizophrenia fall into five general categories (Table 3.1):

Positive symptoms of psychosis include hallucinations (auditory, visual, olfactory, gustatory), and delusions (a variety of types, which are

Table 3.1 CLINICAL FEATURES OF SCHIZOPHRENIA

Positive symptoms	Negative symptoms	Disorganized symptoms	Cognitive deficits	Psychosocial impairments
Delusions	Avolition	Inappropriate affect	Impaired executive functioning, working memory, processing speed, sensory processing Dyskinesias	Social, occupational, and self-care dysfunction
Hallucinations	Affective flattening	Disorganized speech		
Paranoia	Alogia	Odd behavior		
Unusual thought content	Poverty of thought			

listed below; Table 3.2). Auditory hallucinations are the most common of the hallucinatory symptoms. Delusions are typically classified as either *bizarre* or *non-bizarre*, which the DSM defines as depending on whether the belief is possible. For instance, a delusion about a radio residing in an individual's brain would be considered a bizarre delusion, whereas the belief that the government is monitoring an individual's behavior would be considered non-bizarre. Dysregulation of the mesolimbic dopamine system is thought to contribute to altered appraisal of sensory stimuli and aberrant attribution of salience (Howes & Kapur, 2009). Hallucinations and delusions are considered the result of an "aberrant salience network," which includes the anterior insula and anterior cingulate (Palaniyappan, Mallikarjun, Joseph, White, & Liddle, 2011). This network recruits neural systems to identify and process salient information from a myriad of internal and external stimuli. Auditory hallucinations have also been shown to be associated with abnormalities in corollary discharge—the normal neural responses in the brain to self-generated vocalizations (Ford & Mathalon, 2004; Mathalon & Ford, 2008).

Table 3.2 POSITIVE SYMPTOMS

Positive symptoms	Definition	Types	Neurobiological underpinnings
Hallucinations	Perception of stimuli that are not present	Auditory, visual, olfactory, gustatory	Dysregulation of subcortical dopamine Abnormal corollary discharge
Delusions	Fixed false beliefs	Paranoid, bizarre, non-bizarre, somatic, grandiose, religious, referential, guilt	Aberrant salience brain network

Negative symptoms of psychosis include avolition (reduction in motivation), anergia (reduction in activity), alogia (reduction of speech), flat affect (reduction of emotional expression), anhedonia (reduction of pleasure), asociality, and decreased ideational richness. Negative symptoms are often misunderstood as depression, but the course varies significantly. Major depressive disorder is an episodic illness, whereas individuals with negative symptoms experience more longstanding and stable symptoms. While less is known about the neurobiological underpinning of negative symptoms, recent attention has focused on neural systems that subserve reward and emotion processing (Gold et al., 2012) as well as on psychological models highlighting the role of defeatist beliefs (Beck, Grant, Huh, Perivoliotis, & Chang, 2013).

Disorganized symptoms of psychosis include disorganized communication, disorganized thinking, and disorganized behavior. Examples include communication that is difficult to follow due to nonsensical thought patterns, an expression of affect that is inappropriate for the context, and wearing many layers of clothing on a warm day. Neuroimaging findings implicate deficits in prefrontal activation and cognitive control in the expression of disorganized symptoms (Becker, Cicero, Cowan, & Kerns, 2012; Yoon et al., 2012)

Impaired cognition: Even though the symptoms of the illness are dramatic and are what most clinicians focus on, it is now axiomatic that schizophrenia is a neurocognitive disorder, one that is characterized by impairments in a wide range of cognitive function, ranging from the earliest stages of information processing, to higher-level abilities to abstract, to self-reflect, and to engage in meta-cognition. These various areas of cognitive dysfunction are accompanied by abnormalities in their neural system correlates. Moreover, patients exhibit a fair amount of cognitive heterogeneity, and different patients will often have different patterns of impairment. Nonetheless, the following findings are common: *sensory processing abnormalities* (subtle deficiencies in processing early auditory and visual information); *neuromotor findings* (dyscoordination, slowed and impaired motor sequencing, mild dystonic posturing and dyskinesias); *executive dysfunction,* sometimes also called *impaired cognitive control* (deficits in attention and working memory; problems with inhibition of pre-potent responses; impaired abstraction, reasoning, planning); *memory deficits* (impairments in episodic memory—e.g., autobiographical events; semantic memory—meanings and associations); and fear-extinction learning (Rajji et al., 2013).

Reduced psychosocial functioning: One of the central features of schizophrenia is a reduction, at least initially, in social and educational/vocational functioning. Too often, individuals with schizophrenia are unemployed, have failed to achieve academic or vocational milestones, and are socially isolated. Several factors put individuals at particular risk for poor functional outcome: poor premorbid functioning, younger age of onset, greater severity of cognitive deficits, and prominent negative and depressive symptoms (Bowie et al., 2010; Green, Hellemann, Horan, Lee, & Wynn, 2012; Milev, Ho, Arndt, & Andreasen, 2005). Indeed, cognitive deficits and negative symptom severity are greater determinants of long-term outcome than the more dramatic positive symptoms. Poor functional outcome is often correlated with impairments in prefrontal cortical functioning (Lesh, Niendam, Minzenberg, & Carter, 2011).

What Is the Onset and Course of the Illness?

As with almost every other aspect of schizophrenia, there is a large amount of variability in the onset and course of the illness. Most individuals will exhibit some kind of a *clinical prodrome* in their adolescence that often goes unrecognized, but in retrospect can be seen as heralding the onset of a break with reality. Late adolescence and early adulthood is the peak period for onset of the first episode, but often there are indications of incipient psychiatric illness earlier in adolescence, before the first full-blown psychosis. This is typically followed by a prodromal stage characterized by ongoing mood and anxiety symptoms, worsening functional status, and attenuated psychotic symptoms. This prodromal phase may be brief and acute or may proceed slowly and gradually for several years.

After recovery from the first episode, individuals will often go on to have further exacerbations, especially if they are not able to engage in adequate treatment, and these usually occur during the first five years of illness. Finally, for most, there is stabilization, followed by small but steady gains towards recovery, especially when well-tailored treatment is provided. Growing evidence indicates unequivocally that the earlier and more vigorously we intervene in schizophrenia, the better the short- and long-term outcome.

At present, in individuals with a first episode of psychosis, a good long-term outcome occurs in 42%, an intermediate outcome in 35%, and a poor outcome in 27%, and a large portion of the variance in outcome is determined by the availability of targeted, early interventions (Nordentoft, Jeppesen, Petersen, Bertelsen, & Thorup, 2009).

As briefly mentioned earlier, typical prodromal features that are present before the first episode include social withdrawal, decline in school/work performance, "depressive" symptoms, irritability, decreased emotional expressivity, and attenuated psychotic-like symptoms that the person recognizes as

Table 3.3 CLINICAL HIGH-RISK CRITERIA FROM THE STRUCTURED INTERVIEW FOR PRODROMAL SYNDROMES

Prodromal syndrome	Attenuated positive symptom syndrome	Genetic risk and deterioration	Brief intermittent psychotic syndrome
Symptom characteristics	At least 1 attenuated positive symptom, including unusual thought content; persecutory ideation; grandiosity; perceptual disturbances; disorganized communication	First-degree relative with a psychotic disorder AND either 1) a 30% drop or more in global functioning over the past month compared to 12 months ago OR 2) meets criteria for schizotypal personality disorder	The experience of a brief psychotic intensity positive symptom that only lasts for several minutes per day but no more than an hour at a time
Frequency	At least 1x/week	N/A	Less than 4 days/week
Onset	Within the past year, or an experience of symptoms' worsening over the past year	N/A	Within the past three months

problematic (but is often fearful to reveal). Recent advances have been made to identify individuals in the prodromal phase based on operationalized "clinical high risk" (CHR) criteria, which are defined by the presence of attenuated psychotic symptoms and/or genetic risk and functional deterioration (Miller et al., 2002) (Table 3.3). Approximately 35% of individuals defined using these CHR criteria will develop a psychotic disorder within two and a half years (Cannon et al., 2008), providing a unique window into the pathophysiology of psychosis onset. Additionally, the CHR criteria ushers in the possibility of truly preventive or preemptive interventions aimed at delaying or even preventing the onset of psychosis. While biomarkers of a heightened risk for conversion are currently under study, and include brain volumetric changes and EEG abnormalities, they have not entered clinical practice.

ETIOLOGY AND PATHOPHYSIOLOGY OF SCHIZOPHRENIA

Genetic Risk Factors

Schizophrenia carries a strong genetic component, with various genetic risk factors accounting for about 80% of the liability for the illness (Cannon,

Kaprio, Lönnqvist, Huttunen, & Koskenvuo, 1998). This was shown by the mid-twentieth century through family studies, where the risk of schizophrenia is ~15% in first-degree relatives; through twin studies, where the monozygotic concordance rate is 50%; and through adoption studies, where babies born to mothers with schizophrenia but adopted away at birth still show an increased risk of the disorder (Tsuang, Stone, & Faraone, 2001; Wicks, Hjern, & Dalman, 2010).

More recently, the genetic architecture of schizophrenia has been the subject of great debate. The predominant view for many years has been the "common disease, common variant" hypothesis, in which schizophrenia results from a large number of common variants of individually small effect. However, there has also been increasing evidence for the "common disease, rare variant" hypothesis, which involves extreme genetic heterogeneity from many rare, but highly penetrant mutations (Gejman, Sanders, & Kendler, 2011). The latest genome wide association studies (GWAS) and genome-wide copy number variant (CNV) studies show that the truth lies between these two extremes, and indicate that schizophrenia involves a spectrum of allelic variation from common to rare (Mowry & Gratten, 2013). Some examples of interesting candidate genes include: neuroregulin, important in neuronal growth; dysbindin, important for synaptic vesicle function; NRXN1 = neurexin 1, a cell adhesion molecule necessary for proper synaptic function; an intron of *MIR137*, a microRNA involved in neuronal maturation and adult neurogenesis; and a region spanning the major histocompatability complex, which has a prominent role in the development of host defense and immunity.

Another interesting recent development is the discovery of shared polygenic variation between schizophrenia and bipolar disorder at four individual loci, suggesting that some aspects of shared neurobiological liability exist between these two disorders (*ANK3, CACNA1C, ITIH3-ITIH4* and *ZNF804A*). Links have also been at four specific loci (regions on chromosomes 3p21 and 10q24 and single-nucleotide polymorphisms (SNPs) within two L-type voltage-gated calcium channel subunits, CACNA1C and CACNB2) between schizophrenia, bipolar disorder, major depressive disorder, and attention-deficit hyperactivity disorder (Cross-Disorder Group of the Psychiatric Genomics Consortium, 2013). Also, shared rare CNVs have been found between schizophrenia and other neurodevelopmental disorders, including autism spectrum disorders, intellectual disability (ID), developmental delay and epilepsy (Cross-Disorder Group of the Psychiatric Genomics Consortium, 2013). For example, deletions in 2p16.3 (*NRXN1*), 1q21.1, and 15q13.3 have all been identified in autism spectrum disorders and ID in addition to schizophrenia (Stefansson et al., 2008).

What may be inherited in schizophrenia from most, if not all, of these genetic variants are subtle impairments in normal patterns of neuronal migration and function, resulting in an increased risk for neural network "disconnectivity" and a liability to some forms of cognitive dysfunction, such as working-memory impairment (Camchong, MacDonald, Bell, Mueller, & Lim, 2011). Research shows that genetic vulnerability interacts with prenatal and perinatal insults in schizophrenia in a way that is especially detrimental to the genetically at-risk fetus. For example, infants with a genetic risk for schizophrenia are much more likely to show deleterious long-term effects of perinatal hypoxia than infants without this genetic risk (Cannon et al., 2000).

A substantial proportion of first-degree relatives of patients with schizophrenia carry a predisposing genotype without full phenotypic expression (but sometimes showing a subtle, attenuated phenotype). They can nonetheless pass on the susceptibility to schizophrenia to their offspring. However, as was shown in a Finnish study, when the offspring of a patient with schizophrenia is adopted away and raised in a psychologically healthy family, his/her risk for developing schizophrenia was only 5%, whereas if he/she was adopted away and raised in a psychologically stressful family, the risk was approximately 30% (Tienari et al., 2004). Thus, psychological trauma and stress also play a role in the expression of the illness in those who are genetically susceptible.

Environmental Risk Factors

Although schizophrenia is highly heritable disorder, with various genes accounting for a large portion of the liability, the remaining variance is attributed to environmental insults occurring during the prenatal and perinatal period (Brown, 2011). These include:

Gestational factors: High maternal weight gain, maternal respiratory or rubella infection, influenza infection, gestational diabetes, malnutrition during pregnancy.

Obstetric complications: Complications of pregnancy (bleeding during pregnancy, rhesus incompatibility, preeclampsia); abnormal fetal growth and development (fetal hypoxia, low birth weight, congenital malformations, reduced head circumference); complications of delivery (asphyxia, uterine atonia, emergency C-section).

The current model of pathogenesis (Figure 3.1) posits that genetic factors interact with these early environmental insults, with the result that at-risk individuals are highly vulnerable to a range of later environmental

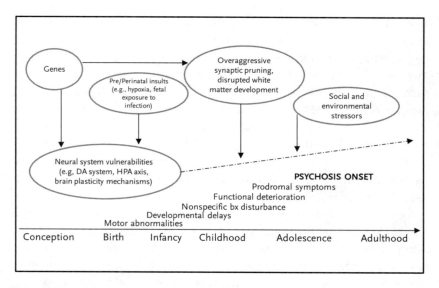

Figure 3.1:
Neurodevelopmental model of schizophrenia (adapted and modified by permission of Tyrone Cannon, PhD). Key: DA = dopamine, HPA = hypothalamic-pituitary-adrenal.

stressors, such as childhood physical and sexual abuse, being bullied, the effects of cannabis use, and psychosocial trauma (urban poverty, immigration). This interaction of genes and exogenous insults leads to aberrations in brain development and neural network functioning, which are not typically evident until adolescence or very early adulthood, when brain maturation is nearing completion (Andreasen 2010; Hoffman & McGlashan 1997). At that point, usually as a response to some specific environmental or interpersonal stressors, such as moving away to college or experiencing a bad break-up, the individual (who may until then have had no observable symptoms or only mild, non-specific symptoms), experiences a catastrophic disruption in normal cognitive operations and neuromodulatory function—what we call *psychosis*. A number of studies have shown an association between stressors and psychotic relapse in individuals with established illness, and there is growing evidence of a link between stress and attenuated psychosis during the prodromal phase. Understanding schizophrenia as a neurodevelopmental disorder characterized by decreased efficiency and abnormal connectivity in cortical and subcortical neural networks—rendering them particularly vulnerable to the deleterious effects of stress—sheds light on why emerging interventions that help an individual respond more adaptively to stressful stimuli, or that target abnormal neural system processing, may help ameliorate the early course of illness.

Models of Pathophysiology in Schizophrenia

In healthy neural development, the maximal proliferation of neuronal synapses and the peak synaptic density occur at ~2 years of age, which is then followed by a steady drop in synaptic density during childhood and a steep decline in adolescence (Spear, 2003). This process is "synaptic pruning," which can be thought of as a sculpting of the cortex in response to experience in order to support increased efficiency of neural network processing, particularly in prefrontal regions (Spear, 2003). As the prefrontal cortex undergoes synaptic pruning, there is an increased ability to solve abstract and complex problems, with enhanced capacities for reasoning, planning, and inhibitory control (Spear, 2003). Several studies suggest that abnormal synaptic pruning may contribute to the onset of psychosis in adolescence (Andreasen et al., 2011; McGlashan & Hoffman, 2000). At present it is not known with certainty which specific gene products or molecular/cellular processes are associated with abnormal synapse pruning and synaptic functioning in schizophrenia, but the net effect is a reduction in gray matter volume in key brain regions. For example, in a recent meta-analysis on clinical high-risk patients, those who later converted to psychosis showed baseline decreases in gray matter in frontal and temporal areas (Fusar-Poli et al., 2012).

Another important process in neurodevelopment is increased white matter density. Starting in adolescence and leading into early adulthood, the hippocampus and frontal lobe undergo substantial myelination, which is also driven by experience-dependent plasticity mechanisms in the brain (or, simply put, adaptive learning). Again, in schizophrenia, accumulating evidence suggests that this process is disrupted; the net result is that decreased white matter density impairs the fast and efficient integration of information processing both within and across cortical zones, and contributes to cognitive impairment and risk for psychosis (Dwork, Mancevski, & Rosoklija, 2007). For example, clinical high-risk patients do not show the normal increase in white matter with age, and this is associated with poor functional outcome (Carletti et al., 2012; Karlsgodt, Niendam, Bearden, & Cannon, 2009). In the largest longitudinal study to date, young individuals with schizophrenia showed decreases in multiple gray and white matter regions, which were most pronounced two years after the first episode of psychosis (Andreasen et al., 2011).

The *stress-vulnerability model of schizophrenia* posits that a range of environmental stressors interact with these underlying neurobiological vulnerabilities in at-risk individuals to trigger the onset of psychosis (Nuechterlein & Dawson, 1984; Walker & Diforio, 1997). The primary mechanism proposed to underlie this process is dysfunction of the hypothalamic-pituitary-adrenal (HPA) axis, the primary neurobiological stress response system in mammals. Findings from several human and animal studies indicate that persistently elevated glucocorticoid levels can be neurotoxic, and the hippocampus might be especially sensitive to these effects (Walker, Mittal, & Tessner, 2008). Exposure to repeated stressors increases glutamate in the prefrontal cortex and the hippocampus, and results in altered subcortical dopamine levels (Moghaddam, 2002). Studies examining HPA functioning in schizophrenia demonstrate the following:

1) Baseline HPA axis activity (without explicit exposure to stress), especially in those not on psychotropic medications, shows higher adrenocorticotropic hormone (ACTH) and cortisol than healthy comparison subjects (Walker & Diforio, 1997);
2) Dysregulated response to pharmacological challenge of the negative feedback loop (Walker et al., 2008), and
3) Maladaptive cortisol response to laboratory stress tests, suggesting an important pathway by which environmental insults increase the risk for schizophrenia.

THE DEVELOPMENT OF TARGETED TREATMENTS

Overall, the emerging picture in schizophrenia is one of a brain that has undergone aberrant patterns of neurodevelopment, with reduced functional connectivity among key neural systems and reduced efficiency in its cognitive and socio-affective operations and a heightened response to stressors. This suggests that, in order to prevent a deteriorating course, early interventions must be designed to address and, if possible, "correct" the abnormal neural system functioning before the individual has undergone what might be irreversible maladaptive changes in his/her cortical representational systems.

Given that CHR patients have been found to report even higher stress levels than first-episode psychosis patients (Pruessner et al., 2011), reducing stress and improving coping is a critical target for preemptive interventions. New areas of research are starting to focus on the natural plasticity of the HPA axis during adolescent development, with the aim of developing interventions during the prodromal phase that promote resiliency to stress. Some examples include cognitive therapy approaches that help individuals reappraise their interpretation of stressful stimuli in a more adaptive manner; behavioral stress-reduction techniques that teach individuals to take an active role in reducing their exposure and physiological response to stressors; family therapy to reduce stressful familial interactions and increase family support; and cognitive training exercises that aim to improve the accuracy and fidelity of the processing of cognitive and socio-affective stimuli and increase the brain's "cognitive resilience" to data in its environment. We will discuss two of these—cognitive therapy and cognitive training—in more detail below, after a brief review of novel, emerging psychopharmacological approaches.

The Current and Future Pharmacological Treatment Landscape for Schizophrenia

Until very recently, antipsychotic medications have been the backbone of treatment for schizophrenia, as early as the first episode, and sometimes even prescribed in the prodrome (Van Os & Kapur, 2009). Antipsychotics function by suppressing the dopamine D2 receptor. The "first-generation" antipsychotics (e.g., chloropromazine, haloperidol), which date back to the 1950s, frequently induce troublesome extrapyramidal side effects due to their brain-wide dopamine-blocking effects. In the past 15 years, "second generation" antipsychotics have been introduced (ziprasidone, risperidone, olanzapine, quetiapine, etc.); these medications have a somewhat broader neuroreceptor profile, affecting serotonin receptors as well as dopamine receptors, and are effective for positive symptoms while avoiding motor system side effects. Unfortunately, they induce considerable weight gain, diabetes, and metabolic syndrome (Agid, Kapur, & Remington, 2008; Leucht et al., 2009). Aripiprazole, which is a partial D2 receptor agonist, is sometimes considered a "third generation" antipsychotic with its own unique mechanism of action and side effect profile; because it does not induce complete D2 receptor blockade with all of the potential deleterious effects this implies for normal neuromodulatory function in the brain, some feel that it may be a preferable medication for younger individuals. Another treatment option that is under active study for younger patients is the use of long-acting injection (LAI) antipsychotics. LAIs reduce the risk of relapse and improve cognitive performance compared to oral treatments (Bartzokis et al., 2011). In general, treatment programs for early psychosis emphasize a thoughtful algorithm of medication prescription that uses the lowest possible dose due to increased sensitivity to side effects (Moore et al., 2007). Treatment-refractory patients are often offered clozapine, which can be highly effective, but involves a risk of potentially serious side effects such as agranulocytosis, significant anticholinergic burden, and cognitive effects (Meltzer, 2013).

Many antipsychotic medications, in fact, including the second-generation agents olanzapine, quetiapine, and clozapine, have anticholinergic side effects both peripherally and centrally; anticholinergic burden is association with poorer cognitive performance at baseline and a reduced response to computerized cognitive training (Minzenberg, Poole, Benton, & Vinogradov, 2004; Sophia Vinogradov et al., 2009). In addition, higher exposure to antipsychotic medications, especially during the first few years of illness, is associated with reduced gray matter volume (Ho, Andreasen, Ziebell, Pierson, & Magnotta, 2011; Radua et al., 2012). Because of the numerous serious side effects associated with antipsychotic medications, as well as the fact that they do not address the functionally important negative and cognitive symptoms of schizophrenia, there is now a small but growing realization that the field needs to consider a fundamental paradigm shift in its approach to medication management of the illness. This includes both a greater and more rigorous use of behavioral treatments, as well as the use of novel pharmacological agents currently under development.

Some of the emerging areas of medication development include adjunctive treatments targeting the negative cognitive and social symptoms of schizophrenia. Glycine transport (GlyT1) inhibitors have proved effective in the mitigation of positive and negative symptoms when combined with traditional antipsychotic treatment (Lane et al., 2010) by regulating glycine concentration at N-methyl-D-aspartate (NMDA) receptors that require glycine as a co-agonist. Alpha 7 nicotinic receptor (a7 nAChR) agonists, another adjunctive treatment, were developed based on findings of altered receptor function (Martin, Kem, & Freedman, 2004), and their use has been associated with improvements in cognition (Freedman et al., 2008). The use of Minocycline, a second-generation tetracycline antibiotic, has improved cognitive functioning in recent-onset schizophrenia (Levkovitz et al., 2010), possibly because of its neuroprotective and anti-inflammatory effects. Interestingly, high-dose omega-3 essential fatty acids, which are also believed to confer anti-inflammatory and neuroprotective effects, were found to significantly reduce the rates of conversion to psychosis in a sample of 81 young CHR patients (4.9% conversion rate in those taking 1.2g/day of omega-3 polyunsaturated fatty acids vs. 27.5% conversion rate in the placebo group); (Amminger & McGorry, 2012). Administration of erythropoietin (EPO) alongside traditional antipsychotics has also improved cognition in chronic schizophrenia (Ehrenreich et al., 2007), and has delayed cortical gray matter loss (Wüstenberg et al., 2011). Finally,

Oxytocin, an endogenously produced hormone, has improved social cognition and lessened paranoia (Feifel et al., 2010; Pedersen et al., 2011), and also shows antipsychotic-like effects in animal models of schizophrenia (Caldwell, Stephens, & Young, 2009).

An as-of-yet untested treatment is the combination of these pro-cognitive agents with cognitive training (cognitive training is discussed in more detail below). One recently posited combination involves the use of nicotinic acetylcholine receptor (nAChR) agonists with the cognitive training programs produced by PositScience (Hahn, Gold, & Buchanan, 2013). In their article, Hahn et al. suggest that nicotinic agonists' ability to facilitate early sensory processing would combine well with PositScience's focus on early sensory processing, and would be further enhanced by additional agonist-induced attentional engagement. nAChR agonists have also been implicated in the neuroplastic changes that are the targeted mechanism of cognitive gains in these training programs (Buccafusco, Letchworth, Bencherif, & Lippiello, 2005; Castner et al., 2011), making them an ideal pairing. Another promising treatment is to combine cognitive training with neuromodulation via transcranial direct current stimulation (tDCS). Healthy volunteers receiving tDCS in combination with behavioral inhibition training made greater task improvements than those receiving the behavioral training alone (Ditye, Jacobson, Walsh, & Lavidor, 2012). Several in-depth studies are currently underway.

Finally, Chou et al. suggest that one of the reasons for the limited effect of cognition-enhancing agents as studied to date is the lack of constructive cognitive challenges present in the lives of most patients. They note that "drugs designed to enhance specific components of neurocognition might not be beneficial unless paired with interventions that access, utilize, and place demands on those components" (Chou, Twamley, & Swerdlow, 2012). This idea reframes the use of cognitive enhancing agents, suggesting they should be administered in concert with learning-based behavioral interventions, to increase effective cognitive reserve and the ability to respond to treatment (Keshavan et al., 2011).

Early Intervention Programs and Cognitive Therapy for Psychosis

A fairly recent but critically important development in the treatment of schizophrenia is the widespread establishment of early detection and intervention programs, which aim to identify clinically at-risk and first-episode patients as quickly as possible and initiate age-appropriate treatment. The goal is to decrease the duration of untreated psychosis (DUP) (Norman,

Lewis, & Marshall, 2005) and apply effective treatment during the "critical period" (Birchwood, Todd, & Jackson, 1998), creating an environment that is less traumatic and disruptive, improving outcomes (Yung & Nelson, 2011). Early intervention programs have sprung up around the world and typically include psychological and psychosocial interventions (family psychoeducation and support, CBT, supported education/employment), pharmacological interventions, nutritional supplements, and basic monitoring and supportive counseling (Stafford, Jackson, Mayo-Wilson, Morrison, & Kendall, 2013).

A key psychological treatment used in many early intervention programs is cognitive therapy (CT), which has as its aim the development of more adaptive coping skills and the enhancement of stress resilience. CT for psychosis addresses the relationship between thoughts, feelings, and behaviors, with a particular focus on assisting clients to examine, and ultimately alter, their interpretation of a situation. The main goal of this cognitive restructuring is distress reduction as a result of the client's learning skills to interpret and assess stressful situations in a more adaptive, resilient, and helpful manner. Within this approach, skills are also taught to assist the client in recognizing and managing personal stressors, thus targeting an individual's stress responsivity.

A bevy of both behavioral and neuroimaging data have shown that CT for psychosis is an effective treatment, affecting positive and negative symptoms, mood, and overall functioning (Furmark et al., 2002; Goldapple et al., 2004; Kumari et al., 2011; Wykes, Steel, Everitt, & Tarrier, 2008). CT's efficacy in preventing the conversion of CHR individuals, however, has been less consistent. To date, only six studies of CT's effects on CHR youth have been conducted, and all six are limited by methodological issues (choice of control, sample size, attrition, etc.) (Addington et al., 2011; Bechdolf et al., 2012; McGorry et al., 2002; Morrison et al., 2004, 2012; Yung et al., 2011). In the largest trial of cognitive therapy to date, Morrison and his group did not find any significant difference in between-group conversion rates of 288 participants receiving either CT or monitoring (Morrison et al., 2012). While this finding is somewhat disconcerting, CT had a highly significant impact on the severity of positive symptoms in the CHR youths (p = 0.005).

Cognitive therapy does potentially have a greater effect in preventing conversion to psychosis when functioning within a multi-element program (Bechdolf et al., 2012). When adding in computerized cognitive training, social skills training, and multifamily psychoeducation, Bechdolf et al. found a trend level (p = 0.08) change in conversion rate at 12 months, and a significant (p = 0.02) improvement at 24 months.

Computerized Cognitive Training for Impaired Neural System Functioning

Computerized cognitive training that targets the neural system impairments of schizophrenia is another emerging behavioral treatment that is under study. A large number of cognitive remediation or cognitive training approaches have been studied over the years; they have included therapist-guided strategy coaching, pen-and-pencil exercises, educational software, and computer-based drill and practice methods. In two meta-analyses, a large variety of cognitive remediation protocols resulted in modest gains in overall cognitive functioning (effect sizes from .41–.45) with no particular cognitive remediation method proving to be the most effective, raising questions about the specificity of these prior approaches (McGurk, Twamley, Sitzer, McHugo, & Mueser, 2007; Wykes, Huddy, Cellard, McGurk, & Czobor, 2011). More recent developments have focused on the neuroscience behind cognitive remediation, emphasizing the use of carefully designed computerized training approaches that target specific neural impairments relevant to schizophrenia (Vinogradov, Fisher, & de Villers-Sidani, 2012).

One computerized cognitive training software package, CogPack (Marker, 1987), has been used with individuals at clinical high risk for psychosis. In their 2011 pilot study, Rauchensteiner et al. (2011) delivered 10 sessions of CogPack over a four-week period to 10 CHR individuals, and compared them with 16 patients with chronic schizophrenia also receiving CogPack. Between-group analyses revealed greater improvement in verbal memory, and on 3 out of 8 CogPack exercises in the CHR group. A second study of CogPack in CHR youth was conducted by Bechdolf et al. (2012), as previously discussed. Over 100 individuals received 25 sessions of cognitive therapy, plus 15 sessions of group skills training, plus 12 sessions of cognitive training using the CogPack software package, along with 3 multifamily psychoeducation sessions, compared to a control group receiving supportive counseling. At the completion of the intervention, only 3.2% of participants in the active treatment arm had converted to psychosis, compared to 16.9% in the control arm. These data, despite some limitations (sample size, uncertainty regarding relative contribution) paint a promising picture for the effectiveness of multimodal treatment approaches for clinical high-risk youth that include cognitive training.

In the treatment of recent-onset schizophrenia, both therapist-guided paper and pencil tasks (Wykes et al., 2007), as well as another multimodal program, cognitive enhancement therapy (CET) (Eack et al., 2009), have been used. Wykes et al. (2007) administered 40 hour-long sessions of either cognitive remediation, or treatment as usual, to 40 young, primarily in-patients with adolescent-onset schizophrenia. The sessions focused on memory, complex planning, and problem solving, using paper/pencil tasks and the guidance of a therapist. Three primary outcome measures were selected, one of which showed a significant change in response to CRT: cognitive flexibility. There was no effect on any secondary measures or psychosocial functioning.

CET, used by Eack et al. (2009), combines 60 hours of computerized cognitive training using CogRehab (Bracy, 1995), with 45 90-minute sessions of social cognitive group exercises. After one year of treatment, improvements on cognitive measures were not observed compared to an enriched supportive-therapy control. After two years, however, moderate cognitive improvement was observable. At both assessments, gains on measures of social cognition, cognitive style, social adjustment, and symptoms were evident. After a one-year follow-up was conducted, gains on social and symptom measures were maintained, and the cognitive gains made during active training were significantly associated with improvement in functional outcome (Eack, Greenwald, Hogarty, & Keshavan, 2010). Additional MRI conducted at the one-year follow-up also showed greater gray matter preservation in the CET group, with an association between gray matter retention in the left parahippocampal and fusiform gyrus, greater gray matter increases in the left amygdala, and improved cognition (Eack et al., 2010).

More recently, the Vinogradov group has focused on the use of highly intensive computerized cognitive training that is explicitly developed on principles from basic neuroscience, and that targets specific neural system dysfunction in schizophrenia (Fisher, Holland, Merzenich, & Vinogradov, 2009; Vinogradov et al., 2012). In a double-blind randomized controlled trial (RCT), chronic schizophrenia participants were either enrolled in a computer games condition or administered 50 hours of training in auditory processing and auditory/verbal working memory. The cognitive training group made significant gains in verbal learning (effect size of 0.86), verbal memory (0.89), verbal working memory (0.58), and global cognition (0.86) compared to the control group (Fisher et al., 2009). Participants showed a significant increase in serum brain-derived neurotrophic (BDNF) levels compared to control subjects, and adaptive changes in neural activation patterns as assayed by magnetoencephalography (Dale et al., 2010; Vinogradov et al., 2009). A subsequent functional magnetic resonance imaging (fMRI) study after 30 additional hours of training revealed an improvement in cortical activation patterns that was associated both with better cognitive performance and with better psychosocial functioning at six months' follow-up (Subramaniam et al., 2012). Overall, the pattern of change was consistent with restoration of functioning in key distributed neural systems, and demonstrated that these patterns of improvement were correlated by real-world behavioral gains. A study using 40 hours of this form of cognitive training in first-episode patients found significant increases in global cognition, verbal memory, and problem-solving. More importantly, this was the first study to deliver cognitive training on a laptop computer and to allow participants to do the exercises on their own schedule at home, indicating a potentially new treatment tool that is stigma-free and consistent with the recovery model (Fisher et al., 2014).

CONCLUSIONS AND FUTURE DIRECTIONS

The shifting landscape for schizophrenia treatment in the past 15 years has been dramatic. Indeed, only recently, the director of the National Institute of Mental Health challenged the field to focus on "preemption"—envisioning a future in which early detection and interventions will prevent individuals from ever developing the illness in the first place (Insel, 2010). And while prevention may not be possible for all, recovery is now seen as the primary treatment goal, especially for those who are early in the course of illness. Early-detection methods at this point in time consist primarily of behavioral indicators; however, exciting endeavors are underway to identify predictive biomarkers of risk, based on an understanding of the biology of schizophrenia.

Treatment approaches are now slowly shifting from palliative approaches to curative ones. Traditional D2 antagonist antipsychotic medications are no longer seen as the mainstay of treatment, and novel psychopharmacological agents are under development to specifically target the features of schizophrenia that cause the greatest disability: cognitive deficits and negative symptoms (amotivation and anhedonia, in particular). Aggressive application of psychosocial interventions, including family psychoeducation and supported educational or supported employment services, are now considered a cornerstone of treatment. Moreover, the innovative emerging use of cognitive training and adaptive psychological therapies indicate that it is possible to harness the brain's intrinsic plasticity mechanisms and normalize the abnormal neural system functioning in schizophrenia. While it is unlikely that there will be a single silver bullet for the illness, the treatment armamentarium is growing rapidly, with the promise of helping every individual achieve a maximally satisfying life—an outcome that Kraepelin would have deemed impossible.

DISCLOSURES

Dr. Schlosser is an Assistant Professor in the Department of Psychiatry at the University of California, San Francisco. Dr. Schlosser directs the Digital Research and Interventions for Volitional Enhancement (DRIVE) lab, an NIMH-funded research program (K23 MH097795-01; R34 MH13061-01; NIH UL1 TR0000004). Dr. Schlosser reports no conflicts to disclose.

Mr. Garrett is Dr. Sophia Vinogradov's laboratory manager. He reports no conflicts to disclose.

Dr. Vinogradov is a Professor in Residence and the Vice Chair of the University of California, San Francisco, Department of Psychiatry. Additionally, she is Associate Chief of Staff for Mental Health at the San Francisco Veterans Medical Center and directs an NIMH-funded research program. Dr. Vinogradov is a paid consultant on an NIMH BROG-SPAN grant to Brain Plasticity Institute, which has a commercial interest in the cognitive training software. Dr. Vinogradov holds a patent entitled "A Computerized Neuro-Plasticity Based Training Module to Remediate Social Cognitive Deficits" with other members of the Brain Plasticity Institute.

REFERENCES

Addington, J., Epstein, I., Liu, L., French, P., Boydell, K. M., & Zipursky, R. B. (2011). A randomized controlled trial of cognitive behavioral therapy for individuals at clinical high risk of psychosis. *Schizophrenia Research*, *125*(1), 54–61. doi:10.1016/j.schres.2010.10.015

Agid, O., Kapur, S., & Remington, G. (2008). Emerging drugs for schizophrenia. *Expert Opinion on Emerging Drugs*, *13*(3), 479–495. doi:10.1517/14728214.13.3.479

Alaräisänen, A., Miettunen, J., Räsänen, P., Fenton, W., Koivumaa-Honkanen, H.-T. J., & Isohanni, M. (2009). Suicide rate in schizophrenia in the Northern Finland 1966 birth cohort. *Social Psychiatry and Psychiatric Epidemiology*, *44*(12), 1107–1110. doi:10.1007/s00127-009-0033-5

Amminger, G. P., & McGorry, P. D. (2012). Update on omega-3 polyunsaturated fatty acids in early-stage psychotic disorders. *Neuropsychopharmacology*, *37*(1), 309–310. doi:10.1038/npp.2011.187

Andreasen, N. C. (2010). The lifetime trajectory of schizophrenia and the concept of neurodevelopment. *Dialogues in Clinical Neuroscience*, *12*(3), 409–415.

Andreasen, N. C., Nopoulos, P., Magnotta, V., Pierson, R., Ziebell, S., & Ho, B.-C. (2011). Progressive brain change in schizophrenia: A prospective longitudinal study of first-episode schizophrenia. *Biological Psychiatry*, *70*(7), 672–679. doi:10.1016/j.biopsych.2011.05.017

Bartels, S. J., Clark, R. E., Peacock, W. J., Dums, A. R., & Pratt, S. I. (2003). Medicare and Medicaid costs for schizophrenia patients by age cohort compared with costs for depression, dementia, and medically ill patients. *The American journal of geriatric psychiatry: official journal of the American Association for Geriatric Psychiatry*, *11*(6), 648–657.

Bartzokis, G., Lu, P. H., Amar, C. P., Raven, E. P., Detore, N. R., Altshuler, L. L., . . . Nuechterlein, K. H. (2011). Long acting injection versus oral risperidone in first-episode schizophrenia: Differential impact on white matter myelination trajectory. *Schizophrenia Research*, *132*(1), 35–41. doi:10.1016/j.schres.2011.06.029

Bechdolf, A., Wagner, M., Ruhrmann, S., Harrigan, S., Putzfeld, V., Pukrop, R., . . . Klosterkötter, J. (2012). Preventing progression to first-episode psychosis in early initial prodromal states. *The British Journal of Psychiatry: The Journal of Mental Science*, *200*(1), 22–29. doi:10.1192/bjp.bp.109.066357

Beck, A. T., Grant, P. M., Huh, G. A., Perivoliotis, D., & Chang, N. A. (2013). Dysfunctional attitudes and expectancies in deficit syndrome schizophrenia. *Schizophrenia Bulletin*, *39*(1), 43–51. doi:10.1093/schbul/sbr040

Becker, T. M., Cicero, D. C., Cowan, N., & Kerns, J. G. (2012). Cognitive control components and speech symptoms in people with schizophrenia. *Psychiatry Research*, *196*(1), 20–26. doi:10.1016/j.psychres.2011.10.003

Birchwood, M., Todd, P., & Jackson, C. (1998). Early intervention in psychosis. The critical period hypothesis. *The British Journal of Psychiatry. Supplement*, *172*(33), 53–59.

Bowie, C. R., Depp, C., McGrath, J. A., Wolyniec, P., Mausbach, B. T., Thornquist, M. H., . . . Pulver, A. E. (2010). Prediction of real-world functional disability in chronic mental disorders: A comparison of schizophrenia and bipolar disorder. *The American Journal of Psychiatry*, *167*(9), 1116–1124. doi:10.1176/appi.ajp.2010.09101406

Bracy, O. (1995). Cogrehab Software. Indianapolis, Indiana: Psychological Software Services.

Brown, A. S. (2011). The environment and susceptibility to schizophrenia. *Progress in Neurobiology*, *93*(1), 23–58. doi:10.1016/j.pneurobio.2010.09.003

Buccafusco, J. J., Letchworth, S. R., Bencherif, M., & Lippiello, P. M. (2005). Long-lasting cognitive improvement with nicotinic receptor agonists: Mechanisms of pharmacokinetic-pharmacodynamic discordance. *Trends in Pharmacological Sciences*, *26*(7), 352–360. doi:10.1016/j.tips.2005.05.007

Caldwell, H. K., Stephens, S. L., & Young, W. S., 3rd. (2009). Oxytocin as a natural antipsychotic: A study using oxytocin knockout mice. *Molecular Psychiatry*, *14*(2), 190–196. doi:10.1038/sj.mp.4002150

Camchong, J., MacDonald, A. W., 3rd, Bell, C., Mueller, B. A., & Lim, K. O. (2011). Altered functional and anatomical connectivity in schizophrenia. *Schizophrenia Bulletin*, *37*(3), 640–650. doi:10.1093/schbul/sbp131

Cannon, T. D., Kaprio, J., Lönnqvist, J., Huttunen, M., & Koskenvuo, M. (1998). The genetic epidemiology of schizophrenia in a Finnish twin cohort. A population-based modeling study. *Archives of General Psychiatry*, *55*(1), 67–74.

Cannon, T. D., Rosso, I. M., Hollister, J. M., Bearden, C. E., Sanchez, L. E., & Hadley, T. (2000). A prospective cohort study of genetic and perinatal influences in the etiology of schizophrenia. *Schizophrenia Bulletin*, *26*(2), 351–366.

Cannon, T. D., Cadenhead, K., Cornblatt, B., Woods, S. W., Addington, J., Walker, E., . . . Heinssen, R. (2008). Prediction of psychosis in youth at high clinical risk: A multisite longitudinal study in North America. *Archives of General Psychiatry*, *65*(1), 28–37.

Carletti, F., Woolley, J. B., Bhattacharyya, S., Perez-Iglesias, R., Fusar Poli, P., Valmaggia, L., . . . McGuire, P. K. (2012). Alterations in white matter evident before the onset of psychosis. *Schizophrenia Bulletin*. doi:10.1093/schbul/sbs053

Castner, S. A., Smagin, G. N., Piser, T. M., Wang, Y., Smith, J. S., Christian, E. P., . . . Williams, G. V. (2011). Immediate and sustained improvements in working memory after selective stimulation of α7 nicotinic acetylcholine receptors. *Biological psychiatry, 69*(1), 12–18. doi:10.1016/j.biopsych.2010.08.006

Chou, H.-H., Twamley, E., & Swerdlow, N. R. (2012). Towards medication-enhancement of cognitive interventions in schizophrenia. *Handbook of Experimental Pharmacology,* (213), 81–111. doi:10.1007/978-3-642-25758-2_4

Cross-Disorder Group of the Psychiatric Genomics Consortium. (2013). Identification of risk loci with shared effects on five major psychiatric disorders: A genome-wide analysis. *The Lancet.* doi:10.1016/S0140-6736(12)62129-1

Dale, C. L., Findlay, A. M., Adcock, R. A., Vertinski, M., Fisher, M., Genevsky, A., . . . Vinogradov, S. (2010). Timing is everything: Neural response dynamics during syllable processing and its relation to higher-order cognition in schizophrenia and healthy comparison subjects. *International Journal of Psychophysiology, 75*(2), 183–193.

Ditye, T., Jacobson, L., Walsh, V., & Lavidor, M. (2012). Modulating behavioral inhibition by tDCS combined with cognitive training. *Experimental Brain Research. Experimentelle Hirnforschung. Expérimentation Cérébrale, 219*(3), 363–368. doi:10.1007/s00221-012-3098-4

Dwork, A. J., Mancevski, B., & Rosoklija, G. (2007). White matter and cognitive function in schizophrenia. *The International Journal of Neuropsychopharmacology/Official Scientific Journal of the Collegium Internationale Neuropsychopharmacologicum (CINP), 10*(4), 513–536. doi:10.1017/S1461145707007638

Eack, S. M., Greenwald, D. P., Hogarty, S. S., Cooley, S. J., DiBarry, A. L., Montrose, D. M., & Keshavan, M. S. (2009). Cognitive enhancement therapy for early-course schizophrenia: Effects of a two-year randomized controlled trial. *Psychiatric Services (Washington, D.C.), 60*(11), 1468–1476. doi:10.1176/appi.ps.60.11.1468

Eack, S. M., Hogarty, G. E., Cho, R. Y., Prasad, K. M. R., Greenwald, D. P., Hogarty, S. S., & Keshavan, M. S. (2010). Neuroprotective effects of cognitive enhancement therapy against gray matter loss in early schizophrenia: Results from a 2-year randomized controlled trial. *Archives of General Psychiatry, 67*(7), 674–682. doi:10.1001/archgenpsychiatry.2010.63

Eack, Shaun M, Greenwald, D. P., Hogarty, S. S., & Keshavan, M. S. (2010). One-year durability of the effects of cognitive enhancement therapy on functional outcome in early schizophrenia. *Schizophrenia Research, 120*(1–3), 210–216. doi:10.1016/j.schres.2010.03.042

Ehrenreich, H., Hinze-Selch, D., Stawicki, S., Aust, C., Knolle-Veentjer, S., Wilms, S., . . . Krampe, H. (2007). Improvement of cognitive functions in chronic schizophrenic patients by recombinant human erythropoietin. *Molecular psychiatry, 12*(2), 206–220. doi:10.1038/sj.mp.4001907

Feifel, D., Macdonald, K., Nguyen, A., Cobb, P., Warlan, H., Galangue, B., . . . Hadley, A. (2010). Adjunctive intranasal oxytocin reduces symptoms in schizophrenia patients. *Biological Psychiatry, 68*(7), 678–680. doi:10.1016/j.biopsych.2010.04.039

Fisher, M., Loewy, R., Carter, A., Lee, A., Ragland, J. D., Niendam, T., Schlosser, D. A., Pham, L., & Vinogradov, S. (2014). Neuroplasticity-based auditory training via laptop computer improves cognition in young individuals with recent onset schizophrenia. *Schizophrenia Bulletin,* In Press.

Fisher, M., Holland, C., Merzenich, M. M., & Vinogradov, S. (2009). Using neuroplasticity-based auditory training to improve verbal memory in schizophrenia. *The American Journal of Psychiatry, 166*(7), 805–811. doi:10.1176/appi.ajp.2009.08050757

Ford, J. M., & Mathalon, D. H. (2004). Electrophysiological evidence of corollary discharge dysfunction in schizophrenia during talking and thinking. *Journal of Psychiatric Research, 38*(1), 37–46.

Freedman, R., Olincy, A., Buchanan, R. W., Harris, J. G., Gold, J. M., Johnson, L., . . . Kem, W. R. (2008). Initial phase 2 trial of a nicotinic agonist in schizophrenia. *The American Journal of Psychiatry, 165*(8), 1040–1047. doi:10.1176/appi. ajp.2008.07071135

Furmark, T., Tillfors, M., Marteinsdottir, I., Fischer, H., Pissiota, A., Långström, B., & Fredrikson, M. (2002). Common changes in cerebral blood flow in patients with social phobia treated with citalopram or cognitive-behavioral therapy. *Archives of General Psychiatry, 59*(5), 425–433.

Fusar-Poli, P., Deste, G., Smieskova, R., Barlati, S., Yung, A. R., Howes, O., . . . Borgwardt, S. (2012). Cognitive functioning in prodromal psychosis: A meta-analysis. *Archives of General Psychiatry, 69*(6), 562–571. doi:10.1001/ archgenpsychiatry.2011.1592

Gejman, P. V., Sanders, A. R., & Kendler, K. S. (2011). Genetics of schizophrenia: New findings and challenges. *Annual Review of Genomics And Human Genetics, 12,* 121–144. doi:10.1146/annurev-genom-082410-101459

Gold, J. M., Waltz, J. A., Matveeva, T. M., Kasanova, Z., Strauss, G. P., Herbener, E. S., . . . Frank, M. J. (2012). Negative symptoms and the failure to represent the expected reward value of actions: Behavioral and computational modeling evidence. *Archives of General Psychiatry, 69*(2), 129–138. doi:10.1001/ archgenpsychiatry.2011.1269

Goldapple, K., Segal, Z., Garson, C., Lau, M., Bieling, P., Kennedy, S., & Mayberg, H. (2004). Modulation of cortical-limbic pathways in major depression: Treatment-specific effects of cognitive behavior therapy. *Archives of General Psychiatry, 61*(1), 34–41. doi:10.1001/archpsyc.61.1.34

Goldstein, J. M., Tsuang, M. T., & Faraone, S. V. (1989). Gender and schizophrenia: Implications for understanding the heterogeneity of the illness. *Psychiatry Research, 28*(3), 243–253.

Green, M. F., Hellemann, G., Horan, W. P., Lee, J., & Wynn, J. K. (2012). From perception to functional outcome in schizophrenia: Modeling the role of ability and motivation. *Archives of General Psychiatry, 69*(12), 1216–1224. doi:10.1001/ archgenpsychiatry.2012.652

Hahn, B., Gold, J. M., & Buchanan, R. W. (2013). The potential of nicotinic enhancement of cognitive remediation training in schizophrenia. *Neuropharmacology, 64,* 185–190. doi:10.1016/j.neuropharm.2012.05.050

Harrison, G., Hopper, K., Craig, T., Laska, E., Siegel, C., Wanderling, J., . . . Wiersma, D. (2001). Recovery from psychotic illness: A 15- and 25-year international follow-up study. *The British Journal of Psychiatry: The Journal of Mental Science, 178,* 506–517.

Ho, B.-C., Andreasen, N. C., Ziebell, S., Pierson, R., & Magnotta, V. (2011). Long-term antipsychotic treatment and brain volumes. *Archives of General Psychiatry, 68*(2), 128–137. doi:10.1001/archgenpsychiatry.2010.199

Hoffman, R. E., & McGlashan, T. H. (1997). Synaptic elimination, neurodevelopment, and the mechanism of hallucinated "voices" in schizophrenia. *The American Journal of Psychiatry, 154*(12), 1683–1689.

Howes, O. D., & Kapur, S. (2009). The dopamine hypothesis of schizophrenia: Version III— the final common pathway. *Schizophrenia Bulletin, 35*(3), 549–562. doi:10.1093/ schbul/sbp006

Insel, T. R. (2010). Rethinking schizophrenia. *Nature, 468*(7321), 187–193. doi:10.1038/nature09552

Jablensky, A. (1997). The 100-year epidemiology of schizophrenia. *Schizophrenia Research, 28*(2-3), 111–125.

Karlsgodt, K. H., Niendam, T. A., Bearden, C. E., & Cannon, T. D. (2009). White matter integrity and prediction of social and role functioning in subjects at ultra-high risk for psychosis. *Biological Psychiatry, 66*(6), 562–569. doi:10.1016/j.biopsych.2009.03.013

Keshavan, M. S., Eack, S. M., Wojtalik, J. A., Prasad, K. M. R., Francis, A. N., Bhojraj, T. S., . . . Hogarty, S. S. (2011). A broad cortical reserve accelerates response to cognitive enhancement therapy in early course schizophrenia. *Schizophrenia Research, 130*(1-3), 123–129. doi:10.1016/j.schres.2011.05.001

Kraepelin, E. (1919). *Dementia Praecox and Paraphrenia.* R. M. Barclay, translator. Huntington, NY: Robert E. Kreiger Publishing Co., Inc., 1999.

Kumari, V., Fannon, D., Peters, E. R., Ffytche, D. H., Sumich, A. L., Premkumar, P., . . . Kuipers, E. (2011). Neural changes following cognitive behaviour therapy for psychosis: A longitudinal study. *Brain: A Journal of Neurology, 134*(Pt 8), 2396–2407. doi:10.1093/brain/awr154

Lane, H.-Y., Lin, C.-H., Huang, Y.-J., Liao, C.-H., Chang, Y.-C., & Tsai, G. E. (2010). A randomized, double-blind, placebo-controlled comparison study of sarcosine (N-methylglycine) and D-serine add-on treatment for schizophrenia. *The International Journal of Neuropsychopharmacology/Official Scientific Journal of The Collegium Internationale Neuropsychopharmacologicum (Cinp), 13*(4), 451–460. doi:10.1017/S1461145709990939

Lesh, T. A., Niendam, T. A., Minzenberg, M. J., & Carter, C. S. (2011). Cognitive control deficits in schizophrenia: Mechanisms and meaning. *Neuropsychopharmacology, 36*(1), 316–338. doi:10.1038/npp.2010.156

Leucht, S., Corves, C., Arbter, D., Engel, R. R., Li, C., & Davis, J. M. (2009). Second-generation versus first-generation antipsychotic drugs for schizophrenia: A meta-analysis. *Lancet, 373*(9657), 31–41. doi:10.1016/S0140-6736(08)61764-X

Levkovitz, Y., Mendlovich, S., Riwkes, S., Braw, Y., Levkovitch-Verbin, H., Gal, G., . . . Kron, S. (2010). A double-blind, randomized study of minocycline for the treatment of negative and cognitive symptoms in early-phase schizophrenia. *The Journal of Clinical Psychiatry, 71*(2), 138–149. doi:10.4088/JCP.08m04666yel

Marker, K. R. (1987). *COGPACK. The Cognitive Training Package Manual.* Marker Software: Heidelberg & Ladenburg. Retrieved March 2012, from www.marker-software.com.

Martin, L. F., Kem, W. R., & Freedman, R. (2004). Alpha-7 nicotinic receptor agonists: Potential new candidates for the treatment of schizophrenia. *Psychopharmacology, 174*(1), 54–64. doi:10.1007/s00213-003-1750-1

Mathalon, D. H., & Ford, J. M. (2008). Corollary discharge dysfunction in schizophrenia: Evidence for an elemental deficit. *Clinical Eeg and Neuroscience: Official Journal of the Eeg and Clinical Neuroscience Society (Encs), 39*(2), 82–86.

McEvoy, J. P., Meyer, J. M., Goff, D. C., Nasrallah, H. A., Davis, S. M., Sullivan, L., . . . Lieberman, J. A. (2005). Prevalence of the metabolic syndrome in patients with schizophrenia: Baseline results from the Clinical Antipsychotic Trials of Intervention Effectiveness (CATIE) schizophrenia trial and comparison with national estimates from NHANES III. *Schizophrenia Research, 80*(1), 19–32. doi:10.1016/j.schres.2005.07.014

McGlashan, T. H., & Hoffman, R. E. (2000). Schizophrenia as a disorder of developmentally reduced synaptic connectivity. *Archives of General Psychiatry, 57*(7), 637–648.

McGorry, P. D., Yung, A. R., Phillips, L. J., Yuen, H. P., Francey, S., Cosgrave, E. M., . . . Jackson, H. (2002). Randomized controlled trial of interventions designed to reduce the risk of progression to first-episode psychosis in a clinical sample with subthreshold symptoms. *Archives of General Psychiatry, 59*(10), 921–928.

McGrath, J. J., & Richards, L. J. (2009). Why schizophrenia epidemiology needs neurobiology—and vice versa. *Schizophrenia Bulletin, 35*(3), 577–581. doi:10.1093/schbul/sbp004

McGurk, S. R., Twamley, E. W., Sitzer, D. I., McHugo, G. J., & Mueser, K. T. (2007). A meta-analysis of cognitive remediation in schizophrenia. *American Journal of Psychiatry, 164*(12), 1791–1802.

Meltzer, H. Y. (2013). Update on typical and atypical antipsychotic drugs. *Annual Review of Medicine, 64*, 393–406. doi:10.1146/annurev-med-050911-161504

Milev, P., Ho, B.-C., Arndt, S., & Andreasen, N. C. (2005). Predictive values of neurocognition and negative symptoms on functional outcome in schizophrenia: A longitudinal first-episode study with 7-year follow-up. *The American Journal of Psychiatry, 162*(3), 495–506. doi:10.1176/appi.ajp.162.3.495

Miller, T. J., McGlashan, T. H., Rosen, J. L., Somjee, L., Markovich, P. J., Stein, K., & Woods, S. W. (2002). Prospective diagnosis of the initial prodrome for schizophrenia based on the Structured Interview for Prodromal Syndromes: Preliminary evidence of interrater reliability and predictive validity. *The American Journal of Psychiatry, 159*(5), 863–865.

Minzenberg, M. J., Poole, J. H., Benton, C., & Vinogradov, S. (2004). Association of anticholinergic load with impairment of complex attention and memory in schizophrenia. *American Journal of Psychiatry, 161*(1), 116–124.

Moghaddam, B. (2002). Stress activation of glutamate neurotransmission in the prefrontal cortex: Implications for dopamine-associated psychiatric disorders. *Biological Psychiatry, 51*(10), 775–787.

Moore, T. A., Buchanan, R. W., Buckley, P. F., Chiles, J. A., Conley, R. R., Crismon, M. L., . . . Miller, A. L. (2007). The Texas Medication Algorithm Project antipsychotic algorithm for schizophrenia: 2006 update. *The Journal of Clinical Psychiatry, 68*(11), 1751–1762.

Morrison, A. P., French, P., Stewart, S. L. K., Birchwood, M., Fowler, D., Gumley, A. I., . . . Dunn, G. (2012). Early detection and intervention evaluation for people at risk of psychosis: Multisite randomised controlled trial. *BMJ (Clinical Research Ed.), 344*, e2233.

Morrison, A. P., French, P., Walford, L., Lewis, S. W., Kilcommons, A., Green, J., . . . Bentall, R. P. (2004). Cognitive therapy for the prevention of psychosis in people at ultra-high risk: Randomised controlled trial. *The British Journal of Psychiatry: The Journal of Mental Science, 185*, 291–297. doi:10.1192/bjp.185.4.291

Mowry, B. J., & Gratten, J. (2013). The emerging spectrum of allelic variation in schizophrenia: Current evidence and strategies for the identification and functional characterization of common and rare variants. *Molecular Psychiatry, 18*(1), 38–52. doi:10.1038/mp.2012.34

Nasrallah, H. A., & Newcomer, J. W. (2004). Atypical antipsychotics and metabolic dysregulation: Evaluating the risk/benefit equation and improving the standard of care. *Journal of Clinical Psychopharmacology, 24*(5 Suppl 1), S7–14.

Nordentoft, M., Jeppesen, P., Petersen, L., Bertelsen, M., & Thorup, A. (2009). The rationale for early intervention in schizophrenia and related disorders. *Early Intervention in Psychiatry, 3 Suppl 1*, S3–7. doi:10.1111/j.1751-7893.2009.00123.x

Norman, R. M. G., Lewis, S. W., & Marshall, M. (2005). Duration of untreated psychosis and its relationship to clinical outcome. *The British Journal of Psychiatry. Supplement, 48*, s19–23. doi:10.1192/bjp.187.48.s19

Nuechterlein, K. H., & Dawson, M. E. (1984). A heuristic vulnerability/stress model of schizophrenic episodes. *Schizophrenia Bulletin, 10*(2), 300–312.

Palaniyappan, L., Mallikarjun, P., Joseph, V., White, T. P., & Liddle, P. F. (2011). Reality distortion is related to the structure of the salience network in schizophrenia. *Psychological Medicine, 41*(8), 1701–1708. doi:10.1017/S0033291710002205

Pedersen, C. A., Gibson, C. M., Rau, S. W., Salimi, K., Smedley, K. L., Casey, R. L., . . . Penn, D. L. (2011). Intranasal oxytocin reduces psychotic symptoms and improves Theory of Mind and social perception in schizophrenia. *Schizophrenia Research, 132*(1), 50–53. doi:10.1016/j.schres.2011.07.027

Pompili, M., Lester, D., Innamorati, M., Tatarelli, R., & Girardi, P. (2008). Assessment and treatment of suicide risk in schizophrenia. *Expert Review of Neurotherapeutics, 8*(1), 51–74. doi:10.1586/14737175.8.1.51

Pruessner, M., Iyer, S. N., Faridi, K., Joober, R., & Malla, A. K. (2011). Stress and protective factors in individuals at ultra-high risk for psychosis, first episode psychosis and healthy controls. *Schizophrenia Research, 129*(1), 29–35. doi:10.1016/j.schres.2011.03.022

Radua, J., Borgwardt, S., Crescini, A., Mataix-Cols, D., Meyer-Lindenberg, A., McGuire, P. K., & Fusar-Poli, P. (2012). Multimodal meta-analysis of structural and functional brain changes in first episode psychosis and the effects of antipsychotic medication. *Neuroscience and Biobehavioral Reviews, 36*(10), 2325–2333. doi:10.1016/j.neubiorev.2012.07.012

Rajji, T. K., Voineskos, A. N., Butters, M. A., Miranda, D., Arenovich, T., Menon, M., . . . Mulsant, B. H. (2013). Cognitive performance of individuals with schizophrenia across seven decades: A study using the MATRICS Consensus Cognitive Battery. *The American Journal of Geriatric Psychiatry: Official Journal of the American Association for Geriatric Psychiatry, 21*(2), 108–118. doi:10.1016/j.jagp.2012.10.011

Rauchensteiner, S., Kawohl, W., Ozgurdal, S., Littmann, E., Gudlowski, Y., Witthaus, H., . . . Juckel, G. (2011). Test-performance after cognitive training in persons at risk mental state of schizophrenia and patients with schizophrenia. *Psychiatry Research, 185*(3), 334–339. doi:10.1016/j.psychres.2009.09.003

Riecher-Rössler, A., & Häfner, H. (2000). Gender aspects in schizophrenia: Bridging the border between social and biological psychiatry. *Acta Psychiatrica Scandinavica. Supplementum, 407*, 58–62.

Robinson, D. G., Woerner, M. G., McMeniman, M., Mendelowitz, A., & Bilder, R. M. (2004). Symptomatic and functional recovery from a first episode of schizophrenia or schizoaffective disorder. *The American Journal of Psychiatry, 161*(3), 473–479.

Spear, L. P. (2003). Neurodevelopment during adolescence. In D. Cicchetti & E. Walker (Eds.), *Neurodevelopmental Mechanisms in Psychopathology* (pp. 62–83). New York: Cambridge University Press.

Stafford, M. R., Jackson, H., Mayo-Wilson, E., Morrison, A. P., & Kendall, T. (2013). Early interventions to prevent psychosis: Systematic review and meta-analysis. *British Medical Journal (Clinical Research Ed.), 346*, f185.

Stefansson, H., Rujescu, D., Cichon, S., Pietiläinen, O. P. H., Ingason, A., Steinberg, S., . . . Buizer-Voskamp, J. E. (2008). Large recurrent microdeletions associated with schizophrenia. *Nature, 455*(7210), 232–236. doi:10.1038/nature07229

Subramaniam, K., Luks, T. L., Fisher, M., Simpson, G. V., Nagarajan, S., & Vinogradov, S. (2012). Computerized cognitive training restores neural activity within the reality monitoring network in schizophrenia. *Neuron, 73*(4), 842–853. doi:10.1016/j.neuron.2011.12.024

Tienari, P., Wynne, L. C., Sorri, A., Lahti, I., Läksy, K., Moring, J., . . . Wahlberg, K.-E. (2004). Genotype-environment interaction in schizophrenia-spectrum disorder. Long-term follow-up study of Finnish adoptees. *The British Journal of Psychiatry: The Journal of Mental Science, 184*, 216–222.

Tsuang, M. T., Stone, W. S., & Faraone, S. V. (2001). Genes, environment and schizophrenia. *The British Journal of Psychiatry. Supplement, 40*, s18–24.

Van Os, J., & Kapur, S. (2009). Schizophrenia. *Lancet, 374*(9690), 635–645. doi:10.1016/S0140-6736(09)60995-8

Vinogradov, S., Fisher, M., Holland, C., Shelly, W., Wolkowitz, O., & Mellon, S. H. (2009). Is serum brain-derived neurotrophic factor a biomarker for cognitive enhancement in schizophrenia? *Biological Psychiatry, 66*(6), 549–553.

Vinogradov, S., Fisher, M., & De Villers-Sidani, E. (2012). Cognitive training for impaired neural systems in neuropsychiatric illness. *Neuropsychopharmacology, 37*, 43–76. doi:10.1038/npp.2011.251

Vinogradov, S., Fisher, M., Warm, H., Holland, C., Kirshner, M. A., & Pollock, B. G. (2009). The cognitive cost of anticholinergic burden: Decreased response to cognitive training in schizophrenia. *The American Journal of Psychiatry, 166*(9), 1055–1062. doi:10.1176/appi.ajp.2009.09010017

Walker, E. F., & Diforio, D. (1997). Schizophrenia: A neural diathesis-stress model. *Psychological Review, 104*(4), 667–685.

Walker, E., Mittal, V., & Tessner, K. (2008). Stress and the hypothalamic pituitary adrenal axis in the developmental course of schizophrenia. *Annual Review of Clinical Psychology, 4*, 189–216. doi:10.1146/annurev.clinpsy.4.022007.141248

Wicks, S., Hjern, A., & Dalman, C. (2010). Social risk or genetic liability for psychosis? A study of children born in Sweden and reared by adoptive parents. *The American Journal of Psychiatry, 167*(10), 1240–1246. doi:10.1176/appi.ajp.2010.09010114

World Health Organization. (2001). The World Health Report 2001. Mental health: New understanding, new hope. Geneva: World Health Organization.

Wüstenberg, T., Begemann, M., Bartels, C., Gefeller, O., Stawicki, S., Hinze-Selch, D., . . . Ehrenreich, H. (2011). Recombinant human erythropoietin delays loss of gray matter in chronic schizophrenia. *Molecular Psychiatry, 16*(1), 26–36, 1. doi:10.1038/mp.2010.51

Wykes, T., Huddy, V., Cellard, C., McGurk, S. R., & Czobor, P. (2011). A meta-analysis of cognitive remediation for schizophrenia: Methodology and effect sizes. *The American Journal of Psychiatry, 168*(5), 472–85. doi:10.1176/appi.ajp.2010.10060855

Wykes, T., Reeder, C., Landau, S., Everitt, B., Knapp, M., Patel, A., & Romeo, R. (2007). Cognitive remediation therapy in schizophrenia: Randomised controlled trial. *British Journal of Psychiatry, 190*, 421–7.

Wykes, Til, Steel, C., Everitt, B., & Tarrier, N. (2008). Cognitive behavior therapy for schizophrenia: Effect sizes, clinical models, and methodological rigor. *Schizophrenia Bulletin, 34*(3), 523–537. doi:10.1093/schbul/sbm114

Yoon, J. H., Nguyen, D. V., McVay, L. M., Deramo, P., Minzenberg, M. J., Ragland, J. D., . . . Carter, C. S. (2012). Automated classification of fMRI during cognitive control identifies more severely disorganized subjects with schizophrenia. *Schizophrenia Research*, *135*(1-3), 28–33. doi:10.1016/j.schres.2012.01.001

York, G. K., & Steinberg, D. A. (2006). An introduction to the life and work of John Hughlings Jackson with a catalogue raisonné of his writings. *Medical History. Supplement*, 26, 3–157.

Yung, A. R., & Nelson, B. (2011). Young people at ultra-high risk for psychosis: A research update. *Early Intervention in Psychiatry*, *5 Suppl 1*, 52–57. doi:10.1111/j.1751-7893.2010.00241.x

Yung, A. R., Phillips, L. J., Nelson, B., Francey, S. M., PanYuen, H., Simmons, M. B., . . . McGorry, P. D. (2011). Randomized controlled trial of interventions for young people at ultra-high risk for psychosis: 6-month analysis. *The Journal of Clinical Psychiatry*, *72*(4), 430–440. doi:10.4088/JCP.08m04979ora

CHAPTER 4

Neurodevelopmental and Neurobiological Aspects of Major Depressive Disorder

From Theory to Therapy

BLAKE J. RAWDIN, DANIEL LINDQVIST, NICOLE BUSH, STEVEN HAMILTON, RUHEL BOPARAI, R. SCOTT MACKIN, VICTOR I. REUS, SYNTHIA H. MELLON, AND OWEN M. WOLKOWITZ

INTRODUCTION

Major depressive disorder (MDD) affects more than 15% of the U.S. population at some point in their lives (Kessler, Berglund, et al., 2003) and is estimated to become the second leading cause of disability worldwide by the year 2020, second to only ischemic heart disease (Murray & Lopez, 1996). Despite its prevalence and economic and health costs, the underlying causes of MDD, and even its proper nosology, are unclear. The fifth edition of the *Diagnostic and Statistical Manual* (DSM-V) (American Psychiatric Association, 2013) defines MDD according to observable or subjectively reportable symptoms rather than according to biologically based criteria. In order to diagnose a patient with major depressive disorder, the clinician must find that at least five of the following criteria are present in the patient during the same two-week period, and they must represent a change from previous functioning: depressed mood, diminished interest or pleasure, significant weight loss or gain, insomnia or hypersomnia, psychomotor agitation or retardation, fatigue or loss of energy, feelings of worthlessness, diminished ability to think or concentrate, indecisiveness, and death thoughts/suicidal ideation—with at least one of the first two symptoms present.

Despite the single diagnostic label, it is possible that MDD is not a homogenous condition, but may comprise several different syndromes with unique (and sometimes shared) pathophysiological mechanisms (Maj, 2005). Currently available treatments fail to bring about full remission in many patients, suggesting that new models of MDD pathogenesis, leading to new treatment targets, may be required. In this chapter, we explore certain biological mediators that may be dysregulated in MDD and that may contribute to the depressed state itself, to medical conditions that often accompany MDD, and even to the possibility of an acceleration of aging processes in MDD. Defining MDD along new biological lines could contribute to the development of new targeted treatments and could help us reconceptualize MDD as a multisystem bodily disorder rather than one confined to the mind or the brain. In this chapter, we review neurodevelopmental and other aspects of depression from the perspectives of neuroimaging, genetics and epigenetics, and older and newer biochemical theories of depressive pathogenesis and treatment.

NEUROIMAGING: NEUROANATOMICAL AND NEUROPHYSIOLOGICAL FEATURES

Accumulating evidence suggests the involvement of neuroanatomical and neurophysiological abnormalities in major depression, although findings vary between studies, probably as a function of subtypes of depression, the age and gender of the subjects, age of onset, chronicity of depression, and other factors. Most studies, especially those studying recurrent unipolar depression using high-resolution scanners, have shown significantly smaller hippocampal volumes in depression, ranging from approximately 8–18% smaller volume (Videbech & Ravnkilde, 2004). Lifetime duration of depression (especially untreated depression) is generally associated with hippocampal volume diminution (Sheline, Sanghavi, et al., 1999), although some studies have reported smaller hippocampal volumes even in young first-episode depressed subjects (Cole, Costafreda, et al., 2011), raising the question of whether volume changes are neurodevelopmental or degenerative. Causes of this possible hippocampal volume loss are not known but may involve impaired neurogenesis, synaptic pruning, glial cell loss, or even fluid shifts.

Depression in the elderly, or late life depression (LLD), may present with additional neuroanatomical abnormalities. While the etiology of LLD is a complex interaction of psychological, medical, disability, and psychosocial factors (Holley 2006), there is also evidence that subcortical white matter abnormalities and cortical atrophy are significant. Most but not all studies of LLD have focused on associations of cerebrovascular disease and depressive symptoms, such as vascular depression (Alexopoulos, Meyers, et al., 1997). These studies have produced relatively consistent findings of ischemic white matter abnormalities in the deep white matter tracts and periventricular areas (Thomas, Kalaria, et al., 2004; Teodorczuk, O'Brien, et al., 2007). Reduced white matter integrity in these patients may be associated with poor response to antidepressant medication (Alexopoulos, Kiosses, et al., 2002). There are also reports of cortical atrophy, especially in frontal brain regions, and to a lesser extent, in parietal and temporal regions, and it is most probably caused by neuronal loss (Ballmaier, Toga, et al., 2004; Egger, Schocke, et al., 2008).

A particularly exciting development in the study of MDD is the identification of putative depressogenic circuits or tracts within the brain, which may lead to new approaches to treatment. Functional MRI (fMRI) and positron emission tomography (PET) have shown correlations between depressive symptoms and hypermetabolism of the subgenual cingulate cortex and amygdala along with hypometabolism of the dorsal prefrontal cortex and striatum leading to hypotheses of a depression circuit (Krishnan & Nestler, 2010; Hamani, Mayberg, et al., 2011). Substantiating the importance of this circuit, pioneering work by Mayberg and others has demonstrated significant antidepressant effects of deep-brain stimulation of a major point of intersection of this circuit, the subgenual anterior cingulate cortex (Hamani, Mayberg, et al., 2011). Neural systems analyses have highlighted the importance of these and related structures in certain networks that may be dysregulated in MDD, such as the executive, default-mode, and salience networks, which also may be amenable to specific forms of treatment (Ressler & Mayberg, 2007; Hamilton, Chen, et al., 2013).

GENETICS

The evidence for a genetic contribution to MDD comes from the study of twins, with resulting estimates of broad heritability on the order of 37% to 43% (Sullivan, Neale, et al., 2000). Linkage studies, which involve the genetic analysis of pedigrees in which members are affected or unaffected with the trait of interest, have been used to identify genetic determinants of MDD. A number of studies provide supportive evidence for genetic loci for MDD on several chromosomes, which have been difficult to reproduce in other samples (Levinson 2006; Shyn & Hamilton, 2010). An exception involves two separate linkage studies where both samples supported the involvement of a single region of chromosome 3 (Breen, Webb, et al., 2011; Pergadia, Glowinski, et al., 2011), which may involve a gene highlighted by genome-wide studies of MDD (Hamilton, 2011). Linkage efforts in MDD have not led to replicable gene candidates, although the studies performed to date represent an important effort.

The genome-wide association study (GWAS), a method analyzing hundreds of thousands to upwards of 1 million bi-allelic single nucleotide polymorphisms across the genome, constituted a significant advance in human genetics. For MDD, there are now a number of published GWAS, although none of them individually reports significant findings using the stringent criteria for genome-wide statistical significance. A meta-analysis of these reports, totaling more than 9,200 MDD cases and 9,500 controls, the largest study of MDD, again yielded no finding meeting a strong threshold for significance (Ripke, Wray, et al., 2013). It is likely that the relatively low heritability of MDD, accompanied by the presumed etiological heterogeneity, generate low power to detect a genetic effect with the current sample sizes. In parallel, studies of structural variants (Rucker, Breen, et al., 2013) and future exome- and genome-wide sequencing efforts may reveal rare genomic contributors to MDD, providing a more complete description of the genetic architecture of MDD.

An alternative to the genome-wide association and linkage approaches described above focuses on a single gene or group of genes, representing a hypothesis informed by biological plausibility based on insights from animal models, clinical observations, or existing pharmacological treatments. There have been hundreds of candidate-gene studies of MDD, typically focusing on genes related to monoamine signaling, neuroendocrine mediators, neurotrophic proteins, and inflammatory effectors. A meta-analysis of such studies, where at least three independent papers examined the same polymorphism, suggested significant, but modest, support for association between MDD and *APOE* (apolipoprotein E), *GNB3* (guanine nucleotide-binding protein, beta 3), *MTHFR* (methylene tetrahydrofolate reductase), and *SLC6A4* (serotonin transporter) (Lopez-Leon, Janssens, et al., 2008)

While candidate-gene studies of MDD have allowed investigators to test favored hypotheses about the neurobiological origins of the disorder, these best-supported genes, like *APOE, GNB3*, and *MTHFR*, have the most obscure mechanistic connection to depression. Additionally, these genes contribute only small amounts of risk, suggesting that many unidentified loci may influence the predisposition to MDD. Nonetheless, investigators have pursued genetic correlations between depression and genes related to stress and resilience (Krishnan & Nestler, 2010). A potential explanation for a lack of replication of MDD genetic findings is insufficient consideration of gene–environment (or G × E) interactions. For example, numerous studies have demonstrated that single nucleotide polymorphism (SNP) genotypes in the corticotropin-releasing hormone receptor gene (*CRHR1*) are associated with depression or depressive symptoms, but only when examined by stratifying by environmental factors like childhood adversity (Bradley, Binder, et al., 2008; Grabe, Schwahn, et al., 2010; Ressler, Bradley, et al., 2010; Kranzler, Feinn, et al., 2011). A more established literature involving a possible G × E effect was reported by Caspi et al.(2003), in an investigation of the length of a polymorphism (5-HTTLPR) in a region upstream of the serotonin transporter (Caspi, Sugden, et al., 2003). These authors found that in 847 prospectively studied Australian Caucasians from age 3 to 26 years, the number of stressful life events was significantly correlated with probability of developing MDD when one or two copies of the short S allele of 5-HTTLPR were present. Subsequent research has been reported, with multiple meta-analyses that support (Munafo, Durrant, et al., 2009; Risch, Herrell, et al., 2009; Karg, Burmeister, et al., 2011) or do not support this finding, suggesting the importance of study-specific methodology in interpreting these data. G × E interaction studies are still relatively few in number, however, and this is probably due, in part, to difficulties inherent in standardizing or quantifying disparate life experiences, as well as to the challenges posed by extra instances of multiple-hypothesis testing.

NEUROBIOLOGY OF ADVERSE CHILDHOOD EVENTS AND RISK FOR DEPRESSION

Nervous, endocrine, and immune systems are not fully matured at birth, and developmental neuroscience has demonstrated periods of particular plasticity of the brain throughout development in which experiences may have profound effects on organisms' risk for depression (see Andersen & Teicher, 2008). The biological embedding of early experience (Hertzman, 1999) appears to begin *in utero*, through fetal programming (Barker, 1998). Prenatal maternal stress, which exposes the fetus to stress peptides and hormones, exerts meaningful influences on offspring stress physiology and behavior, placing them at increased risk for emotional and cognitive impairment (Sandman, Davis, et al., 2011).

Adverse experiences during early childhood increase risk for depression, as well as a host of other psychiatric, physical, and addictive diseases, later in life (see, for review, Danese & McEwen, 2012; or Heim & Binder, 2012), suggesting as much as a four-fold risk of depression for individuals who experienced multiple early-life adversities (Felitti, Anda, et al., 1998). Little is understood about the mechanisms for these effects, but recent evidence points to several biological pathways, including upregulation (Cicchetti & Rogosch, 2001; Tarullo & Gunnar, 2006; Miller, Chen, et al., 2007; Chen, Cohen, et al., 2010) or downregulation (Carlson & Earls, 1997; Gunnar & Vazquez, 2001; Dozier, Manni, et al., 2006; Bush, Obradovic, et al., 2011) of the HPA axis (perhaps depending upon the chronicity and severity of the early adversity), increased inflammatory cytokines (Kiecolt-Glaser, Gouin, et al., 2011), and disrupted cardiovascular regulatory stress-response systems (McEwen 2000; Evans & Kim, 2007; McEwen 2007).

Animal studies also suggest that early life stress can contribute to lasting disruptions in brain development as well. A particularly compelling example is the finding that two weeks of isolation post-weaning in mice led to alteration in prefrontal cortex function and myelination that persisted even after the mice were reintroduced into a social environment (Makinodan, Rosen, et al., 2012). Evidence from human research is also accumulating, yet it is not well understood what kinds of experiences are important in the development of higher-order association cortex or how fundamental aspects of brain plasticity play out in humans. Some exceptions are findings that children of high socioeconomic status (SES), who on average are exposed to fewer stressors and greater access to physical, nutritional, and educational resources than low SES children, showed more activity/greater responsivity in the prefrontal cortex than did their low SES peers when confronted with a novel or unexpected stimulus (Kishiyama, Boyce, et al., 2009; Sheridan, Sarsour, et al., 2012). Such adversity-related functional differences in prefrontal cortex response are likely to affect cognitions, behavior, and emotion that the prefrontal cortex is involved in regulating, and may contribute to depressive symptomatology. These effects of early-life adversity have been shown to last through adulthood, as evidenced by findings that childhood SES (Staff, Murray, et al., 2012) and childhood abuse (Vythilingam et al., 2002) predicted reduced MRI-derived hippocampal volume in adulthood.

One of the best empirical examples of the effects of early-life stress (ELS) on developmental trajectories of depression is found in the recent work of Burghy et al. (Burghy, Stodola, et al., 2012), which integrates biomarkers across systems and developmental periods. Using longitudinal data, they found that exposure to high levels of family stress in infancy predicted higher levels of cortisol in preschool, which was then linked to reduced connections (resting-state functional connectivity, fcMRI) between the amygdala, or threat center of the brain, and the ventromedial prefrontal cortex, a part of the brain responsible for emotional regulation. Moreover, these intermediate biological changes in cortisol and brain activity predicted levels of adolescent anxiety and depression at age 18. That this evidence was found in females only, and not the males in the sample, is not entirely surprising, given the sex-based differences in depression during adolescence.

To summarize, ELS (such as parental loss, physical or emotional neglect or abuse) predisposes to adult depression (Breier, Kelsoe, et al., 1988; Chapman, Whitfield, et al., 2004) as well as to limbic-hypothalamic-pituitary-adrenal (LHPA) axis hyper-reactivity to stress (Breier, Kelsoe, et al., 1988; Heim, Plotsky, et al., 2004), increased allostatic load (McEwen 2000; Grassi-Oliveira, Ashy, et al., 2008), diminished hippocampal volume (although this is controversial; Vythilingam, Heim, et al., 2002), lower brain serotonin transporter binding potential (Miller, Kinnally, et al., 2009), and a myriad of adult physical diseases (Anda, Felitti, et al., 2006). Childhood adversity also predisposes to alterations in many of the mediators presented in our model of stress/depression/illness/cell aging, such as: inflammation (Kiecolt-Glaser, Gouin et al. 2011; Pace, Mletzko, et al., 2006), oxidative stress (Barnes & Ozanne, 2011), neurotrophic factors (Roth, Lubin, et al., 2009), neurosteroids (Avital, Ram, et al., 2006), glucose/insulin/insulin-like growth factor (IGF-1) regulation (Thomas, Hypponen, et al., 2008), telomerase activity (Wolkowitz, Epel, et al., 2009), and telomere length (Price, Kao, et al., 2013; Shalev 2012). In fact, several instances of neurobiological changes thought to typify MDD may actually be more attributable to early-life adversity (Vythilingam, Heim, et al., 2002; Heim, Plotsky, et al., 2004), which is over-represented among individuals with MDD, than to the MDD itself.

Despite all the evidence for the effects of ELS on neurobiological functioning and later psychopathology, it is important to note that many individuals exposed to ELS are quite resilient and do not evidence symptoms of depression. A multitude of resiliency factors, ranging from genetics, to positive social relationships (e.g., Gunnar 1998; Kaufman, Yang, et al., 2006), to the quality of the family's adaptation to the adversity (Breier, Kelsoe, et al., 1988) have been shown to protect individuals exposed to early life stressors from the increased risk for depression.

EPIGENETICS OF DEPRESSION

One explanation for the very long-lasting effects of such adversity (or the buffering of such) involves epigenetic modifications (Weaver, Cervoni, et al., 2004; McGowan, Sasaki, et al., 2009). Epigenetics, which focuses on non-genomic alterations of gene expression, provides a mechanism for understanding such findings, through alteration of DNA methylation and subsequent silencing of gene expression or through physical changes in DNA packaging into histones (Schroeder, Krebs, et al., 2010). At least one locus of epigenetic change that has been characterized is the glucocorticoid receptor (GR) promoter region. Consequent to epigenetic methylation of the GR promoter region (causing diminished GR expression), affected individuals may become glucocorticoid (GC)-resistant, show decreased negative feedback onto the LHPA axis, increased stress responses, chronic hypercortisolemia, poor memory, and hippocampal atrophy (Weaver, Cervoni, et al., 2004; McGowan, Sasaki, et al., 2009). Retrospective data have shown decreased levels of GR expression in the hippocampus of suicide victims with a history of childhood abuse, in comparison to those without such history and to controls (Labonte, Yerko, et al., 2012). Such findings are strengthened by findings from prospective data demonstrating that prenatal exposure to third-trimester maternal depression was associated with increased methylation of the glucocorticoid receptor gene at three months of age in the newborn child (Oberlander, Weinberg, et al., 2008), and that parental stressors (presumably reflecting household stresses) during the child's first few years of life were predictive of differential DNA methylation in the child across the genome during adolescence (Essex, Thomas Boyce, et al., 2013).

BIOCHEMICAL MODELS OF DEPRESSION

Biogenic Amines

The biogenic amine hypothesis of MDD posits that low intra-synaptic levels of biogenic amines (norepinephrine, dopamine, or serotonin) are a causal factor in MDD. This hypothesis has been investigated for several decades, with variable results (Charney, 1998; Hindmarch, 2002). It was initially based on two observations of mood elevation in depressed patients treated with iproniazid, an anti-tuberculosis drug that has monoamine oxidase–inhibiting (MAO-I) effects, and mood worsening in patients treated with catecholamine-depleting drugs. Deriving from this theory, nearly all current antidepressant drugs were developed to increase intra-synaptic biogenic amine levels. Surprisingly, there is a lack of compelling data that intra-synaptic biogenic amine concentrations are actually low in MDD (Charney, 1998; Hindmarch, 2002). The closest evidence of direct involvement of biogenic amines in MDD was provided by Delgado and colleagues who found that acute catecholamine or serotonin depletion rapidly reversed the antidepressant effects of catecholaminergic or serotonergic antidepressants, respectively (Delgado, 2000). Even this finding, however, speaks more to antidepressant mechanisms than to the intrinsic pathophysiology of MDD.

Evidencing the inadequacy of the biogenic amine hypothesis and of the drugs based on it, a sizable number of depressed patients obtain only partial or no relief in response to traditional antidepressants. In the largest naturalistic study to date, the Sequenced Treatment Alternatives to Relieve Depression (STAR*D) study found that after two adequate antidepressant treatment trials, only 37% of patients achieved remission if they stayed in treatment. The cumulative remission rate following four different consecutive treatments trials was only 67%. As discussed below, the sharp treatment focus on biogenic amines may have led to the neglect of other pharmacological strategies that could target different loci of pathology and help treat patients with different subtypes of depression (see Table 4.1). In fact, many traditional biogenic amine-based antidepressants have other, non-monoaminergic actions, some of which address other sites of theorized biochemical pathology, as discussed below.

Table 4.1 POSSIBLY DAMAGING AND PROTECTIVE MEDIATORS IN MAJOR DEPRESSION

Potentially Damaging Mediators	Potentially Protective Mediators
Increased	*Decreased*
• Hyperactive LHPA axis and hypercortisolemia (with net hypercortisolism or hypocortisolism)	• Neurosteroids (e.g., DHEA* and allopregnanolone)
• Synaptic glutamate and excitotoxicity	• Insulin sensitivity
• Intracytoplasmic calcium	• Intracellular glucose
• Free radicals with oxidative stress	• Antioxidants
• Inflammatory cytokines	• Anti-inflammatory/immunomodulatory cytokines**
	• Neurotrophic factors (e.g., BDNF)
	• Telomerase***

Key: LHPA, limbic-hypothalamic-pituitary-adrenal; DHEA, dehydroepiandrosterone; BDNF, brain-derived neurotrophic factor.
*Evidence is mixed as to whether DHEA concentrations are elevated or lowered in depression.
**Evidence is mixed as to whether the anti-inflammatory/immunomodulatory cytokine, IL-10, is elevated or lowered in depression.
***Evidence is mixed as to whether telomerase activity is elevated or lowered in states of chronic stress and depression.

Limbic-Hypothalamic-Pituitary-Adrenal Axis

Cortisol

Elevated hypothalamic-pituitary-adrenal axis (LHPA) axis activity has been reported in depressed individuals (especially in those with severe, melancholic, psychotic, or inpatient depression), although considerable variability exists between studies, between individuals, and even within individuals over time, and some depressed individuals are even hypo-cortisolemic (Fries, Hesse, et al., 2005). The physiological significance of increased circulating GC levels remains unknown, and it is debatable whether hyper-cortisolemia results in hyper-cortisolism at the individual cell level, or, rather, in hypo-cortisolism due to down-regulation of the GR (often referred to as GC resistance; Raison & Miller, 2003). Specifically, even in the presence of elevated circulating cortisol levels, diminished GR sensitivity to cortisol could result in insufficient levels of cortisol entering the nucleus and interacting with the DNA (Raison & Miller, 2003). Thus, determination of net intracellular GC activity in depressed individuals has remained elusive. Chronic hyper-cortisolemia, in particular, has been proposed by Sapolsky and others to result in a biochemical cascade, which can culminate in cell endangerment or cell death in certain cells, including cells in the hippocampus (Sapolsky, 2000). In the simplest description of this model, GC excess engenders a state of intracellular glucoprivation (insufficient intracellular glucose energy stores) in certain cells such as glial cells, impairing the ability of glia and other cells to clear synaptic glutamate. The resulting excitotoxicity results in excessive influx and release of calcium into the cytoplasm, which contributes to oxidative damage, proteolysis, and cytoskeletal damage. Unchecked, these processes can culminate in diminished cell viability or cell death (Figure 4.1). Furthermore, since the hippocampus plays a role in negative feedback onto the LHPA axis, progressive loss of hippocampal neurons may compromise its braking activity, engendering a positive, rather than negative, feedback loop onto cortisol release (Sapolsky, 2000).

A widely studied method of assessing LHPA activity in MDD has been the dexamethasone suppression test (DST), which assesses sensitivity of pituitary GRs to negative feedback. The DST was initially proposed as laboratory test for melancholia (Carroll, Feinberg, et al., 1981). After much investigation, however, it was found to lack sufficient sensitivity and specificity to be clinically useful for diagnosing MDD (Mossner, Mikova, et al., 2007). This lack of sensitivity suggests that many individuals with MDD do not have prominent LHPA axis disturbances, and the lack of specificity

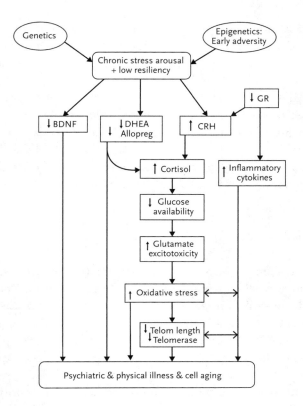

Figure 4.1:
Model of multiple pathways leading to psychiatric and physical illness and cell aging. In conjunction with genetic and epigenetic moderators, elevated cortisol levels, associated with down-regulation of glucocorticoid receptor (GC) function (GC resistance) may result in altered immune function, leading to excessive synthesis of proinflammatory cytokines. Changes in glucocorticoid-mediated activities also result in genomic changes (altered levels of certain neurotransmitters, neurotrophins, and other mediators), as well as dysregulation of the limbic-hypothalamic-pituitary adrenal (LHPA) axis that might contribute to neuroendangerment or neurotoxicity, perhaps leading to depressive or cognitive symptoms. Dysregulation of the LPHA axis can also lead to intracellular glucose deficiency, glutamatergic hyperactivity, increased cellular calcium concentrations, mitochondrial damage, free-radical generation, and increased oxidative stress. This cascade of events, coupled with a milieu of increased inflammatory cytokines, may lead to accelerated cellular aging via effects on the telomere/telomerase maintenance system. Dysregulation of normal compensatory mechanisms, such as increased neurosteroid or neurotrophin production, may further result in the inability to reduce cellular damage, and thereby exacerbate destructive processes. This juxtaposition of enhanced destructive processes with diminished protective/ restorative processes may culminate in cellular damage, apoptosis, and physical disease.
Key: Allopreg, allopregnanolone; BDNF, brain-derived neurotrophic factor; CRH, cortico-trophin releasing hormone; DHEA, dehydroepiandrosterone; GR, glucocorticoid receptor.

Limited portions of this chapter, including Figure 4.1, have been reproduced, with the kind permission of the publishers, Les Laboratoires Servier, from a previously published article by the same author: Wolkowitz O, Reus VI, Mellon SH. Of sound mind and body: depression, disease, and accelerated aging. *Dialogues Clin Neurosci* 2011;13:25–39. Copyright Les Laboratoires Servier, 2011.

raises the possibility that specific *trans-diagnostic* symptoms may be related to LHPA axis dysregulation (Reus, 1982). Nonetheless, persistent DST non-suppression following clinical recovery is correlated with early relapse and poor outcome on follow-up (Ribeiro, Tandon, et al., 1993), suggesting that LHPA axis normalization (or resensitization of hypothalamic and pituitary GRs) is a prerequisite for more abiding recovery. Indeed, many traditional antidepressant medications increase GR levels in animals, rendering them more sensitive to glucocorticoid negative feedback (Holsboer & Barden, 1996), and antidepressant drugs inhibit the glucocorticoid-induced gene transcription (Budziszewska, Jaworska-Feil, et al., 2000).

Neurosteroids

Neurosteroids are a class of steroid hormone that is synthesized in the gonads and adrenal cortex as well as *in situ* in the brain. Neurosteroids have rapid, generally non-genomically mediated, effects in the brain and elsewhere. Although circulating cortisol concentrations are often elevated in depression, CSF concentrations of the potent GABAA receptor agonist neurosteroid, allopregnanolone, are decreased in unmedicated depressives (Uzunova, Sheline, et al., 1998), and CSF levels of allopregnanolone increase with treatment in direct proportion to the antidepressant effect (Uzunova, Sheline, et al., 1998). One mechanism by which certain selective serotonin reuptake inhibitor (SSRI) antidepressants rapidly increase allopregnanolone synthesis involves modulation of neurosteroidogenic enzymes (Griffin & Mellon, 1999) and this may contribute to their anxiolytic effects and to their rapid efficacy in treating PMDD (Guidotti & Costa, 1998) Another neurosteroid, dehydroepiandrosterone (DHEA) and its sulfate, DHEA-S, may also be involved in MDD pathophysiology (fully reviewed in Maninger, Mellon, et al., 2009). This and allopregnanolone are further discussed below in the section on novel treatment approaches to MDD.

Brain-Derived Neurotrophic Factor (BDNF)

The neurotrophin hypothesis of depression (Duman, 2004) emphasizes the centrality of neurogenesis and neuronal plasticity in the pathophysiology and treatment of depression. It posits that diminished hippocampal BDNF activity, caused by stress or excessive GCs, impairs the ability of stem cells in the subgranular layer of the dentate gyrus in the hippocampus (as well as cells in the subventricular zone, projecting to the prefrontal cortex) to remain viable and to proliferate into mature cells. It is not known whether diminished neurogenesis can cause depression, but it does seem relevant to the mechanism of action of antidepressants (Groves, 2007). Unmedicated patients with MDD have decreased hippocampal concentrations of BDNF (Groves, 2007), and over 20 studies have documented decreased serum concentrations of BDNF; this is now one of the most consistently replicated biochemical findings in major depression (Sen, Duman, et al., 2008). A role of BDNF in antidepressant mechanisms of action is supported by findings that hippocampal neurogenesis (in animals) and serum BDNF concentrations (in depressed humans) increase with antidepressant treatment (Groves, 2007), and that hippocampal neurogenesis and intact BDNF expression are required for behavioral effects of antidepressants in animals (Santarelli, Saxe, et al., 2003). Interestingly, traditional antidepressants generally increase serum BDNF levels in depressed patients, calling into question the centrality of their effects on biogenic amine neurotransmission (Groves, 2007).

Inflammation/Immune Dysfunction

The inflammatory hypothesis of MDD posits that excessive inflammation contributes to depressive symptomatology. This hypothesis is based on several lines of evidence:

(1) Rodents administered pro-inflammatory cytokines or lipopolysaccharide (LPS) exhibit sickness behavior and depressive-like behavior, which may resemble certain (but not all) aspects of MDD (Dantzer & Kelley, 2007).

(2) Interferon-alpha treatment in medically ill patients may induce a depressive syndrome, and this syndrome can be treated or prevented by traditional antidepressants (Capuron, Hauser, et al., 2002).

(3) Many, but not all, studies, have found elevated pro-inflammatory cytokine levels in MDD (Dowlati, Herrmann, et al., 2010). These cytokine elevations may normalize with successful antidepressant treatment (Hannestad, DellaGioia, et al., 2011).

(4) Anti-inflammatory drugs may have antidepressant effects in some patients (discussed further below).

Dysregulation of the LHPA axis contributes to immune dysregulation in depression, and immune dysregulation, in turn, can activate the HPA axis and precipitate depressive symptoms (Raison & Miller, 2003). Immune dysregulation may also be an important pathway by which MDD heightens the risk of serious medical co-morbidity (Kiecolt-Glaser & Glaser, 2002; Bauer, Jeckel, et al., 2009; Epel 2009). Several major pro-inflammatory cytokines, such as IL-1β, IL-2, IL-6 and TNF-α, may be elevated in depression, either basally or in response to mitogen stimulation or acute stress (Raison & Miller, 2003; Dhabhar, Burke, et al., 2009; Dowlati, Herrmann, et al., 2010). Conversely, certain anti-inflammatory or immunomodulatory cytokines, such as IL-1 receptor antagonist and IL-10, may be decreased or dysregulated (Dhabhar, Burke, et al., 2009). Indeed, the ratio of pro-inflammatory to anti-inflammatory/immunomodulatory cytokines may be disturbed in depression and could result in net increased inflammatory activity (Dhabhar, Burke, et al., 2009) as well as in oxidative stress.

Oxidative Stress

Stress and increased LHPA axis activity can also induce oxidative stress (as discussed briefly above) and decrease antioxidant defenses (Irie, Miyata, et al., 2005; Wolkowitz, Epel, et al., 2008; Epel, 2009). Oxidative stress often increases with aging and various disease states, while antioxidant and anti-inflammatory activities decrease, resulting in a heightened likelihood of cellular damage and of a senescent phenotype (Joseph, Shukitt-Hale, et al., 2005; Epel, 2009). The co-occurrence of oxidative stress and inflammation (the so-called evil twins of brain aging; Joseph, Shukitt-Hale, et al., 2005) may also be seen in depression (Rawdin, Mellon, et al., 2013) and can be especially detrimental. Oxidative stress occurs when the production of oxygen free radicals (and other oxidized molecules) exceeds the capacity of the body's antioxidants to neutralize them. Oxidative stress damages DNA, protein, lipids, and other macromolecules in many tissues, with telomeres (discussed below) and the brain being particularly sensitive. Elevated plasma and/or urine oxidative stress markers (e.g., increased F2-isoprostanes and 8-hydroxydeoxyguanosine [8-OHdG], along with decreased anti-oxidant compounds, such as vitamin C, vitamin E and co-enzyme Q) have been reported in individuals with MDD or chronic psychological stress, and the concentration of peripheral oxidative stress markers is positively correlated with the severity and chronicity of depression (Irie, Miyata, et al., 2005; Forlenza & Miller, 2006). Many traditional antidepressants decrease oxidative stress (Cumurcu, Ozyurt, et al., 2009), again calling into question the centrality of their monoaminergic effects.

Glutamate

Glutamate is the predominant excitatory neurotransmitter of the central nervous system, present at approximately 60% of synapses. It acts upon a number of different receptors, including N-methyl-D-aspartate receptors (NMDARs). While critical for normal functioning, excess glutamate activity and extrasynaptic NMDAR activity, particularly in the prefrontal cortex and hippocampus, can be neurotoxic. Excess glutamate release may cause a surge in intracellular free calcium resulting in excitotoxicity through activation of various kinases and proteases that cause cytoskeletal damage, protein misfolding, and free radicals. Glutamatergic and NMDAR dysfunction have been associated with depression (Pittenger, Sanacora, et al., 2007; Marsden, 2011). Certain antidepressants (selective serotonin reuptake inhibitors [SSRIs] and tricyclic antidepressants [TCAs], for example) have been shown to act as NMDAR antagonists, and ketamine (as will be discussed in greater detail in the treatment section below), an NMDAR antagonist, appears to have rapid antidepressant effects (McNally, Bhagwagar, et al., 2008; Marsden, 2011).

Cell Aging: Telomere Length and Telomerase

MDD has been referred to as a disease with accelerated biological aging (Heuser, 2002; Wolkowitz, Epel, et al., 2008; Wolkowitz, Epel, et al., 2010; Wolkowitz, Reus, et al., 2011). One index of biological (as opposed to just chronological) age is telomere length (TL), often assessed in peripheral leukocytes (Aviv, 2004; Epel, Blackburn, et al., 2004; Blackburn, Greider, et al., 2006; Epel, Lin, et al., 2006; Effros, 2009; Epel, 2009). Telomeres are DNA-protein complexes that cap the ends of linear DNA strands, protecting DNA from damage. Telomeres may shorten during repeated mitoses in somatic cells (including leukocytes) or as a result of cumulative exposure to certain genotoxic environments (Wolkowitz, Mellon, et al., 2012; Wolkowitz, Reus, et al., 2011; von Zglinicki, 2002) (Figure 4.1). Therefore, telomere shortening can index excessive cell turnover (e.g., during repeated episodes of immune activation) or excessive exposure to inflammation or oxidation, as may be seen in depression and chronic stress. When telomeres reach a critically short length, cells become susceptible to apoptosis and death. Recent studies have suggested that chronically stressed (Epel, Blackburn, et al., 2004; Epel, Lin, et al., 2006) or depressed (Lindqvist, Epel, et al., in review) individuals have premature leukocyte telomere shortening, indicating accelerated cell aging, although inconsistencies exist in the MDD literature (reviewed in Lindqvist, in review; Malan, Hemmings, et al., 2011;

Surtees, Wainwright, et al., 2011; Rius-Ottenheim, Houben, et al., 2012; Shaffer, Epel, et al., 2012). Generally, studies that utilized rigorous diagnostic criteria and included individuals with more severe or more long-standing depression or psychological stress, revealed shorter leukocyte TL (LTL) (reviewed in Lindqvist, in review). The estimated magnitude of the acceleration of biological aging in the studies reporting shortened LTL was not trivial, approximating 9–17 additional years of chronological aging in chronically stressed individuals and 6–10 years in depressed individuals (reviewed in Wolkowitz, Reus, et al., 2011). LTL shortening is not a specific biomarker of stress or MDD, as it is also observed in other psychiatric and medical conditions (Shalev, Entringer, et al., 2013). Interestingly, individuals with histories of ELS (including individuals exposed *in utero* to excessive maternal stress—Shalev, Entringer, et al., 2013) also have shortened LTL (Price, Kao, et al., 2013). The importance of accelerated telomere shortening for understanding co-morbid medical illnesses and premature mortality in depressed individuals is highlighted by studies in non-depressed populations showing significantly increased medical morbidity and earlier mortality in those with shortened telomeres (Cawthon, Smith, et al., 2003). Thus, cell aging (as manifest by shortened telomeres) may provide a conceptual link between depression and its associated medical co-morbidities and shortened life span (Aviv, 2004; Bauer, Jeckel, et al., 2009; Epel, 2009).

A major enzyme responsible for protecting, repairing, and lengthening telomeres is telomerase (Blackburn, Greider, et al., 2006). In one study in which LTL shortening was reported in stressed caregivers, telomerase activity in peripheral blood mononuclear cells (PBMCs) was significantly diminished (Epel, Blackburn, et al., 2004), but, in another study (in which caregivers were generally more depressed), telomerase activity was significantly *increased* (Damjanovic, Yang, et al., 2007). Wolkowitz et al. also reported, in a small pilot study, significantly increased telomerase activity in unmedicated depressed individuals (Wolkowitz, Mellon, et al., 2012). It is possible that increased telomerase activity, in the face of shortened telomeres, is an attempted compensatory response to telomere shortening (Damjanovic, Yang, et al., 2007; Wolkowitz, Mellon, et al., 2012) and may facilitate antidepressant responses (Zhou, Hu, et al., 2011).

NOVEL MECHANISM-BASED TREATMENT CONSIDERATIONS

The limited utility of traditional antidepressants may be related to MDD being a heterogeneous condition. To the extent that the alternative hypotheses reviewed in this chapter are related to the pathophysiology of MDD, new treatments targeting novel mechanisms should be feasible. Indeed, as noted throughout this chapter, many current antidepressants exhibit effects distinct from biogenic amine mechanisms (Table 4.2). In the remainder of this chapter, we review accumulating data on novel drug classes that target specific hypothesized mechanisms, and that may have different patterns of efficacy and tolerability than currently available antidepressants. We conclude this section with a brief discussion of nonpharmacological interventions that may also target these newly considered mechanisms in MDD.

Corticotrophin Releasing Hormone (CRH) and Corticotrophin Releasing Hormone Receptor (CRH-R) Antagonists

Treatments aimed at decreasing LHPA axis actions are being investigated as novel antidepressants. Many of these studies were small-scale

Table 4.2 POTENTIAL MECHANISM-BASED
THERAPEUTIC INTERVENTIONS

Biochemical Mediator	Potential Treatment Interventions
Stress vulnerability	Stress reduction, meditation, lifestyle changes
Epigenetic changes	Epigenetic reprogramming
LHPA axis dysregulation	Antidepressants upregulate GR function
Hypercortisolemia	CRH antagonists
	Cortisol antagonists and GR antagonists or agonists
Glucose/insulin dysregulation	Insulin receptor sensitizers
Glutamate/excitotoxicity	Glutamate antagonists
Oxidative stress	Antidepressants have antioxidant effects
	Antioxidants
Intracellular calcium	Calcium blockers
Inflammation	Antidepressants have anti-inflammatory effects
	Anti-inflammatory drugs, TNF-α antagonists, etc.
Decreased counter-regulatory	SSRIs increase allopregnanolone synthesis
neurosteroids	DHEA administration
Decreased BDNF	Antidepressants (esp. SSRIs) increase BDNF concentrations
	Environmental enrichment
	Exercise
	Dietary restriction
	BDNF administration via novel routes or vectors
Cell aging (telomeres, telomerase)	Telomerase activation
	Exercise? Dietary restriction

Key: LHPA, limbic-hypothalamic-pituitary-adrenal; GC, glucocorticoid; GR, glucocorticoid receptor; CRH, corticotrophin-releasing hormone; DHEA, dehydroepiandrosterone; BDNF brain-derived neurotrophic factor; TNF, tumor necrosis factor; SSRI, selective serotonin reuptake inhibitor.

and were considered proof of concept studies or safety studies; thus, firm conclusions cannot yet be made. One approach has been to block corticotrophin releasing hormone (CRH)-1 receptors. Although preclinical data support the view that such CRH-1 receptor antagonists are useful in the treatment of depression, currently no controlled studies are available that demonstrate their clinical efficacy in depressed patients (Schule, Baghai, et al., 2009), and several trials were curtailed due to toxicity of the agents employed.

Anti-Glucocorticoids

To the extent cortisol dysregulation is etiologically involved in MDD, treatments that primarily normalize cortisol activity, even if they have no direct effect on biogenic amines, should treat depression. The most convincing evidence of this is from patients with Cushing's syndrome, whose psychiatric symptoms responded promptly to adrenalectomy, pituitary adenoma resection, or treatment with cortisol-inhibiting or cortisol-antagonizing drugs (reviewed in Wolkowitz, Burke, et al., 2009). A sizable number of studies have also utilized cortisol biosynthesis-inhibiting drugs or cortisol receptor-antagonist drugs in MDD. In each of the double-blind studies of cortisol biosynthesis inhibitors—e.g., metyrapone, aminoglutethimide, and ketoconazole—antidepressant effects were reported in at least some patients (reviewed in Wolkowitz, Burke, et al., 2009). Wolkowitz, Reus, et al. (1999) found that the hyper-cortisolemic, but not the non-hyper-cortisolemic, patients showed antidepressant effects, but this study was too small to draw meaningful conclusions. More recent studies have investigated possible antidepressant effects of mifepristone (RU-486) in the treatment of depression, particularly psychotic depression, which is often characterized by elevated cortisol levels. This drug has demonstrated positive effects in some small, double-blind, placebo-controlled studies. However, three recently completed Phase III trials failed to significantly separate mifepristone from placebo in MDD (Gallagher, Malik, et al., 2008). It is plausible that the glucocorticoid antagonism approach may have merit in selected, but perhaps not all, depressed individuals.

Dehydroepiandrosterone (DHEA)

Double-blind treatment trials have demonstrated significant antidepressant effects of orally administered DHEA, both as a sole agent and as an antidepressant adjunct, in treatment-resistant patients (reviewed in Maninger, Wolkowitz, et al., 2009). However, the magnitude of these effects relative to standard antidepressants has not been studied, and parameters of dosing, length of treatment, and long-term safety have not been adequately investigated. In several studies, antidepressant efficacy was unrelated to pre-treatment levels of circulating DHEA or DHEA-sulfate (DHEA[S]) levels, suggesting that the antidepressant effect was not simply due to replacing a deficient hormone. The mechanisms for DHEA's efficacy have been reviewed elsewhere, but include possible cortisol-antagonizing effects (Maninger, Wolkowitz, et al., 2009).

Allopregnanolone

Several lines of evidence, reviewed above and elsewhere (Schule, Eser, et al., 2011), have piqued interest in allopregnanolone or synthetic neurosteroids like ganaxolone as possible antidepressant treatments (Reddy 2010). We are unaware of any published trials of these compounds in humans as antidepressants, although ganaxolone is being tested as an anticonvulsant due to its GABA-ergic effect.

Antioxidants and Anti-inflammatory Treatments

As mentioned above, SSRIs have both anti-inflammatory and antioxidant properties (Khanzode, Dakhale, et al., 2003; Behr, Moreira, et al., 2012). Evidence suggests SSRIs may dampen serum levels of certain inflammatory cytokines, such as IL-6, IL-1β and tumor-necrosis factor (TNF-α) (Hannestad, DellaGioia, et al., 2011), while also reducing oxidative stress levels (Cumurcu, Ozyurt, et al., 2009). Evidence is lacking, however, that antidepressant-associated lowering of inflammatory cytokine levels parallels improvements in depressive symptoms, and to further complicate matters, other classes of antidepressants (e.g., serotonin-norepinephrine reuptake inhibitors [SNRIs]) actually appear to be associated with pro-inflammatory changes, perhaps due to norepinephrine's effects on immune cells (Thayer & Sternberg, 2010; Hannestad, DellaGioia, et al., 2011). Though few studies have yet tested the antidepressant effects of anti-inflammatories, the studies that have been completed are promising (Muller, Schwarz, et al., 2006; Akhondzadeh, Jafari, et al., 2009). It is possible that anti-inflammatory therapies may only be effective in depressed individuals with elevated inflammatory markers at baseline (Raison, Rutherford, et al., 2013).

Though we currently lack randomized controlled trials (RCTs) demonstrating efficacy, antioxidant therapies hold promise as treatments in depression. N-acetylcysteine (NAC) is a precursor of glutathione, a potent antioxidant, which is able to cross the blood–brain barrier (Berk, Ng, et al., 2008). Interestingly, NAC may also be involved in the glutamate system and have anti-inflammatory properties (Berk, Ng, et al., 2008). So far, an eight-week open-label study of NAC in bipolar patients showed a significant reduction in depressive symptoms. While a small follow-up RCT of this same trial to test the efficacy of NAC as maintenance therapy was unable to show a statistical difference, 37% of the NAC subjects had depression relapse, versus 48% in the placebo group (Berk, Copolov, et al., 2008).

Other agents with both anti-inflammatory and antioxidant properties that have some limited evidence for efficacy are zinc (Lai, Moxey, et al., 2012), vitamin D (Anglin, Samaan, et al., 2013), and curcumin (Lopresti, Hood, et al., 2012). Additionally, recent investigations of minocycline, an antibiotic with both antioxidant and anti-inflammatory effects, raise the possibility of efficacy in depression, and further investigation is under way (Dean, Data-Franco, et al., 2012). High-quality RCTs are needed, but initial findings suggest there may be a role for anti-inflammatory and anti-oxidant treatments either as monotherapy or as adjuvants, particularly for patients with elevated inflammatory and antioxidant biomarkers.

Glutamate Antagonists

A particularly exciting development has been the demonstration of acute antidepressant effects of NMDAR antagonists, such as ketamine and riluzole, in certain patients (Price, Nock, et al., 2009; Larkin & Beautrais, 2011; Ibrahim, Diazgranados, et al., 2012; Zarate, Brutsche, et al., 2012). Ketamine appears to take effect rapidly, though its effects may only be short-lived. To date, few studies have monitored efficacy or patient safety beyond two weeks.

Nutrition and Supplementation

Inadequate nutrition may be a risk factor for unipolar depression (Tolmunen, Hintikka, et al., 2004; Rao, Asha, et al., 2008), and preliminary data suggest that a Mediterranean diet, rich in B vitamins and omega-3 fatty acids, may help reduce the incidence of depression (Sanchez-Villegas, Delgado-Rodriguez, et al., 2009; Kiecolt-Glaser, 2010; Bloch & Hannestad,

2012). One study, in particular, showed that a Mediterranean diet supplemented with nuts resulted in significantly higher levels of plasma BDNF at 36 months among patients with baseline depression (Sanchez-Villegas, Galbete, et al., 2011). A recent randomized controlled trial of omega-3 fatty acids suggests that this intervention lowers oxidative stress as measured by F2-isoprostanes, as well as certain inflammatory markers in overweight, sedentary adults, and is additionally associated with longer leukocyte telomeres (Kiecolt-Glaser, Epel, et al., 2012). Other complementary and alternative treatments to treating depression exist but do not have known connections to the mechanisms discussed in this chapter; e.g., 5-methyltetrahydrofolate (5-MTHF), S-adenosyl methionine (SAMe), and St. John's wort (Larzelere, Campbell, et al., 2010).

Non-pharmacological Approaches

To the extent that altered stress hormone secretion underlies or perpetuates depressive symptoms, behavioral interventions that normalize the hormonal milieu should also prove therapeutic (Cohen, 2000; Drugan et al., 1994; Sapolsky, 1993). In fact, behavioral approaches to decreasing stress and arousal might prove superior in the long run to the pharmacological approaches outlined above, since pharmacological strategies may clamp hormonal activity at either a low or high state and thereby reduce responsiveness to environmental demands (Sterling & Eyer, 1988). Behavioral techniques, on the other hand, have the potential to increase flexibility and adaptability (Sterling & Eyer, 1988). In addition, various non-pharmacological approaches that have demonstrated antidepressant efficacy may also engage some of the novel biological targets described in this chapter. Since these are not a major focus of this chapter, several promising non-pharmacological treatment approaches that influence the reviewed biological targets will be briefly reviewed here for the interested reader.

- *Mindfulness*: Research on mindfulness-based interventions indicates that telomerase activity increases in proportion to mindfulness-based positive psychological changes (Jacobs, Epel, et al., 2011; Daubenmier, Lin, et al., 2012).
- *Exercise*: Though some of the research on exercise and physical activity is troubled by methodological weaknesses, exercise, particularly aerobic-type, may be effective for the treatment of depression and for relapse prevention. The most recent Cochrane Review of exercise for

depression found exercise to have a positive effect; however, when considering only high-quality studies, the effect size was small. It is possible that the beneficial effects of exercise are at least partly related to changes in cortisol (Puterman, O'Donovan, et al., 2011), BDNF (and neurogenesis) (Hillman, Erickson, et al., 2008), and cell aging (Hillman, Erickson, et al., 2008; Krauss, Farzaneh-Far, et al., 2011).

- *Cognitive behavior therapy (CBT) and other psychotherapies*: While various psychotherapies are effective in the treatment of depression, both alone and in combination with medications, many of the biological mediators and mechanisms involved have yet to be elucidated. Limited data suggest psychotherapy was less effective than medication for depressed patients with elevated C-reactive protein (CRP) (Thase, Simons, et al., 1993). Poorer response to CBT for major depression has also been associated with elevated LHPA activity, as measured by urinary cortisol and dexamethasone-suppression testing (Thase, Dube, et al., 1996). However, in other populations, CBT has helped dampen stress reactivity (Facchinetti, Tarabusi, et al., 2004). As far as CBT and other psychotherapies precipitate cognitive reframing and reappraisals, they can help regulate corticolimbic circuitry (Stein, 2008). Research suggests that CBT produces changes in medial prefrontal cortex and ventral anterior cingulate cortex activation during self-referential processing of emotional stimuli, and the degree of these changes correlates with improvements in depressive symptoms (Yoshimura, Okamoto, et al., 2013).

SUMMARY

In this chapter, we have reviewed current neuroanatomical, genetic and epigenetic, developmental, and biochemical findings in major depression. We have also explored certain novel treatments with discrete and specific pharmacological actions, as they relate to the neurobiology of depression. Depression at this time remains a syndrome, as defined by symptoms, not biology or pathophysiology. Therefore, these novel agents operate on pathways distinct from those of traditional antidepressants. Moreover, we speculate these treatments will have a varying spectrum of action that will affect various depressive subgroups and symptoms differently. Further research is needed in order to better evaluate targeted treatments for depression based on distinct underlying pathologies.

DISCLOSURES

None of the authors has conflicts to disclose.

Send correspondence to Dr. Owen M. Wolkowitz: 401 Parnassus Avenue, San Francisco, California, 94143-0984; telephone: (415) 476-7433; email: owen.wolkowitz@ucsf.edu.

REFERENCES

Akhondzadeh, S., Jafari, S., et al. (2009). Clinical trial of adjunctive celecoxib treatment in patients with major depression: a double blind and placebo controlled trial. *Depression & Anxiety, 26*(7), 607–611.

Alexopoulos, G. S., Kiosses, D. N., et al. (2002). Frontal white matter microstructure and treatment response of late-life depression: a preliminary study. *American Journal of Psychiatry, 159*(11), 1929–1932.

Alexopoulos, G. S., Meyers, B. S., et al. (1997). "Vascular depression" hypothesis. *Archives of General Psychiatry, 54*(10), 915–922.

American Psychiatric Association (2013). Diagnostic and Statistical Manual of Mental Disorders: DSM-5, Fifth edition. Arlington, VA: American Psychiatric Association.

Anda, R. F., Felitti, V. J., et al. (2006). The enduring effects of abuse and related adverse experiences in childhood: A convergence of evidence from neurobiology and epidemiology. *European Archives of Psychiatry & Clinical Neuroscience, 256*(3), 174–186.

Andersen, S. L., & Teicher, M. H. (2008). Stress, sensitive periods and maturational events in adolescent depression. *Trends in Neurosciences, 31*(4), 183–191.

Anglin, R. E., Samaan, Z., et al. (2013). Vitamin D deficiency and depression in adults: systematic review and meta-analysis. *British Journal of Psychiatry, 202*, 100–107.

Avital, A., Ram, E., et al. (2006). Effects of early-life stress on behavior and neurosteroid levels in the rat hypothalamus and entorhinal cortex. *Brain Research Bulletin, 68*(6), 419–424.

Aviv, A. (2004). Telomeres and human aging: facts and fibs. *Science of Aging Knowledge Environment, 2004*(51), pe43.

Ballmaier, M., Toga, A. W., et al. (2004). Anterior cingulate, gyrus rectus, and orbitofrontal abnormalities in elderly depressed patients: an MRI-based parcellation of the prefrontal cortex. *American Journal of Psychiatry, 161*(1), 99–108.

Barker, D. J. (1998). In utero programming of chronic disease. *Clinical Science (London), 95*(2), 115–128.

Barnes, S. K., & Ozanne, S. E. (2011). Pathways linking the early environment to long-term health and lifespan. *Progress in Biophysics & Molecular Biology, 106*, 323–336.

Bauer, M. E., Jeckel, C. M., et al. (2009). The role of stress factors during aging of the immune system. *Annals of the New York Academy of Science, 1153*: 139–152.

Behr, G. A., Moreira, J. C., et al. (2012). Preclinical and clinical evidence of antioxidant effects of antidepressant agents: implications for the pathophysiology of major depressive disorder. *Oxidative Medicine & Cellular Longevity, 2012*: 609421.

Berk, M., Copolov, D. L., et al. (2008). N-acetyl cysteine for depressive symptoms in bipolar disorder—a double-blind randomized placebo-controlled trial. *Biological Psychiatry, 64*(6), 468–475.

Berk, M., Ng, F., et al. (2008). Glutathione: a novel treatment target in psychiatry. *Trends in Pharmacological Science, 29*(7), 346–351.

Blackburn, E. H., Greider, C. W., et al. (2006). Telomeres and telomerase: the path from maize, Tetrahymena and yeast to human cancer and aging. *Nature Medicine, 12*(10), 1133–1138.

Bloch, M. H., & Hannestad, J. (2012). Omega-3 fatty acids for the treatment of depression: systematic review and meta-analysis. *Molecular Psychiatry, 17*(12), 1272–1282.

Bradley, R. G., Binder, E. B., et al. (2008). Influence of child abuse on adult depression: moderation by the corticotropin-releasing hormone receptor gene. *Archives of General Psychiatry, 65*(2), 190–200.

Breen, G., Webb, B. T., et al. (2011). A genome-wide significant linkage for severe depression on chromosome 3: the depression network study. *American Journal of Psychiatry, 168*(8), 840–847.

Breier, A., Kelsoe, Jr., J. R., et al. (1988). Early parental loss and development of adult psychopathology. *Archives of General Psychiatry, 45*(11), 987–993.

Budziszewska, B., Jaworska-Feil, L., et al. (2000). Antidepressant drugs inhibit glucocorticoid receptor-mediated gene transcription—a possible mechanism. *British Journal of Pharmacology, 130*(6), 1385–1393.

Burghy, C. A., Stodola, D. E., et al. (2012). Developmental pathways to amygdala-prefrontal function and internalizing symptoms in adolescence. *Nature Neuroscience, 15*(12), 1736–1741.

Bush, N. R., Obradovic, J., et al. (2011). Kindergarten stressors and cumulative adrenocortical activation: The first straws of allostatic load? *Development & Psychopathology, 23*(4), 1089–1106.

Capuron, L., Hauser, P., et al. (2002). Treatment of cytokine-induced depression. *Brain, Behavior & Immunity, 16*(5), 575–580.

Carlson, M., & Earls, F. (1997). Psychological and neuroendocrinological sequelae of early social deprivation in institutionalized children in Romania. *Annals of the New York Academy of Sciences, 807*: 419–428.

Carroll, B. J., Feinberg, M., et al. (1981). A specific laboratory test for the diagnosis of melancholia. Standardization, validation, and clinical utility. *Archives of General Psychiatry, 38*(1), 15–22.

Caspi, A., Sugden, K., et al. (2003). Influence of life stress on depression: moderation by a polymorphism in the 5-HTT gene. *Science, 301*(5631), 386–389.

Cawthon, R. M., Smith, K. R., et al. (2003). Association between telomere length in blood and mortality in people aged 60 years or older. *Lancet, 361*(9355), 393–395.

Chapman, D. P., Whitfield, C. L., et al. (2004). Adverse childhood experiences and the risk of depressive disorders in adulthood. *Journal of Affective Disorders, 82*(2), 217–225.

Charney, D. S. (1998). Monoamine dysfunction and the pathophysiology and treatment of depression. *Journal of Clinical Psychiatry, 59*(suppl 14), 11–14.

Chen, E., Cohen, S., et al. (2010). How low socioeconomic status affects 2-year hormonal trajectories in children. *Psychological Science, 21*(1), 31–37.

Cicchetti, D., & Rogosch, F. A. (2001). The impact of child maltreatment and psychopathology on neuroendocrine functioning. *Development & Psychopathology, 13*(4), 783–804.

Cohen, J. I. (2000). Stress and mental health: a biobehavioral perspective. *Issues in Mental Health Nursing, 21*(2), 185–202.

Cole, J., Costafreda, S. G., et al. (2011). Hippocampal atrophy in first episode depression: a meta-analysis of magnetic resonance imaging studies. *Journal of Affective Disorders, 134*(1–3), 483–487.

Cumurcu, B. E., Ozyurt, H., et al. (2009). Total antioxidant capacity and total oxidant status in patients with major depression: impact of antidepressant treatment. *Psychiatry & Clinical Neurosciences, 63*(5), 639–645.

Damjanovic, A. K., Yang, Y., et al. (2007). Accelerated telomere erosion is associated with a declining immune function of caregivers of Alzheimer's disease patients. *Journal of Immunology, 179*(6), 4249–4254.

Danese, A., & McEwen, B. S. (2012). Adverse childhood experiences, allostasis, allostatic load, and age-related disease. *Physiology & Behavior, 106*(1), 29–39.

Dantzer, R., & Kelley, K. W. (2007). Twenty years of research on cytokine-induced sickness behavior. *Brain, Behavior & Immunity, 21*(2), 153–160.

Daubenmier, J., Lin, J., et al. (2012). Changes in stress, eating, and metabolic factors are related to changes in telomerase activity in a randomized mindfulness intervention pilot study. *Psychoneuroendocrinology, 37*(7), 917–928.

Dean, O. M., Data-Franco, J., et al. (2012). Minocycline: therapeutic potential in psychiatry. *Central Nervous System Drugs, 26*(5), 391–401.

Delgado, P. (2000). Depression: the case for a monoamine deficiency. *Journal of Clinical Psychiatry, 61*(suppl 6), 7–11.

Dhabhar, F. S., Burke, H. M., et al. (2009). Low serum IL-10 concentrations and loss of regulatory association between IL-6 and IL-10 in adults with major depression. *Journal of Psychiatric Research, 43*(11), 962–969.

Dowlati, Y., Herrmann, N., et al. (2010). A meta-analysis of cytokines in major depression. *Biological Psychiatry, 67*(5), 446–457.

Dozier, M., Manni, M., et al. (2006). Foster children's diurnal production of cortisol: An exploratory study. *Child Maltreatment, 11*(2), 189–197.

Drugan, R. C., Basile, A. S., Ha, J. H., & Ferland, R. J. (1994). The protective effects of stress control may be mediated by increased brain levels of benzodiazepine receptor agonists. *Brain Research, 661*(1–2), 127–136.

Duman, R. S. (2004). Role of neurotrophic factors in the etiology and treatment of mood disorders. *Neuromolecular Medicine, 5*(1), 11–25.

Effros, R. B. (2009). Kleemeier Award Lecture 2008—the canary in the coal mine: telomeres and human healthspan. *Journals of Gerontology Series A: Biological Sciences & Medical Sciences, 64*(5), 511–515.

Egger, K., Schocke, M., et al. (2008). Pattern of brain atrophy in elderly patients with depression revealed by voxel-based morphometry. *Psychiatry Research, 164*(3), 237–244.

Epel, E. S. (2009). Psychological and metabolic stress: a recipe for accelerated cellular aging? *Hormones (Athens), 8*(1), 7–22.

Epel, E. S., Blackburn, E. H., et al. (2004). Accelerated telomere shortening in response to life stress. *Proceedings of the National Academy of Sciences, USA, 101*(49), 17312–17315.

Epel, E. S., Lin, J., et al. (2006). Cell aging in relation to stress arousal and cardiovascular disease risk factors. *Psychoneuroendocrinology, 31*(3), 277–287.

Essex, M. J., Thomas Boyce, W., et al. (2013). Epigenetic vestiges of early developmental adversity: Childhood stress exposure and DNA methylation in adolescence. *Child Development, 84*(1), 58–75.

Evans, G. W., & Kim, P. (2007). Childhood poverty and health: Cumulative risk exposure and stress dysregulation. *Psychological Science, 18*(11), 953–957.

Facchinetti, F., Tarabusi, M., et al. (2004). Cognitive-behavioral treatment decreases cardiovascular and neuroendocrine reaction to stress in women waiting for assisted reproduction. *Psychoneuroendocrinology, 29*(2), 162–173.

Felitti, V. J., Anda, R. F., et al. (1998). Relationship of childhood abuse and household dysfunction to many of the leading causes of death in adults. The Adverse Childhood Experiences (ACE) study. *American Journal of Preventive Medicine, 14*(4), 245–258.

Forlenza, M. J., & Miller, G. E. (2006). Increased serum levels of 8-hydroxy-2'-deoxyguanosine in clinical depression. *Psychosomatic Medicine, 68*(1), 1–7.

Fries, E., Hesse, J., et al. (2005). A new view on hypocortisolism. *Psychoneuroendocrinology, 30*(10), 1010–1016.

Gallagher, P., Malik, N., et al. (2008). Antiglucocorticoid treatments for mood disorders. *Cochrane Database of Systematic Reviews* (1), CD005168.

Grabe, H. J., Schwahn, C., et al. (2010). Childhood maltreatment, the corticotropin-releasing hormone receptor gene and adult depression in the general population. *American Journal of Medical Genetics Part B: Neuropsychiatric Genetics, 153B*(8), 1483–1493.

Grassi-Oliveira, R., Ashy, M., et al. (2008). Psychobiology of childhood maltreatment: effects of allostatic load? *Revista Brasileira de Psiquiatria, 30*(1), 60–68.

Griffin, L. D., & Mellon, S. H. (1999). Selective serotonin reuptake inhibitors directly alter activity of neurosteroidogenic enzymes. *Proceedings of the National Academy of Sciences, 96*(23), 13512–13517.

Groves, J. O. (2007). Is it time to reassess the BDNF hypothesis of depression? *Molecular Psychiatry, 12*(12), 1079–1088.

Guidotti, A., & Costa, E. (1998). Can the antidysphoric and anxiolytic profiles of selective serotonin reuptake inhibitors be related to their ability to increase brain allopregnanolone availability? *Biological Psychiatry, 44*(865–873).

Gunnar, M. R. (1998). Quality of early care and buffering of neuroendocrine stress reactions: Potential effects on the developing human brain. *Preventive Medicine: An International Journal Devoted to Practice & Theory, 27*(2), 208–211.

Gunnar, M. R., & Vazquez, D. M. (2001). Low cortisol and a flattening of expected daytime rhythm: potential indices of risk in human development. *Developmental Psychopathology, 13*(3), 515–538.

Hamani, C., Mayberg, H., et al. (2011). The subcallosal cingulate gyrus in the context of major depression. *Biological Psychiatry, 69*(4), 301–308.

Hamilton, J. P., Chen, M. C., et al. (2013). Neural systems approaches to understanding major depressive disorder: an intrinsic functional organization perspective. *Neurobiology of Disease, 52*, 4–11.

Hamilton, S. P. (2011). A new lead from genetic studies in depressed siblings: assessing studies of chromosome 3. *American Journal of Psychiatry, 168*(8), 783–789.

Hannestad, J., N. Della Gioia, et al. (2011). The effect of antidepressant medication treatment on serum levels of inflammatory cytokines: a meta-analysis. *Neuropsychopharmacology, 36*(12), 2452–2459.

Heim, C., & Binder, E. B. (2012). Current research trends in early life stress and depression: Review of human studies on sensitive periods, gene–environment interactions, and epigenetics. *Experimental Neurology, 233*(1), 102–111.

Heim, C., Plotsky, P. M., et al. (2004). Importance of studying the contributions of early adverse experience to neurobiological findings in depression. *Neuropsychopharmacology, 29*(4), 641–648.

Hertzman, C. (1999). The biological embedding of early experience and its effects on health in adulthood. *Annals of the New York Academy of Science, 896*, 85–95.

Heuser, I. (2002). Depression, endocrinologically a syndrome of premature aging? *Maturitas, 41*(Suppl 1), S19–S23.

Hillman, C. H., Erickson, K. I., et al. (2008). Be smart, exercise your heart: exercise effects on brain and cognition. *Nature Reviews Neuroscience, 9*(1), 58–65.

Hindmarch, I. (2002). Beyond the monoamine hypothesis: mechanisms, molecules and methods. *European Psychiatry, 17*(Suppl 3), 294–299.

Holley, C., Murrell, S. A., & Mast, B. T. (2006). Psychosocial and vascular risk factors for depression in the elderly. *American Journal of Geriatric Psychiatry, 14*(1), 84–90.

Holsboer, F., & Barden, N. (1996). Antidepressants and hypothalamic-pituitary-adrenocortical regulation. *Endocrine Reviews, 17*(2), 187–205.

Ibrahim, L., Diazgranados, N., et al. (2012). Course of improvement in depressive symptoms to a single intravenous infusion of ketamine vs add-on riluzole: results from a 4-week, double-blind, placebo-controlled study. *Neuropsychopharmacology 37*(6), 1526–1533.

Irie, M., Miyata, M., et al. (2005). Depression and possible cancer risk due to oxidative DNA damage. *Journal of Psychiatric Research, 39*(6), 553–560.

Jacobs, T. L., Epel, E. S., et al. (2011). Intensive meditation training, immune cell telomerase activity, and psychological mediators. *Psychoneuroendocrinology, 36*(5), 664–681.

Joseph, J. A., Shukitt-Hale, B., et al. (2005). Oxidative stress and inflammation in brain aging: nutritional considerations. *Neurochem Res 30*(6-7), 927–935.

Karg, K., Burmeister, M., et al. (2011). The serotonin transporter promoter variant (5-HTTLPR), stress, and depression meta-analysis revisited: evidence of genetic moderation. *Archives of General Psychiatry, 68*(5), 444–454.

Kaufman, J., Yang, B.-Z., et al. (2006). Brain-derived neurotrophic factor-5-HHTLPR gene interactions and environmental modifiers of depression in children. *Biological Psychiatry, 59*(8), 673–680.

Kessler, R. C., Berglund, P., et al. (2003). The epidemiology of major depressive disorder: results from the National Comorbidity Survey Replication (NCS-R). *Journal of the American Medical Association, 289*(23), 3095–3105.

Khanzode, S. D., Dakhale, G. N., et al. (2003). Oxidative damage and major depression: the potential antioxidant action of selective serotonin re-uptake inhibitors. *Redox Report, 8*(6), 365–370.

Kiecolt-Glaser, J. K. (2010). Stress, food, and inflammation: psychoneuroimmunology and nutrition at the cutting edge. *Psychosomatic Medicine, 72*(4), 365–369.

Kiecolt-Glaser, J. K., Epel, E. S., et al. (2012). Omega-3 fatty acids, oxidative stress, and leukocyte telomere length: A randomized controlled trial. *Brain, Behavior & Immunity, 28*, 16–24.

Kiecolt-Glaser, J. K., & Glaser, R. (2002). Depression and immune function: central pathways to morbidity and mortality. *Journal of Psychosomatic Research, 53*(4), 873–876.

Kiecolt-Glaser, J. K., Gouin, J. P., et al. (2011). Childhood adversity heightens the impact of later-life caregiving stress on telomere length and inflammation. *Psychosomatic Medicine, 73*(1), 16–22.

Kishiyama, M. M., Boyce, W. T., et al. (2009). Socioeconomic disparities affect prefrontal function in children. *Journal of Cognitive Neuroscience, 21*(6), 1106–1115.

Kranzler, H. R., Feinn, R., et al. (2011). A CRHR1 haplotype moderates the effect of adverse childhood experiences on lifetime risk of major depressive episode in African-American women. *American Journal of Medical Genetics Part B: Neuropsychiatric Genetics, 156B*(8), 960–968.

Krauss, J., Farzaneh-Far, R., et al. (2011). Physical fitness and telomere length in patients with coronary heart disease: findings from the Heart and Soul Study. *PLoS One, 6*(11), e26983.

Krishnan, V., & Nestler, E. J. (2010). Linking molecules to mood: new insight into the biology of depression. *American Journal of Psychiatry, 167*(11), 1305–1320.

Labonte, B., Yerko, V., et al. (2012). Differential glucocorticoid receptor exon 1(B), 1(C), and 1(H) expression and methylation in suicide completers with a history of childhood abuse. *Biological Psychiatry, 72*(1), 41–48.

Lai, J., Moxey, A., et al. (2012). The efficacy of zinc supplementation in depression: systematic review of randomised controlled trials. *Journal of Affective Disorders, 136*(1–2), e31–e39.

Larkin, G. L., & Beautrais, A. L. (2011). A preliminary naturalistic study of low-dose ketamine for depression and suicide ideation in the emergency department. *International Journal of Neuropsychopharmacology, 14*(8), 1127–1131.

Larzelere, M. M., Campbell, J. S., et al. (2010). Complementary and alternative medicine usage for behavioral health indications. *Prim Care, 37*(2), 213–236.

Levinson, D. F. (2006). The genetics of depression: a review. *Biological Psychiatry, 60*(2), 84–92.

Lindqvist, D., Epel, E. S., et al. (2013). Psychiatric disorders and telomere length: Underlying mechanisms linking mental illness with cellular aging. *In review.*

Lopez-Leon, S., Janssens, A. C., et al. (2008). Meta-analyses of genetic studies on major depressive disorder. *Molecular Psychiatry, 13*(8), 772–785.

Lopresti, A. L., Hood, S. D., et al. (2012). Multiple antidepressant potential modes of action of curcumin: a review of its anti-inflammatory, monoaminergic, antioxidant, immune-modulating and neuroprotective effects. *Journal of Psychopharmacology, 26*(12), 1512–1524.

Maj, M. (2005). Psychiatric comorbidity: an artefact of current diagnostic systems? *British Journal of Psychiatry, 186*: 182–184.

Makinodan, M., Rosen, K. M., et al. (2012). A critical period for social experience— Dependent oligodendrocyte maturation and myelination. *Science, 337*(6100), 1357–1360.

Malan, S., Hemmings, S., et al. (2011). Investigation of telomere length and psychological stress in rape victims. *Depression & Anxiety, 28*(12), 1081–1085.

Maninger, N., Mellon, S. H., et al. (2009). Neurobiological and neuropsychiatric effects of dehydroepiandrosterone (DHEA) and DHEA sulfate (DHEAS). *Frontiers in Neuroendocrinology, 30*(1), 65–91.

Maninger, N., Wolkowitz, O. M., et al. (2009). Neurobiological and neuropsychiatric effects of dehydroepiandrosterone (DHEA) and DHEA sulfate (DHEAS). *Frontiers in Neuroendocrinology, 30*(1), 65–91.

Marsden, W. N. (2011). Stressor-induced NMDAR dysfunction as a unifying hypothesis for the aetiology, pathogenesis and comorbidity of clinical depression. *Medical Hypotheses, 77*(4), 508–528.

McEwen, B. (2000). Allostasis and allostatic load: Implications for neuropsychopharmacology. *Neuropsychopharmacology, 22*(2), 108–124.

McEwen, B. S. (2000). Effects of adverse experiences for brain structure and function. *Biological Psychiatry, 48*(8), 721–731.

McEwen, B. S. (2007). Physiology and neurobiology of stress and adaptation: central role of the brain. *Physiological Reviews, 87*(3), 873–904.

McGowan, P. O., Sasaki, A., et al. (2009). Epigenetic regulation of the glucocorticoid receptor in human brain associates with childhood abuse. *Nature Neuroscience, 12*(3), 342–348.

McNally, L., Bhagwagar, Z., et al. (2008). Inflammation, glutamate, and glia in depression: a literature review. *CNS Spectrums, 13*(6), 501–510.

Miller, G. E., Chen, E., et al. (2007). If it goes up, must it come down? Chronic stress and the hypothalamic-pituitary-adrenocortical axis in humans. *Psychological Bulletin, 133*(1), 25–45.

Miller, J. M., Kinnally, E. L., et al. (2009). Reported childhood abuse is associated with low serotonin transporter binding in vivo in major depressive disorder. *Synapse, 63*(7), 565–573.

Mossner, R., Mikova, O., et al. (2007). Consensus paper of the WFSBP Task Force on Biological Markers: biological markers in depression. *World Journal of Biological Psychiatry, 8*(3), 141–174.

Muller, N., Schwarz, M. J., et al. (2006). The cyclooxygenase-2 inhibitor celecoxib has therapeutic effects in major depression: results of a double-blind, randomized, placebo controlled, add-on pilot study to reboxetine. *Molecular Psychiatry, 11*(7), 680–684.

Munafo, M. R., Durrant, C., et al. (2009). Gene X environment interactions at the serotonin transporter locus. *Biological Psychiatry, 65*(3), 211–219.

Murray, C. J. L., & Lopez, A. (1996). *The Global Burden of Disease: a Comprehensive Assessment of Mortality and Disability from Diseases, Injuries, and Risk Factors in 1990 and Projected to 2020.* Boston, MA: Harvard School of Public Health, on behalf of the World Health Organization and the World Bank.

Oberlander, T. F., Weinberg, J., et al. (2008). Prenatal exposure to maternal depression, neonatal methylation of human glucocorticoid receptor gene (NR3C1) and infant cortisol stress responses. *Epigenetics, 3*(2), 97–106.

Pace, T. W., Mletzko, T. C., et al. (2006). Increased stress-induced inflammatory responses in male patients with major depression and increased early life stress. *American Journal of Psychiatry, 163*(9), 1630–1633.

Pergadia, M. L., Glowinski, A. L., et al. (2011). A 3p26-3p25 genetic linkage finding for DSM-IV major depression in heavy smoking families. *American Journal of Psychiatry, 168*(8), 848–852.

Pittenger, C., Sanacora, G., et al. (2007). The NMDA receptor as a therapeutic target in major depressive disorder. *CNS & Neurological Disorders—Drug Targets, 6*(2), 101–115.

Price, L. H., Kao, H. T., et al. (2013). Telomeres and early-life stress: An overview. *Biological Psychiatry, 73*, 15–23.

Price, R. B., Nock, M. K., et al. (2009). Effects of intravenous ketamine on explicit and implicit measures of suicidality in treatment-resistant depression. *Biological Psychiatry, 66*(5), 522–526.

Puterman, E., O'Donovan, A., et al. (2011). Physical activity moderates effects of stressor-induced rumination on cortisol reactivity. *Psychosomatic Medicine, 73*(7), 604–611.

Raison, C. L., & Miller, A. H. (2003). When not enough is too much: the role of insufficient glucocorticoid signaling in the pathophysiology of stress-related disorders. *American Journal of Psychiatry, 160*(9), 1554–1565.

Raison, C. L., Rutherford, R. E., et al. (2013). A randomized controlled trial of the tumor necrosis factor antagonist infliximab for treatment-resistant depression: The role of baseline inflammatory biomarkers. *Archives of General Psychiatry, 70*(1), 31–41.

Rao, T. S., Asha, M. R., et al. (2008). Understanding nutrition, depression and mental illnesses. *Indian Journal of Psychiatry, 50*(2), 77–82.

Rawdin, B. S., Mellon, S. H., et al. (2013). Dysregulated relationship of inflammation and oxidative stress in major depression. *Brain, Behavior & Immunity, 31*, 143–152.

Reddy, D. S. (2010). Neurosteroids: endogenous role in the human brain and therapeutic potentials. *Progress in Brain Research, 186*, 113–137.

Ressler, K. J., Bradley, B., et al. (2010). Polymorphisms in CRHR1 and the serotonin transporter loci: gene x gene x environment interactions on depressive symptoms. *American Journal of Medical Genetics Part B: Neuropsychiatric Genetics, 153B*(3), 812–824.

Ressler, K. J., & Mayberg, H. S. (2007). Targeting abnormal neural circuits in mood and anxiety disorders: from the laboratory to the clinic. *Nature Neuroscience, 10*(9), 1116–1124.

Reus, V. I. (1982). Pituitary-adrenal disinhibition as the independent variable in the assessment of behavioral symptoms. *Biological Psychiatry, 17*(3), 317–325.

Ribeiro, S. C., Tandon, R., et al. (1993). The DST as a predictor of outcome in depression: a meta-analysis. *American Journal of Psychiatry, 150*(11), 1618–1629.

Ripke, S., Wray, N. R., et al. (2013). A mega-analysis of genome-wide association studies for major depressive disorder. *Molecular Psychiatry, 18*(4), 497–511.

Risch, N., Herrell, R., et al. (2009). Interaction between the serotonin transporter gene (5-HTTLPR), stressful life events, and risk of depression: a meta-analysis. *Journal of the American Medical Association, 301*(23), 2462–2471.

Rius-Ottenheim, N., Houben, J. M., et al. (2012). Telomere length and mental well-being in elderly men from the Netherlands and Greece. *Behavior Genetics, 42*(2), 278–286.

Roth, T. L., Lubin, F. D., et al. (2009). Lasting epigenetic influence of early-life adversity on the BDNF gene. *Biological Psychiatry, 65*(9), 760–769.

Rucker, J. J., Breen, G., et al. (2013). Genome-wide association analysis of copy number variation in recurrent depressive disorder. *Molecular Psychiatry, 18*(2), 183–189.

Sanchez-Villegas, A., Delgado-Rodriguez, M., et al. (2009). Association of the Mediterranean dietary pattern with the incidence of depression: the Seguimiento Universidad de Navarra/University of Navarra follow-up (SUN) cohort. *Archives of General Psychiatry, 66*(10), 1090–1098.

Sanchez-Villegas, A., Galbete, C., et al. (2011). The effect of the Mediterranean diet on plasma brain-derived neurotrophic factor (BDNF) levels: the PREDIMED-NAVARRA randomized trial. *Nutritional Neuroscience, 14*(5), 195–201.

Sandman, C. A., Davis, E. P., et al. (2011). Prenatal programming of human neurological function. *International Journal of Peptides, 2011*, 837596.

Santarelli, L., Saxe, M., et al. (2003). Requirement of hippocampal neurogenisis for the behavioral effects of antidepressants. *Science, 301*: 805–809.

Sapolsky, R. M. (1993). Potential behavioral modification of glucocorticoid damage to the hippocampus. *Behavioural Brain Research, 57*(2), 175–182.

Sapolsky, R. M. (2000). The possibility of neurotoxicity in the hippocampus in major depression: a primer on neuron death. *Biological Psychiatry, 48*(8), 755–765.

Schroeder, M., Krebs, M. O., et al. (2010). Epigenetics and depression: current challenges and new therapeutic options. *Current Opinion in Psychiatry, 23*(6), 588–592.

Schule, C., Baghai, T. C., et al. (2009). Hypothalamic-pituitary-adrenocortical system dysregulation and new treatment strategies in depression. *Expert Review of Neurotherapeutics, 9*(7), 1005–1019.

Schule, C., Eser, D., et al. (2011). Neuroactive steroids in affective disorders: target for novel antidepressant or anxiolytic drugs? *Neuroscience, 191*, 55–77.

Sen, S., Duman, R., et al. (2008). Serum brain-derived neurotrophic factor, depression, and antidepressant medications: meta-analyses and implications. *Biological Psychiatry, 64*(6), 527–532.

Shaffer, J. A., Epel, E., et al. (2012). Depressive symptoms are not associated with leukocyte telomere length: Findings from the Nova Scotia Health Survey (NSHS95), a population-based study. *PLoS One, 7*(10), e48318.

Shalev, I. (2012). Early life stress and telomere length: investigating the connection and possible mechanisms: a critical survey of the evidence base, research methodology and basic biology. *Bioessays, 34*(11), 943–952.

Shalev, I., Entringer, S., et al. (2013). Stress and telomere biology: A Lifespan perspective. *Psychoneuroendocrinology, 38*(9), 1835–1842.

Sheline, Y. I., Sanghavi, M., et al. (1999). Depression duration but not age predicts hippocampal volume loss in medically healthy women with recurrent major depression. *Journal of Neuroscience, 19*(12), 5034–5043.

Sheridan, M. A., Sarsour, K., et al. (2012). The impact of social disparity on prefrontal function in childhood. *PLoS ONE, 7*(4), e35744.

Shyn, S. I., & Hamilton, S. P. (2010). The genetics of major depression: moving beyond the monoamine hypothesis. *Psychiatric Clinics of North America, 33*(1), 125–140.

Staff, R. T., Murray, A. D., et al. (2012). Childhood socioeconomic status and adult brain size: Childhood socioeconomic status influences adult hippocampal size. *Annals of Neurology, 71*(5), 653–660.

Stein, D. J. (2008). Emotional regulation: implications for the psychobiology of psychotherapy. *CNS Spectrums, 13*(3), 195–198.

Sterling and Eyer (1988).

Sullivan, P. F., Neale, M. C., et al. (2000). Genetic epidemiology of major depression: review and meta-analysis. *American Journal of Psychiatry, 157*(10), 1552–1562.

Surtees, P. G., Wainwright, N. W., et al. (2011). Life stress, emotional health, and mean telomere length in the European Prospective Investigation into Cancer (EPIC)-Norfolk population study. *Journals of Gerontology Series A: Biological Sciences & Medical Sciences, 66*(11), 1152–1162.

Tarullo, A. R., & Gunnar, M. R. (2006). Child maltreatment and the developing HPA axis. *Hormones & Behavior, 50*(4), 632–639.

Teodorczuk, A., O'Brien, J. T., et al. (2007). White matter changes and late-life depressive symptoms: longitudinal study. *British Journal of Psychiatry, 191*, 212–217.

Thase, M. E., Dube, S., et al. (1996). Hypothalamic-pituitary-adrenocortical activity and response to cognitive behavior therapy in unmedicated, hospitalized depressed patients. *American Journal of Psychiatry, 153*(7), 886–891.

Thase, M. E., Simons, A. D., et al. (1993). Psychobiological correlates of poor response to cognitive behavior therapy: potential indications for antidepressant pharmacotherapy. *Psychopharmacology Bulletin, 29*(2), 293–301.

Thayer, J. F., & Sternberg, E. M. (2010). Neural aspects of immunomodulation: focus on the vagus nerve. *Brain, Behavior & Immunity, 24*(8), 1223–1228.

Thomas, A. J., Kalaria, R. N., et al. (2004). Depression and vascular disease: what is the relationship? *Journal of Affective Disorders, 79*(1-3), 81–95.

Thomas, C., Hypponen, E., et al. (2008). Obesity and type 2 diabetes risk in midadult life: the role of childhood adversity. *Pediatrics, 121*(5), e1240–e1249.

Tolmunen, T., Hintikka, J., et al. (2004). Dietary folate and the risk of depression in Finnish middle-aged men. A prospective follow-up study. *Psychotherapy & Psychosomatics, 73*(6), 334–339.

Uzunova, V., Sheline, Y., et al. (1998). Increase in the cerebrospinal fluid content of neurosteroids in patients with unipolar major depression who are receiving fluoxetine or fluvoxamine. *Proceedings of the National Academy of Sciences, USA, 95*(6), 3239–3244.

Videbech, P., & Ravnkilde, B. (2004). Hippocampal volume and depression: a meta-analysis of MRI studies. *American Journal of Psychiatry, 161*(11), 1957–1966.

von Zglinicki, T. (2002). Oxidative stress shortens telomeres. *Trends in Biochemical Sciences, 27*(7), 339–344.

Vythilingam, M., Heim, C., et al. (2002). Childhood trauma associated with smaller hippocampal volume in women with major depression. *American Journal of Psychiatry, 159*(12), 2072–2080.

Weaver, I. C., Cervoni, N., et al. (2004). Epigenetic programming by maternal behavior. *Nature Neuroscience, 7*(8), 847–854.

Wolkowitz, O. M., Burke, H., et al. (2009). Glucocorticoids: mood, memory and mechanisms. *Annals of the New York Academy of Science* (in press).

Wolkowitz, O. M., Epel, E. S., et al. (2008). When blue turns to grey: do stress and depression accelerate cell aging? *World Journal of Biological Psychiatry, 9*(1), 2–5.

Wolkowitz, O. M., Epel, E. S., et al. (2009). Major Depression and History of Childhood Sexual Abuse Are Related to Increased PBMC Telomerase Activity. Presented at the International Society of Psychoneuroendocrinology Annual Meeting, San Francisco, CA, July 23–26, 2009.

Wolkowitz, O. M., Epel, E. S., et al. (2010). Depression gets old fast: do stress and depression accelerate cell aging? *Depression & Anxiety, 27*(4), 327–338.

Wolkowitz, O. M., Mellon, S. H., et al. (2011). Leukocyte telomere length in major depression: correlations with chronicity, inflammation and oxidative stress— preliminary findings. *PLoS One, 6*(3), e17837.

Wolkowitz, O. M., Mellon, S. H., et al. (2012). Resting leukocyte telomerase activity is elevated in major depression and predicts treatment response. *Molecular Psychiatry, 17*(2), 164–172.

Wolkowitz, O. M., Reus, V. I., et al. (1999). Antiglucocorticoid treatment of depression: Double-blind ketoconazole. *Biological Psychiatry, 45*, 1070–1074.

Wolkowitz, O. M., Reus, V. I., et al. (2011). Of sound mind and body: depression, disease, and accelerated aging. *Dialogues in Clinical Neuroscience, 13*(1), 25–39.

Yoshimura, S., Okamoto, Y., et al. (2013). Cognitive behavioral therapy for depression changes medial prefrontal and ventral anterior cingulate cortex activity associated with self-referential processing. *Social Cognitive & Affective Neuroscience*, [epub ahead of print]

Zarate, C. A., Jr., Brutsche, N. E., et al. (2012). Replication of ketamine's antidepressant efficacy in bipolar depression: a randomized controlled add-on trial. *Biological Psychiatry, 71*(11), 939–946.

Zhou, Q. G., Hu, Y., et al. (2011). Hippocampal telomerase is involved in the modulation of depressive behaviors. *Journal of Neuroscience, 31*(34), 12258–12269.

CHAPTER 5

Attention-Deficit Hyperactivity Disorder

KYLE J. RUTLEDGE, KHYATI BRAHMBHATT,
AND JULIE B. SCHWEITZER

INTRODUCTION

The high prevalence of attention-deficit hyperactivity disorder (ADHD) and the severity of negative outcomes associated with the disorder call for the need for successful interventions. The critical need for new interventions for ADHD is underscored by the lack of lasting effectiveness of the two most common treatments for ADHD, stimulant medication and behavioral therapies (Molina et al., 2009). This chapter reviews standard treatment options (medication and behavioral therapies) for ADHD as well as evidence for new therapeutics in the form of cognitive and working memory training strategies.

SYMPTOMS AND CLINICAL DESCRIPTION

Attention-deficit/hyperactivity disorder is characterized by developmentally inappropriate and significant problems with inattention and/or excessive motor restlessness and impulsivity, presenting across settings (i.e., home and school or home and work). Common inattentive symptoms may include difficulty maintaining attention, poor organizational skills, careless mistakes, excessive distractibility, disorganization, poor planning and follow-through, or forgetfulness. Hyperactive and impulsive symptoms include restlessness, excessive talking, poor self-control, and interrupting. Adolescents and adults are more likely to exhibit hyperactivity as fidgeting or internal feelings of restlessness, rather than the more prominent "running around" associated with an earlier developmental period. The degree to which the symptoms associated with ADHD are targeted for treatment can be situation- and age-dependent, with hyperactive and impulsive symptoms more prominent during early and middle childhood years and the inattentive symptoms most prominent during adulthood. Little is known about how the developmental progression of ADHD affects treatment efficacy; however, the development of brain structures and connectivity that support cognitive control functions (i.e., prefrontal and parietal lobes) during the adolescent through young adult years provides a new window of opportunity for treatments that may not work during earlier developmental periods.

Treatment for ADHD needs to consider the presence of the many associated symptoms and co-occurring disorders associated with ADHD, such as oppositional defiant, learning, mood, anxiety, speech, language, and motor disorders. Higher rates of conduct and substance abuse disorders are associated with ADHD. The fifth edition of the *Diagnostic and Statistical Manual* (DSM-5) now recognizes that individuals with autism can also present with and be diagnosed with ADHD.

ADHD is associated with a number of characteristics that require intervention, including poor social relationships and underachievement in school and work settings. Cognitive deficits associated with the disorder can impact functioning for the person with ADHD, including problems with working memory, planning, variability in response time, and a steeper discounting in the value of delayed rewards, manifested as impulsivity. Until recently, the cognitive impairments in ADHD were often left unaddressed.

EPIDEMIOLOGY

Males are more likely than females to receive a diagnosis of ADHD; however, during adulthood, the diagnosis of ADHD may occur at equal rates in males and females. Willcutt (2012) found that 5.9%–7.1% of children met criteria for ADHD diagnosis in a meta-analysis. The prevalence rates for adults with the disorder decreases slightly, with 5.0% of adults meeting criteria for ADHD based on DSM-IV symptoms (Willcutt, 2012). The "inattentive" presentation is the most commonly diagnosed subtype, based on the use of self, parent, or teacher ratings. Prevalence estimates using a "best-estimate diagnostic procedure" that rely on a combination of rating scales and evaluation procedures suggest that the "combined" presentation is the most frequent presentation.

PARENT TRAINING

Although medications are highly effective in treating ADHD, non-pharmaceutical options should also be considered, given that medication-based treatment options may work better when used in conjunction with non-pharmacological options (Multimodal Treatment of Attention Deficit Hyperactivity Disorder [MTA], 1999), and because many parents are wary of using medication due to misunderstandings, stigma, and a fear of side-effects (Monastra, 2005). Parent training is the only non-pharmaceutical treatment considered to be a well-established treatment option for ADHD, and it is recommended by the National Institute for Health and Clinical Excellence (NICE, 2008).

In parent training, parents and guardians learn about the nature of ADHD and strategies in addressing its sequela, such as how to use rewards and structure in the home environment to reinforce more appropriate behavior, and response cost and/or time-outs to reduce inappropriate behavior. Much of the focus is on making the cues in the environment more salient for the child with ADHD. Parents are encouraged to implement systems that increase communication between the school and home environment (i.e., daily school–home report cards). A majority of the parent training research was based on working with children with conduct disorder or behavior problems rather than ADHD (Kazdin, 1997). However, numerous empirical studies of the treatment have also demonstrated its efficacy in ADHD (see Pelham, Wheeler & Chronis, 1998; Pelham & Fabiano, 2008; Fabiano, Pelham, et al., 2009; Zwi, Jones, Thorgaard, York & Dennis, 2011). Recent studies have illustrated improvements in functioning with a combination of medication and parent training, above and beyond treatment response when medication alone is used (Mikami, Jack, Emeh, & Stephens, 2010; van den Hoofdakker et al., 2007). This contradicts previous studies that failed to show greater improvements with multimodal treatment, compared to the use of medication alone (Abikoff et al., 2004; Multimodal Treatment of Attention Deficit Hyperactivity Disorder [MTA], 1999).

Parent and child characteristics may affect the effectiveness of parent training. For example, genetic predispositions may limit effectiveness of the treatment for a patient, as recent research has demonstrated that the *DAT1* gene in children may moderate their responsiveness to parent training such that children with fewer repeats (zero or one 10-repeat allele) can respond much more favorably to the treatment than those with more long repeats (two 10-repeat alleles) (van den Hoofdakker et al., 2012). The authors point to the role dopamine plays in learning and motivation in their conjectures as to the mechanism of this relationship. Also, low engagement in the intervention will limit its efficacy, and engagement is likely to be lower in high-risk families characterized by qualities such as high stress, low socioeconomic standing, or antisocial child behavior (Kazdin & Mazurick, 1994). However, a recent study demonstrated that engagement from high-risk (specifically, single-mother) families may be improved by addressing problems that interfere with engagement during the visits, and by clarifying misconceptions and expectations regarding treatment (Chacko, Wymbs, Chimiklis, Wymbs, & Pelham, 2012). Other research has shown that fathers are more likely to participate in parent training when the intervention is conducted within a recreational or sports context (Fabiano, Chacko, et al., 2009). Also, mothers with higher levels of ADHD symptoms themselves are likely to be less successful in improving their children's disruptive behaviors following the intervention (Chronis-Tuscano et al., 2011).

The impact of parent training in ADHD may be significantly enhanced when a component emphasizing a family–school partnership is included, such as how cooperation between teachers and parents can be used to better address the precursors and consequences of ADHD behaviors in children (e.g., MTA, 1999; Sheridan et al., 2001; Hechtman et al., 2004; Pfiffner et al., 2007; Owens et al., 2008; Power, 2012); however, there are still some limitations in how well the parent training can improve behavior in the classroom setting. A recent advancement in the modality of parent training delivery was recently successfully achieved in a pilot randomized-controlled study that demonstrated parent training could be achieved when delivered electronically over videoconferencing procedures. Xie et al. (2013) found that parent training improved child ADHD, oppositional and anxious behaviors (as rated by parents and teachers in a combined score), as well as parent discipline practices equally well, whether the treatment was delivered face-to-face or over a videoconference format. Parents also indicated high satisfaction with both the face-to-face and the videoconference formats.

Unfortunately, at this point, the neurobiological mechanisms of ADHD are not considered in the development of behavioral and parent training treatments for the disorder. The development of future treatments should try to integrate information the neuroscience field has learned about altered reward-processing in ADHD in the basal ganglia and dopamine system and in cognitive control-associated brain structures (i.e., anterior cingulate and prefrontal cortex) (Fassbender & Schweitzer, 2006) so that more precise and effective treatments can be developed. For example, new findings on temporal difference error learning in neuroscience support the use and timing of novel rewards when designing behavioral treatment plans.

COMPLEMENTARY AND ALTERNATIVE MEDICINE

Although a majority of research examining treatment in ADHD focuses on the effects of medication, a wealth of studies have explored complementary and alternative medicine.

Diet and Exercise

One field that has emerged has focused on the potential benefits of restrictive diets. A variety of diets focusing on limiting or increasing the consumption of certain foods, additives, or compounds have been put forward (see Bader & Adesman, 2012, for a review). For example, while met with much controversy, initial findings suggested restricting the intake of artificial food coloring may help with some ADHD symptoms; though these synthetic food additives should not be considered to be a cause of the symptoms but rather a stimulus with downstream consequences that could push an individual with already high levels of ADHD symptoms over the diagnostic threshold (see Arnold et al., 2012, for a review). Future research is needed to support these findings, however, before restriction of additives can be recommended. Caffeine consumption may lead to minor improvements in children with ADHD, though these effects are coupled with risks and side effects.

Supplementation of omega-3 fatty acids is the most studied non-pharmacological treatment in ADHD, with individual studies reporting conflicting findings. Omega-3 fatty acid is entirely diet-derived, as humans cannot synthesize it *de novo*. Omega-3s have been shown to play an anti-inflammatory role and alter cell membrane fluidity. This ability is thought to underlie its effect on neurotransmitters like dopamine and serotonin. A meta-analysis (Bloch & Qawasmi, 2011) on the acid looked at 10 trials that used ADHD rating scales as endpoints and incorporated a double-blind randomized controlled trial (RCT) design. The results found that six trials showed no benefit, two demonstrated some benefit, and two showed significant benefits. The meta-analysis concluded that, overall, omega-3 fatty acids had a significant but modest efficacy in treating ADHD, with an effect size of 0.31 (Bloch & Qawasmi, 2011). Overall, using omega-3 fatty acid is very well tolerated, with few side effects. In summary, given the relatively low effect size of omega-3 fatty acids in treating ADHD compared to those of other pharmacotherapeutic options, it should be considered as an adjunctive treatment only. None of the alternative therapies yields effects as impressive as those found for pharmacotherapy; therefore, dietary changes or supplements meant to target ADHD symptoms should not be considered to be risk-free alternatives to medication, but rather adjuncts that need to be closely monitored.

A 2011 review explored studies examining the effects of exercise, concluding that there is some evidence that exercise can benefit behavioral and cognitive outcomes in children with ADHD (Gapin, Labban, & Etnier, 2011). The authors suggest that exercise may be beneficial for both medicated and non-medicated children in attenuating behavioral symptoms. They posit (Berwid & Halperin, 2012) ways in which physical exercise can lead to improvements in brain structure and function as a basis for its effects in ADHD. Additional work needs to be conducted to further explore the potential for this this low-risk, non-invasive intervention in ADHD.

Neurofeedback

Neurofeedback, or electroencephalogram (EEG) biofeedback, is based on the relationship between arousal and brain waves observable through EEG (Lofthouse, Arnold, Hersch, Hurt, & DeBeus, 2012). Individuals with ADHD often display a trend toward slower wave patterns (see Lofthouse et al., 2012, for a review), and as a result, neurofeedback has shown promise as a treatment option for the disorder, with many studies yielding a medium effect size in reduction in inattentive and hyperactive/impulsive symptoms (Lofthouse, Arnold, Hersch, et al., 2012). While the mechanism of change is not known, it has been theorized that wave patterns reflect resting state, or default mode, central nervous system activity, and training to normalize aberrant wave manifestations from underlying structures induces shifts in network activity toward more stable neural functioning (Legarda, McMahon, & Othmer, 2011).

Despite the positive effects from this treatment option, and its abundant use in many clinics across the country, evidence for its clinical efficacy is lacking. A majority of the neurofeedback studies did not randomize participants to treatment comparison groups (see Moriyama et al., 2012, for a review). Recent studies using randomized controlled trials have demonstrated moderate effect sizes, though these trials have not demonstrated effects as high as those in the non-randomized trials (Skokauskas et al., 2011), and blinded studies have not shown the same positive effects (see Lofthouse, Arnold, & Hurt, 2012, for a review). In light of these findings, and considering the expense and commitment required for the sessions, neurofeedback should be considered to still be in its experimental phase, and not yet a primary treatment for ADHD (see Loo & Makeig, 2012, for more in-depth commentary).

Mindfulness Training

Mindfulness training is an alternative treatment recently gaining in popularity to target a diverse array of child and adolescent clinical populations, including ADHD (see Black et al., 2009, for a review). The training, based in meditation practices, requires individuals to practice self-regulating their attention through a variety of techniques (e.g., focused muscle relaxation, breathing control, focused physical movement) during a number of sessions. There is some potential for the treatment's efficacy, based on findings in training of both the child or adolescent and parent on reducing parent-rated (but not teacher-rated) attention and hyperactive/impulsive ADHD symptoms (van der Oord, Bogels, & Peijnenburg, 2012), as well as some reductions in externalizing problems, internalizing problems, and parental stress as rated by fathers, but not mothers (van de Weijer-Bergsma, Formsma, de Bruin, & Bogels, 2012). These results are preliminary, however, given that the studies had small sample sizes and did not use a random-assignment controlled design.

COGNITIVE TRAINING

Over the past decade, there has been increasing interest in, and availability of, commercially available cognitive training programs to address symptoms associated with ADHD. Some of these programs target the broad category of attention (e.g., Lumosity), whereas others are more limited in their scope and target working memory function (e.g., Cogmed). The primary hypothesis of these training programs is that they are targeting underlying general cognitive functions and that, when these cognitive functions improve, their effects will generalize and improve other behavioral impairments associated with the disorder. The training exercises require repeated practice and become increasingly challenging as the performance improves, or lower the requirements (e.g., span length) if the individual commits errors. Typically, the exercises are performed on a computer, but they may use paper and pencil tools as well.

Attention Training

Two studies compared the effects of general attention training to exercises targeting academic skills (e.g., Kerns et al., 1999; Rabiner et al., 2010).

A combination of objective and nonobjective (i.e., rating scales) measures assessed the presence of any training effects. These studies have shown some modest, positive effects. The Kerns et al. (1999) study had a small sample size, however. In a relatively recent study of first-grade children who exhibited behavior rated one standard deviation or more above their peers in inattentive symptoms by teachers, but not necessarily meeting full criteria for ADHD (Rabiner, et al., 2010), children were randomly assigned to perform visual and auditory attention tasks on the computer for 14 weeks, or to a reading and math skills version of training. An additional wait-list control group was also included for comparison purposes. The sample sizes in this study were moderate. Both the attention and academic interventions resulted in a 50% improvement on teacher ratings of attention. The academic intervention had the added benefit of improving academic functioning. Neither training exercise "normalized" behavior, in that approximately 75% of participants continued to exhibit significantly elevated attention problems on teacher ratings, with attention issues rated at least one standard deviation above the normative mean. The positive effects of the interventions were not maintained into the following year, at which time all participants showed a decline in attentional functioning in the second grade. These results are not wholly without further consideration, however, because even a reduction in attentional symptoms may be significant if it moderates the need for, or lowers the optimal dosage of, medication.

A broader cognitive training program (Oord, Ponsioen, Geurts, Brink, & Prins, 2012) that emphasized the use of "gaming" to provide reinforcement for correct responding on inhibition, cognitive flexibility, and working memory tasks, was compared in effectiveness to a randomized wait-list control group on parent- and teacher-rated measures of ADHD and associated problems for children with ADHD. This program takes into account the need for immediate, salient reward that is associated with ADHD and the underlying impairments found in brain regions (e.g., basal ganglia; Fassbender & Schweitzer, 2006) associated with reward functioning. The authors found significant improvement on parent-rated inattention and hyperactivity/impulsivity symptoms, on subscales of the Behavior Rating Inventory of Executive Functioning (BRIEF; Gioia, Isquith, Guy, & Kenworthy, 2000), and a trend toward improvement on teacher ratings of attention. Children medicated for their ADHD appeared to benefit the most from the training. Ratings suggested significant and large effects of within-subject improvements on parent and teacher measures of ADHD and the rating scale of executive function measures (i.e., BRIEF; Gioia, et al., 2000). While these findings are promising, there are limitations, including the use of the wait-list control design and subjective ratings, no use of objective measures to assess near- or far-transfer effects, and the absence of a control group at the follow-up period.

In addition to examining the clinical effects of attentional training, two studies have examined changes in brain functioning and gray matter volume associated with cognitive training in ADHD (Hoekzema et al., 2011; Hoekzema et al., 2010). In both studies, the cognitive training was compared to a social skills training group. The cognitive training was completed by paper and pencil exercises with a therapist five times per week for 45 minutes for two weeks, and it targeted working memory, attention, planning, and problem-solving processes. The cognitive training program was associated with increases in left orbitofrontal cortex, right middle temporal gyrus, and bilateral inferior frontal gyri activation during the response-inhibition paradigm. During the attention paradigm, the right superior posterior cerebellum activity increased, and the precuneus and the right superior parietal cortex activity decreased after the cognitive training. The social skills training condition was not associated with any significant brain activation pre- or post-treatment, but it was associated with decreased activation in the right superior posterior cerebellum. The cognitive training intervention also was associated with a larger brain volume within the bilateral middle frontal cortex and inferior-posterior cerebellum in comparison to the social skill control condition. These findings are particularly interesting as the regions affected by the cognitive training are regularly found to be smaller in volume in ADHD (Nigg & Casey, 2005).

Working-Memory Training

While attention training seeks to strengthen a broad class of functioning, working-memory training aims to improve a more specific cognitive operation in which the participant is expected to practice recall, rehearsal, and manipulation of increasingly longer spans of information. Published research studies on the effects of working-memory training in ADHD are perhaps the most studied of the cognitive training programs.

From a mechanistic perspective, targeting working-memory functioning in ADHD is logical given that there is well-established evidence of working-memory impairments and the underlying structures that support it in ADHD (Rutledge, van den Bos, McClure, & Schweitzer, 2012). Furthermore, working memory is the most reliable cognitive function to show impairment in ADHD. Theoretically, improvements in working-memory functioning could generalize to other cognitive functions impaired in ADHD, such as attention, resistance to distraction, and higher level processes such as planning, as the processes supporting working-memory functioning are required in these additional cognitive operations. A group of studies with non-placebo comparison groups and relatively small sample sizes in healthy young adults suggests that the neural structures that support working-memory performance, such as the prefrontal cortex, parietal lobe, thalamus, and caudate, and connectivity between anterior and posterior brain regions, are all implicated in ADHD, and are improved by working-memory training (see Rutledge et al., 2012, for further discussion). McNab et al. (2009) published a particularly interesting study in healthy, young adults, demonstrating that working-memory training increases the density of dopamine D1 receptor binding in the prefrontal and parietal cortex. These regions, and the involvement of dopamine, are relevant to ADHD as these brain regions and the neurotransmitter are established as altered in ADHD. Furthermore, the most common treatment for ADHD, stimulant medication, affects dopamine transmission.

The most frequently studied working-memory commercial training program for ADHD is Cogmed (Klingberg, Forssberg, & Westerberg, 2002). The evidence base for the programs that have been tested in ADHD is growing, but the number of randomized, placebo-controlled studies with large sample sizes is still relatively small. Cogmed is a working-memory training program that typically requires about 25 sessions, with five sessions per week over five weeks. A key component of the Cogmed program is the involvement of a coach who is to contact the family once a week to troubleshoot treatment interface (i.e., computer) problems, but even more importantly, to work with the family to maximize motivation in completing the exercises on a regular basis. In the standard, non-research situation, the coach can view the client's progress on each exercise over a web portal. The Cogmed program has a "regular" program and a junior program, with the junior program designed for preschool-aged children, which uses shorter training sessions. In both programs the training is adaptive and dependent on the participant's progress, such that correct responses result in the training trials' increasing in span length and difficulty, and incorrect responses result in decreasing the span length. In studies using a placebo-controlled version, the span length in the placebo condition does not increase in difficulty, but it can then act as a general control for the demands of being in a required session for five weeks. The initial studies of Cogmed by Klingberg and his collaborators (Klingberg, 2010; Klingberg et al., 2005; Klingberg, et al., 2002) included parent and teacher ratings of ADHD and associated symptoms as well as objective task measures. There were improvements on objective measures of functioning, such as the Stroop task (with incongruent trials used only), a reaction time task, head movements, and the Raven's Progressive Matrices, a measure of visuo-spatial functioning sometimes used as a general measure of spatial intellectual functioning. Improvements on some measures were seen for three months after the training ceased. In regard to tasks and ratings that measured far-transfer effects, as noted earlier, there was a significant improvement on parent ADHD ratings for the active treatment group only, but no improvement on teacher ADHD ratings. The use of incongruent trials only as a measure of conflict and response inhibition (versus a mix of congruent and incongruent trials) on the Stroop test has been criticized by some researchers (e.g., Shipstead, Redick, & Engle, 2012).

There have been a few other studies to evaluate Cogmed on functioning in ADHD using objective measures. Holmes et al. (2010) found the training resulted in improvement on the Automated Working Memory Assessment (AWMA). Similar to the earlier studies by Klingberg, they found that the beneficial effects of the cognitive training remained for three to six months after the training had stopped. Green et al. (2012) assessed the effects of Cogmed on two groups of children with ADHD randomized to a placebo-controlled group (i.e., non-adaptive working-memory load) versus a treatment group where the span length was adaptive and grew in length as the child was successful at the game. They found improvements on the Working Memory Index of the Wechsler Intellectual Scale for Children–IV (Wechsler, 2003) and on an observational measure using an analogue classroom task in a laboratory setting to assess off-task behavior. The off-task behavior decreased in the treatment group but did not change in the placebo group. Parent ratings of ADHD symptoms improved for both the placebo and treatment group and therefore were not considered to demonstrate a significant improvement due to the Cogmed training. Based on the improvements seen in the off-task observational measure, the Green et al. (2012) study does provide evidence for far-transfer effects to a clinically important behavior in this study of working-memory training.

A recent study assessed the effects of Cogmed on a group of adolescents with co-morbid ADHD and learning disabilities (Gray et al., 2012). Subjects in this study were randomized to either intense math training or the Cogmed program in a school setting. The participants in the Cogmed training demonstrated improvement on measures directly related to those practiced in the study, (e.g., backward digit span and a spatial span task), but did not show any other significant improvements on other neuropsychological measures or academic tests. The subjects who demonstrated the most improvement on the Cogmed Working Memory Improvement Index score did exhibit higher ratings of improvement on parent ratings of ADHD symptoms. The authors discussed the complexity of trying to address cognitive issues in a population with co-morbid disorders.

Another working-memory training program (see Wong, He, & Chan, 2013) was tested in children with ADHD in a school setting. In this study, subjects were assigned to an active treatment group where they practiced eight working-memory computer games or a waitlist control group. The findings suggested, similar to other studies, improvements on tasks similar to the training games, such as span board and digit span measures; limited improvement on parent measures; and no improvement on teacher measures of ADHD or executive functioning. Furthermore, it appears that the control group actually improved their performance to a greater degree on the Stroop task of inhibition than did the treatment group.

In summary, there is some support for cognitive training programs; however, there is a great need for replication of these studies and the use of randomized, placebo-controlled designs using objective measures in larger samples. Ultimately, we may also find that subgroups of individuals with ADHD may have a more sensitive response to cognitive training. Furthermore, the tepid and in some cases negative results suggest that there is substantial room for improvement in the development of cognitive training programs. At this point, the cognitive training programs lack strong evidence for addressing ADHD symptoms on a consistent, reliable basis. We encourage the further exploration of cognitive training methods to identify how they can be enhanced, given that there are some promising findings.

PSYCHOPHARMACOLOGICAL TREATMENT OF ADHD

Findings of the initial Multimodal Treatment of ADHD (MTA) study (1999) highlighted the central role of medication management in the treatment of ADHD. There continues to be an active effort towards finding newer pharmacological agents with novel mechanisms of action for ADHD. Current medication choices include stimulant and nonstimulant medications, with stimulants being the first-line agents given their superior effect sizes (Faraone, 2003) and long history of successful use in children. The primary advance in medication therapy in the past decade has been in novel delivery systems and the availability of longer-acting drugs.

Stimulant Medications

Stimulant medications can be differentiated into methylphenidate and amphetamine products that are formulated with differing pharmacodynamic and pharmacokinetic properties. Methylphenidate is a modestly potent inhibitor of norepinephrine (NE) and dopamine (DA) reuptake. In contrast to amphetamines, which normalize synaptic DA levels before NE levels, methylphenidate shows a more sustained and comparable reduction of both NE and DA hours after its administration (Heal, Smith, & Findling, 2012) and comparable or superior results to amphetamine salts in clinical practice. The primary therapeutic action for amphetamines is related to their ability to competitively bind with NE transporter and DA transporter receptors and thus increase synaptic monoamine concentrations (Heal et al., 2012). Stimulants are available in shorter-acting and sustained-release formulations, allowing flexibility in dosing frequency and individualization of treatment to attain optimal symptom control while monitoring side effects (see Table 5.1). A recent addition to this group, lisdexamphetamine, is unique in that it is a pro-drug (Jain et al., 2011) that becomes active after first-pass metabolism in the liver, making it a useful pharmacological candidate in patients who have, or are at risk for developing, a co-occurring substance use disorder. Recent additions to stimulant medication formulations are liquid versions (e.g., Liquadd, Procentra, and Quillivant XR).

Common side effects of stimulants include appetite suppression and sleep disturbances, especially with the sustained-release medications. The majority of the children prescribed stimulant medication experience little to no overall growth-slowing, occurring secondary to appetite-reduction, though a small percentage may be more susceptible to this effect. Stimulants have not been shown to worsen tics in most people with tic disorders; the medication may, however, exacerbate tics in individual cases. Treatment with non-stimulant medications may be an option in these cases (Pringsheim & Steeves, 2011). While there were conflicting recommendations regarding cardiac issues with stimulant treatment, current evidence does not support routine need for ECG and is reserved only for patients with preexisting cardiac conditions (O'Keefe, 2008; Olfson et al., 2012). A frequent parental concern is that stimulant treatment may increase addiction to stimulants. There is no support demonstrating that appropriately prescribed stimulant medication increases the risk for substance abuse in persons with ADHD (Wilens, Faraone, Biederman, & Gunawardene, 2003), although the disorder is associated with greater risk for substance abuse disorders (Charach, Yeung, Climans, & Lillie, 2011).

Table 5.1 COMMONLY USED STIMULANT MEDICATIONS

Medications	Avg. Dose Range	Duration of Action	FDA Approval for Age
AMPHETAMINES			
Adderall IR[2]	2.5 mg–40 mg	4–6 hrs	3 yrs of age or above
Dexedrine[1]	5 mg–60 mg	4–6 hrs	6 yrs of age or above
Dextrostat[1]	2.5 mg–40 mg	4–6 hrs	3 yrs of age or above
Adderall XR[2]	5 mg–40 mg	8–10 hrs dual pulse	6 yrs of age or above
Dexedrine Spansules[1]	5 mg–30 mg	6–8 hrs	6 yrs of age or above
Vyvanse[3]	20 mg–70 mg	Up to 12 hrs	
METHYLPHENIDATES			
Ritalin IR	5 mg–60 mg	2–4 hrs	6 yrs of age or above
Methylin (solution/ chewable tablets)	5 mg–60 mg	3–5 hrs	6 yrs of age or above
Focalin[4]	2.5 mg–20 mg	?6 hrs	6 yrs of age or above
Ritalin SR	20 mg–60 mg	3–8 hrs	6 yrs of age or above
Methylin ER	10 mg–40 mg	3–8 hrs	6 yrs of age or above
Metadate ER	20 mg– 60 mg	3–8 hrs	6 yrs of age or above
Focalin XR[4]	5 mg–40 mg	8–12 hrs dual pulse	6 yrs of age or above
Metadate CD	10 mg–60 mg	8–10 hrs dual pulse	6 yrs of age or above
Ritalin LA	10 mg–60 mg	8–10 hrs dual pulse	6 yrs of age or above
Concerta	18 mg–54 mg	10–12 hrs ascending	6 yrs of age or above
Daytrana (transdermal patch)	10 mg–30 mg	Up to 15 hrs	6 yrs of age or above

[1] D-amphetamine salts
[2] Amphetamine mixed salts
[3] Lisdexamphetamine
[4] Dexmethylphenidate (all others d,l methylphenidate)

Non-Stimulant Medication Options

Non-stimulant medications are increasingly used instead of stimulant medication, or as adjunct medications, to reduce side effects associated with stimulant medication. The most commonly prescribed medications include atomoxetine (Durell et al., 2013) and forms of alpha adrenergic agonist agents such as guanfacine. The mechanism of action of atomoxetine fits very well with the neurobiological hypotheses regarding ADHD, including alterations in the noradrenergic system including the locus coeruleus (LC) (Jain et al., 2011; Mefford & Potter, 1989). The regional brain specificity associated with atomoxetine may underlie its lack of side effects compared to those of stimulant medication as well as its lower efficacy, as brain structures or brain functioning not targeted by atomoxetine may be associated

Table 5.2 COMMONLY USED NON-STIMULANT MEDICATIONS

Medication	Avg. Dose Range	Duration of Action	FDA Approval for Age
ATOMOXETINE	0.5 mg/kg/day–1.2 mg/kg/day	24 hrs	6 yrs of age or above
GUANFACINE			
Tenex	0.5 mg–4 mg	Short acting	—
Intuniv	1 mg–4 mg	Long acting	
CLONIDINE			
Catapress/Clonidine	0.05 mg–0.3 mg	Short acting	—
Kapvay	0.1 mg–0.4 mg	Long acting	

with critical mechanisms involved in the pathogenesis of ADHD. Common side effects associated with atomoxetine include gastrointestinal upset and sleep disturbance.

The alpha-2 adrenergic agonists, such as guanfacine, are thought to work both by reducing tonic activity, thus increasing the evoked action potential amplitude, in the locus ceruleus via auto-receptors on the pre-synaptic membrane, and by directly activating autoreceptors in the prefrontal cortex (Stahl, 2010). Common side effects include sedation and possible lowering of blood pressure, with patients presenting with postural hypotension or lightheadedness. Patients need to be warned against abrupt discontinuation of these medications due to concerns about rebound hypertension (Please see Table 5.2 for more details regarding the non-stimulant medications).

Antidepressant medications are prescribed by practitioners for co-morbid depression and when there is concern about abuse of stimulant medications. Buproprion is the most widely used antidepressant for off-label treatment of ADHD, and it has the benefit of lower risk for abuse compared to stimulants; however, its effects are less robust. Tricyclic antidepressants (imipramine, nortriptyline and desipramine) were more frequently prescribed in the past as alternates to stimulant medication for ADHD. They work well in the presence of co-morbid depression or tic disorders with ADHD; however, they have major side effects, including gastrointestinal disturbance and cardiac toxicity, and can be dangerous in overdoses due to corrected QT interval (QTc) changes, limiting their use clinically. Venlafaxine (Effexor) is an antidepressant that blocks the reuptake of both serotonin and norepinephrine in the brain. Uncontrolled studies indicate that venlafaxine can improve ADHD symptoms and may be well suited for use in individuals with co-occurring depressive and anxiety disorders (Lynch,

Lauterborn, & Gall, 2010). Side effects include irritability, insomnia, and gastrointestinal disturbance.

Modafinil is currently approved for use in narcolepsy and sleep apnea, though the exact mechanism of action by which it promotes alertness and wakefulness is not well understood. In animal and human imaging studies, the drug has been shown to impact the dopamine transporter sites in the striatum, but it is not thought to have any effect on adrenergic or catecholamine receptors. Modafinil improved ADHD symptoms in clinical trials with modest but significant efficacy (Biederman et al., 2005); however, it is not FDA-approved for use in children due to concerns that it may elicit Stevens-Johnson syndrome, based on two cases that arose during clinical trial testing.

Cholinergic medications such as acetylcholinesterase inhibitors (tacrine, donepezil, galantamine) are widely used in the treatment of age-related cognitive decline, including Alzheimer's disease. These medications have not been shown to be effective in enhancing cognitive function in healthy subjects. Various open-label studies of donepezil in children (Wilens, Biederman, Wong, Spencer, & Prince, 2000) and a double-blind placebo-controlled study of galantamine in adults (Biederman et al., 2006) failed to show any clear evidence of benefit in ADHD. There may be some benefit in children with co-morbidities such as tic disorders or pervasive developmental disorder. Memantine is an NMDA receptor antagonist that is used in the treatment of Alzheimer's disease and related conditions. At least one study has shown some benefit in children with ADHD (Findling et al., 2007), though the overall efficacy for clinical use remains to be determined. Animal models of memantine suggest there are potential deleterious effects of the medication thus, caution should be used when considering studies and use of the drug in developing populations.

Future Pharmacological Treatments

Numerous other drugs are under investigation for possible use in ADHD. Multiple studies investigating the effects of nicotine on cognition suggest that it has positive effects on attention, working memory, inhibitory control, and other cognitive domains (Heishman, Kleykamp, & Singleton, 2010). While these results provide hope for its role in treating ADHD symptoms, human studies have not shown similar benefits. ABT-418 is a novel cholinergic agent and a nicotinic analog that targets the α4b2 receptor. While there was some evidence for gains in working memory in preclinical studies and some improvement in ADHD symptoms for human adults, the overall effect of nicotine on cognitive performance remains to be established, and it is not considered effective in children with ADHD. However, at a dose of 75 mg daily, the response rate was significantly higher than under placebo and was relatively well tolerated (Wilens et al., 1999). Another compound, ABT-089, a neuronal nicotinic receptor partial agonist, was evaluated in a small sample of adults with ADHD and resulted in dose-dependent improvements in working memory and response inhibition. Additional data so far have failed to establish further evidence to support its use in clinical practice to date.

A new class of compounds known as ampakines is under investigation for ADHD, as they are known to improve attention, alertness, memory, and learning. Ampakines play a key role in memory-formation and communication within and between different regions of the brain. The ampakines boost glutamate transmission, which in turn facilitates memory and learning. Ampakines increase excitatory monosynaptic responses, allowing increased communication rates through the neural network. Recent clinical evaluations of α-amino-3-hydroxy-5-methyl-4-isoxazolepropionic acid receptor (AMPA) compounds for ADHD, however, have been terminated by pharmaceutical companies, raising concerns about its efficacy as target drugs for treatment of ADHD (Lynch, et al., 2010).

Apart from the compounds discussed above, there are various other agents in the development stage or in phase I trials. These agents can be broadly classified under *triple uptake inhibitors* (e.g., Sibutramine), *nicotinic agents* (e.g., lobeline) and *agents with undisclosed mechanisms of action* (e.g., SPN811,812) (Heal et al., 2012). It remains to be seen if any of these other compounds shows further promise. There is also a move toward individualizing treatment by using genetic information and data on P450 enzymetic makeup to guide medication choice to improve outcomes and reduce the number of failed trials before arriving at the appropriate medication. Hopefully, future medications will be developed and integrated into treatment regimens that are more tailored to individuals with ADHD.

CONCLUSION

Effective treatment for many children and adults with ADHD exists; however, there is a strong, and often underappreciated, need for the development of new, targeted, and more effective treatments for persons with ADHD. The majority of treatments used and developed for ADHD are not based on known neurobiological impairments associated with the disorder. Within this scope, cognitive training is the one line of treatment that appears most targeted in its approach, yet it is pharmacological treatment (i.e., stimulant medication) that is the most effective for treating ADHD. The challenges for new treatments for ADHD will be to identify treatments that result in sustained effects, generalize beyond the clinic session, and also prevent worsening severity of symptoms. At this juncture, no recognized treatment for ADHD can meet those challenges. The identification of a biological or genetic marker to help predict treatment response would be of major benefit to the population.

DISCLOSURES

Kyle J. Rutledge, Khyati Brahmbhatt, and Julie B. Schweitzer declare no conflict of interests. Julie Schweitzer receives funding from Shire Pharmaceuticals, the John Merck Fund, the Department of Defense, and the National Institutes of Health. Khyati Brahmbhatt receives funding from Shire Pharmaceuticals.

All correspondence should be directed to Dr. Julie B. Schweitzer: telephone, (916) 703-0450; e-mail, julie.schweitzer@ucdmc.ucdavis.edu; postal address, University of California, Davis MIND Institute, 2825 50th St., Sacramento, California 95817.

REFERENCES

Abikoff, H., Hechtman, L., Klein, R. G., Weiss, G., Fleiss, K., Etcovitch, J.,...Pollack, S. (2004). Symptomatic improvement in children with ADHD treated with long-term methylphenidate and multimodal psychosocial treatment. *Journal of the American Academy of Child & Adolescent Psychiatry, 43*(7), 802–811. doi: 00004583-200407000-00005 [pii]

Arnold, L. E., Lofthouse, N., & Hurt, E. (2012). Artificial food colors and attention-deficit/hyperactivity symptoms: Conclusions to dye for. *Neurotherapeutics, 9*(3), 599–609. doi: 10.1007/s13311-012-0133-x

Bader, A., & Adesman, A. (2012). Complementary and alternative therapies for children and adolescents with ADHD. *Current Opinion in Pediatrics, 24*(6), 760–769. doi: 10.1097/MOP.0b013e32835a1a5f

Berwid, O. G., & Halperin, J. M. (2012). Emerging support for a role of exercise in attention-deficit/hyperactivity disorder intervention planning. *Current Psychiatry Reports, 14*(5), 543–551. doi: 10.1007/s11920-012-0297-4

Biederman, J., Mick, E., Faraone, S., Hammerness, P., Surman, C., Harpold, T.,...Spencer, T. (2006). A double-blind comparison of galantamine hydrogen bromide and placebo in adults with attention-deficit/hyperactivity disorder: A pilot study. *Journal of Clinical Psychopharmacology, 26*(2), 163–166. doi: 10.1097/01.jcp.0000204139.20417.8a

Biederman, J., Swanson, J. M., Wigal, S. B., Kratochvil, C. J., Boellner, S. W., Earl, C. Q.,...Greenhill, L. (2005). Efficacy and safety of modafinil film-coated tablets in children and adolescents with attention-deficit/hyperactivity disorder: Results of a randomized, double-blind, placebo-controlled, flexible-dose study. *Pediatrics*, *116*(6), e777–e784. doi: 10.1542/peds.2005-0617

Black, D. S., Milam, J., & Sussman, S. (2009). Sitting-meditation interventions among youth: A review of treatment efficacy. *Pediatrics*, *124*(3), e532–e541. doi: 10.1542/peds.2008-3434

Bloch, M. H., & Qawasmi, A. (2011). Omega-3 fatty acid supplementation for the treatment of children with attention-deficit/hyperactivity disorder symptomatology: Systematic review and meta-analysis. *Journal of the American Academy of Child & Adolescent Psychiatry*, *50*(10), 991–1000. doi: 10.1016/j.jaac.2011.06.008 S0890-8567(11)00484-9 [pii]

Chacko, A., Wymbs, B. T., Chimiklis, A., Wymbs, F. A., & Pelham, W. E. (2012). Evaluating a comprehensive strategy to improve engagement to group-based behavioral parent training for high-risk families of children with ADHD. *Journal of Abnormal Child Psychology*, *40*(8), 1351–1362. doi: 10.1007/s10802-012-9666-z

Charach, A., Yeung, E., Climans, T., & Lillie, E. (2011). Childhood attention-deficit/ hyperactivity disorder and future substance use disorders: Comparative meta-analyses. *Journal of the American Academy of Child & Adolescent Psychiatry*, *50*(1), 9–21. doi: Http://dx.doi.org/10.1016/j.jaac.2010.09.019

Chronis-Tuscano, A., O'Brien, K. A., Johnston, C., Jones, H. A., Clarke, T. L., Raggi, V. L., ... Seymour, K. E. (2011). The relation between maternal ADHD symptoms & improvement in child behavior following brief behavioral parent training is mediated by change in negative parenting. *Journal of Abnormal Child Psychology*, *39*(7), 1047–1057. doi: 10.1007/s10802-011-9518-2

Durell, T. M., Adler, L. A., Williams, D. W., Deldar, A., McGough, J. J., Glaser, P. E., ... Fox, B. K. (2013). Atomoxetine treatment of attention-deficit/hyperactivity disorder in young adults with assessment of functional outcomes: A randomized, double-blind, placebo-controlled clinical trial. *Journal of Clinical Psychopharmacology*, *33*(1), 45–54. doi: 10.1097/JCP.1090b1013e31827d31828a31823.

Fabiano, G. A., Chacko, A., Pelham, W. E., Jr., Robb, J., Walker, K. S., Wymbs, F., ... Pirvics, L. (2009). A comparison of behavioral parent training programs for fathers of children with attention-deficit/hyperactivity disorder. *Behavioral Therapy*, *40*(2), 190–204. doi: 10.1016/j.beth.2008.05.002

Fabiano, G. A., Pelham, W. E., Jr., Coles, E. K., Gnagy, E. M., Chronis-Tuscano, A., & O'Connor, B. C. (2009). A meta-analysis of behavioral treatments for attention-deficit/hyperactivity disorder. *Clinical Psychology Review*, *29*(2), 129–140. doi: 10.1016/j.cpr.2008.11.001

Faraone, S. (2003). Understanding the effect size of ADHD medications: Implications for clinical care. *Medscape*. September 19, 2003.

Fassbender, C., & Schweitzer, J. B. (2006). Is there evidence for neural compensation in attention deficit hyperactivity disorder? A review of the functional neuroimaging literature. *Clinical Psychology Review*, *26*(4), 445–465. doi: 10.1016/ j.cpr.2006.01.003

Findling, R. L., McNamara, N. K., Stansbrey, R. J., Maxhimer, R., Periclou, A., Mann, A., & Graham, S. M. (2007). A pilot evaluation of the safety, tolerability, pharmacokinetics, and effectiveness of memantine in pediatric patients with attention-deficit/hyperactivity disorder combined type. *Journal of Child & Adolescent Psychopharmacology*, *17*(1), 19–33. doi: 10.1089/cap.2006.0044

Gapin, J. I., Labban, J. D., & Etnier, J. L. (2011). The effects of physical activity on attention deficit hyperactivity disorder symptoms: The evidence. *Preventive Medicine*, *52*(Suppl 1), S70–S74. doi: 10.1016/j.ypmed.2011.01.022

Gioia, G. A., Isquith, P. K., Guy, S. C., & Kenworthy, L. (2000). *BRIEF: Behavior Rating Inventory of Executive Function*. Lutz, FL: Psychological Assessment Resources, Inc.

Gray, S. A., Chaban, P., Martinussen, R., Goldberg, R., Gotlieb, H., Kronitz, R.,...Tannock, R. (2012). Effects of a computerized working memory training program on working memory, attention, and academics in adolescents with severe LD and comorbid ADHD: A randomized controlled trial. *Journal of Child Psychology & Psychiatry*, 53(12), 1277–1284. doi: 10.1111/j.1469-7610.2012.02592.x

Green, C. T., Long, D. L., Green, D., Iosif, A. M., Dixon, J. F., Miller, M. R.,...Schweitzer, J. B. (2012). Will working memory training generalize to improve off-task behavior in children with attention-deficit/hyperactivity disorder? *Neurotherapeutics*, 9(3), 639–648. doi: 10.1007/s13311-012-0124-y

Heal, D., Smith, S., & Findling, R. (2012). ADHD: Current and future therapeutics. In C. Stanford & R. Tannock (Eds.), *Behavioral Neuroscience of Attention Deficit Hyperactivity Disorder and Its Treatment* (Vol. 9, pp. 361–390). Springer Berlin Heidelberg.

Hechtman, L., Abikoff, H., Klein, R. G., Weiss, G., Respitz, C., Kouri, J.,...Pollack, S. (2004). Academic achievement and emotional status of children with ADHD treated with long-term methylphenidate and multimodal psychosocial treatment. *Journal of the American Academy of Child & Adolescent Psychiatry*, 43(7), 812–819. doi: 00004583-200407000-00006 [pii]

Heishman, S. J., Kleykamp, B. A., & Singleton, E. G. (2010). Meta-analysis of the acute effects of nicotine and smoking on human performance. *Psychopharmacology (Berl)*, 210(4), 453–469. doi: 10.1007/s00213-010-1848-1

Hoekzema, E., Carmona, S., Ramos-Quiroga, J. A., Barba, E., Bielsa, A., Tremols, V.,...Vilarroya, O. (2011). Training-induced neuroanatomical plasticity in ADHD: A tensor-based morphometric study. *Human Brain Mapping*, 32(10), 1741–1749. doi: 10.1002/hbm.21143

Hoekzema, E., Carmona, S., Tremols, V., Gispert, J. D., Guitart, M., Fauquet, J.,...Vilarroya, O. (2010). Enhanced neural activity in frontal and cerebellar circuits after cognitive training in children with attention-deficit/hyperactivity disorder. *Human Brain Mapping*, 31(12), 1942–1950. doi: 10.1002/hbm.20988

Holmes, J., Gathercole, S. E., Place, M., Dunning, D. L., Hilton, K. L., & Elliott, J. G. (2010). Working memory deficits can be overcome: Impacts of training and medication on working memory in children with ADHD. *Applied Cognitive Psychology*, 24(6), 827–836. doi: 10.1002/acp.1589

Jain, R., Babcock, T., Burtea, T., Dirks, B., Adeyi, B., Scheckner, B., & Lasser, R. (2011). Efficacy of lisdexamfetamine dimesylate in children with attention-deficit/ hyperactivity disorder previously treated with methylphenidate: A post hoc analysis. *Child & Adolescent Psychiatry & Mental Health*, 5(1), 35.

Kazdin, A. E. (1997). Parent management training: Evidence, outcomes, and issues. *Journal of the American Academy of Child & Adolescent Psychiatry*, 36(10), 1349–1356. doi: 10.1097/00004583-199710000-00016

Kazdin, A. E., & Mazurick, J. L. (1994). Dropping out of child psychotherapy: Distinguishing early and late dropouts over the course of treatment. *Journal of Consulting Clinical Psychology*, 62(5), 1069–1074.

Kerns, K. A., Eso, K., & Thompson, J. (1999). Investigation of a direct intervention for improving attention in young children with ADHD. *Developmental Neuropsychology*, 16, 273–295.

Klingberg, T. (2010). Training and plasticity of working memory. *Trends in Cognitive Science, 14*(7), 317–324. doi: 10.1016/j.tics.2010.05.002

Klingberg, T., Fernell, E., Olesen, P. J., Johnson, M., Gustafsson, P., Dahlstrom, K., ... Westerberg, H. (2005). Computerized training of working memory in children with ADHD—a randomized, controlled trial. *Journal of the American Academy of Child & Adolescent Psychiatry, 44*(2), 177–186. doi: S0890-8567(09)61427-1 [pii] 10.1097/00004583-200502000-00010

Klingberg, T., Forssberg, H., & Westerberg, H. (2002). Training of working memory in children with ADHD. *Journal of Clinical & Experimental Neuropsychology, 24*(6), 781–791. doi: 10.1076/jcen.24.6.781.8395

Legarda, S. B., McMahon, D., & Othmer, S. (2011). Clinical neurofeedback: Case studies, proposed mechanism, and implications for pediatric neurology practice. *Journal of Child Neurology, 26*(8), 1045–1051. doi: 10.1177/0883073811405052

Lofthouse, N., Arnold, L. E., Hersch, S., Hurt, E., & DeBeus, R. (2012). A review of neurofeedback treatment for pediatric ADHD. *Journal of Attention Disorders, 16*(5), 351–372. doi: 10.1177/1087054711427530

Lofthouse, N., Arnold, L. E., & Hurt, E. (2012). Current status of neurofeedback for attention-deficit/hyperactivity disorder. [Review]. *Current Psychiatry Reports, 14*(5), 536–542. doi: 10.1007/s11920-012-0301-z

Loo, S., & Makeig, S. (2012). Clinical utility of EEG in Attention-Deficit/Hyperactivity Disorder: A research update. *Neurotherapeutics.*

Lynch, G., Lauterborn, J., & Gall, C. (2010). Positive modulation of AMPA receptors as a broad spectrum strategy for treating neuropsychiatric disorders. In P. Skolnick (Ed.), *Glutamate-Based Therapies for Psychiatric disorders, Milestones in Drug Therapies.* New York: Springer.

McNab, F., Varrone, A., Farde, L., Jucaite, A., Bystritsky, P., Forssberg, H., & Klingberg, T. (2009). Changes in cortical dopamine D1 receptor binding associated with cognitive training. *Science, 323*(5915), 800–802. doi: 323/5915/800 [pii] 10.1126/science.1166102

Mefford, I. N., & Potter, W. Z. (1989). A neuroanatomical and biochemical basis for attention deficit disorder with hyperactivity in children: A defect in tonic adrenaline mediated inhibition of locus coeruleus stimulation. *Medical Hypotheses, 29*(1), 33–42.

Mikami, A. Y., Jack, A., Emeh, C. C., & Stephens, H. F. (2010). Parental influence on children with attention-deficit/hyperactivity disorder: I. Relationships between parent behaviors and child peer status. *Journal of Abnormal Child Psychology, 38*(6), 721–736. doi: 10.1007/s10802-010-9393-2

Molina, B. S., Hinshaw, S. P., Swanson, J. M., Arnold, L. E., Vitiello, B., Jensen, P. S., ... Houck, P. R. (2009). The MTA at 8 years: Prospective follow-up of children treated for combined-type ADHD in a multisite study. *Journal of the American Academy of Child & Adolescent Psychiatry, 48*(5), 484–500.

Monastra, V. J. (2005). Overcoming the barriers to effective treatment for attention-deficit/hyperactivity disorder: A neuro-educational approach. *International Journal of Psychophysiology, 58*(1), 71–80. doi: 10.1016/j.ijpsycho.2005.03.010

Moriyama, T., Polanczyk, G. V., Caye, A., Banaschewski, T., Brandeis, D., & Rohde, L. A. (2012). Evidence based information on the clinical use of neurofeedback for ADHD. *Neurotherapeutics, 9*, 588–598.

MTA. (1999). A 14-month randomized clinical trial of treatment strategies for attention-deficit/hyperactivity disorder. The MTA Cooperative Group.

Multimodal Treatment Study of Children with ADHD. *Archives of General Psychiatry, 56*(12), 1073–1086.

National Institute for Health and Clinical Excellence (NICE) (2008). Attention deficit hyperactivity disorder: Diagnosis and management of ADHD in children, young people, and adults. www.nice.org.uk/nicemedia/pdf/ADHDConsFullGuideline. pdf, 1-591. Accessed February 28, 2013.

Nigg, J. T., & Casey, B. J. (2005). An integrative theory of attention-deficit/hyperactivity disorder based on the cognitive and affective neurosciences. *Developmental Psychopathology, 17*(3), 785–806. doi: S0954579405050376. 10.1017/ S0954579405050376

O'Keefe, L. (2008). ECGs for all ADHD patients? AAP-AHA release joint "clarification" on AHA recommendation. *AAP News, 29*, 1.

Olfson, M., Huang, C., Gerhard, T., Winterstein, A. G., Crystal, S., Allison, P. D., & Marcus, S. C. (2012). Stimulants and cardiovascular events in youth with attention-deficit/hyperactivity disorder. *Journal of the American Academy of Child & Adolescent Psychiatry, 51*(2), 147–156. doi: Http://dx.doi.org/10.1016/j. jaac.2011.11.008

Oord, S. V., Ponsioen, A. J., Geurts, H. M., Brink, E. L., & Prins, P. J. (2012). A pilot study of the efficacy of a computerized executive functioning remediation training with game elements for children with ADHD in an outpatient setting: Outcome on parent- and teacher-rated executive functioning and ADHD behavior. *Journal of Attention Disorders.* doi: 1087054712453167-10.1177/108 7054712453167

Owens, J. S., Murphy, C. E., Richerson, L., Girio, E. L., & Himawan, L. K. (2008). Science to practice in underserved communities: The effectiveness of school mental health programming. *Journal of Clinical Child & Adolescent Psychology, 37*(2), 434–447. doi: 10.1080/15374410801955912

Pelham, W. E., Jr., & Fabiano, G. A. (2008). Evidence-based psychosocial treatments for attention-deficit/hyperactivity disorder. *Journal of Clinical Child & Adolescent Psychology, 37*(1), 184–214. doi: 792185156 [pii] 10.1080/15374410701818681

Pelham, W. E., Jr., Wheeler, T., & Chronis, A. (1998). Empirically supported psychosocial treatments for attention deficit hyperactivity disorder. *Journal of Clinical Child Psychology, 27*(2), 190–205.

Pfiffner, L. J., Yee Mikami, A., Huang-Pollock, C., Easterlin, B., Zalecki, C., & McBurnett, K. (2007). A randomized, controlled trial of integrated home-school behavioral treatment for ADHD, predominantly inattentive type. *Journal of the American Academy of Child & Adolescent Psychiatry, 46*(8), 1041–1050.

Power, T. J., Mautone, J. A., Soffer, S. L., Clarke, A. T., Marshall, S. A., Sharman, J., . . . Jawad, A. F. (2012). A family-school intervention for children with ADHD: Results of a randomized clinical trial. *Journal of Consulting Clinical Psychology, 80*(4), 611–623. doi: 10.1037/a0028188

Pringsheim, T., & Steeves, T. (2011). Pharmacological treatment for attention deficit hyperactivity disorder (ADHD) in children with comorbid tic disorders. *Cochrane Database System Reviews* (4), CD007990. doi: 10.1002/14651858.CD007990. pub2

Rabiner, D. L., Murray, D. W., Skinner, A. T., & Malone, P. S. (2010). A randomized trial of two promising computer-based interventions for students with attention difficulties. *Journal of Abnormal Child Psychology, 38*(1), 131–142. doi: 10.1007/ s10802-009-9353-x

Rutledge, K. J., van den Bos, W., McClure, S. M., & Schweitzer, J. B. (2012). Training cognition in ADHD: Current findings, borrowed concepts, and future directions. *Neurotherapeutics, 9*(3), 542–558. doi: 10.1007/s13311-012-0134-9

Sheridan, S. M., Eagle, J. W., Cowan, R. J., & Mickelson, W. (2001). The effects of conjoint behavioral consultation: Results of a 4-year investigation. *Journal of School Psychology, 39*(5), 361–385.

Shipstead, Z., Redick, T. S., & Engle, R. W. (2012). Is Working Memory Training Effective? *Psychology Bulletin. 138*, 628–654. doi: 2012-06385-001- 10.1037/a0027473

Skokauskas, N., McNicholas, F., Masaud, T., & Frodl, T. (2011). Complementary medicine for children and young people who have attention deficit hyperactivity disorder. *Current Opinion in Psychiatry, 24*(4), 291–300. doi: 10.1097/YCO.0b013e32834776bd

Stahl, S. M. (2010). Mechanism of action of alpha 2A-adrenergic agonists in attention-deficit/hyperactivity disorder with or without oppositional symptoms. *Journal of Clinical Psychiatry, 71*(3), 223–224. doi: 10.4088/JCP.09bs05899pur

van de Weijer-Bergsma, E., Formsma, A. R., de Bruin, E. I., & Bogels, S. M. (2012). The effectiveness of mindfulness training on behavioral problems and attentional functioning in adolescents with ADHD. *Journal of Child & Family Studies, 21*(5), 775–787. doi: 10.1007/s10826-011-9531-7

van den Hoofdakker, B. J., Nauta, M. H., Dijck-Brouwer, D. A., van der Veen-Mulders, L., Sytema, S., Emmelkamp, P. M., ... Hoekstra, P. J. (2012). Dopamine transporter gene moderates response to behavioral parent training in children with ADHD: A pilot study. *Developmental Psychology, 48*(2), 567–574. doi: 10.1037/a0026564

van den Hoofdakker, B. J., van der Veen-Mulders, L., Sytema, S., Emmelkamp, P. M., Minderaa, R. B., & Nauta, M. H. (2007). Effectiveness of behavioral parent training for children with ADHD in routine clinical practice: A randomized controlled study. *Journal of the American Academy of Child & Adolescent Psychiatry, 46*(10), 1263–1271. doi: 10.1097/chi.0b013e3181354bc2

van der Oord, S., Bogels, S. M., & Peijnenburg, D. (2012). The effectiveness of mindfulness training for children with ADHD and mindful parenting for their parents. *Journal of Child & Family Studies, 21*(1), 139–147. doi: 10.1007/s10826-011-9457-0

Wechsler, D. (2003). *Wechsler Intelligence Scale for Children: Fourth Edition.* San Antonio, TX: The Psychological Corporation.

Wilens, T. E., Biederman, J., Spencer, T. J., Bostic, J., Prince, J., Monuteaux, M. C., ... Polisner, D. (1999). A pilot controlled clinical trial of ABT-418, a cholinergic agonist, in the treatment of adults with attention deficit hyperactivity disorder. *American Journal of Psychiatry, 156*(12), 1931–1937.

Wilens, T. E., Biederman, J., Wong, J., Spencer, T. J., & Prince, J. B. (2000). Adjunctive donepezil in attention deficit hyperactivity disorder youth: Case series. *Journal of Child & Adolescent Psychopharmacology, 10*(3), 217–222. doi: 10.1089/10445460050167322

Wilens, T. E., Faraone, S. V., Biederman, J., & Gunawardene, S. (2003). Does stimulant therapy of attention-deficit/hyperactivity disorder beget later substance abuse? A meta-analytic review of the literature. *Pediatrics, 111*(1), 179–185.

Willcutt, E. G. (2012). The prevalence of DSM-IV attention-deficit/hyperactivity disorder: A meta-analytic review. *Neurotherapeutics, 9*(3), 490–499. doi: 10.1007/s13311-012-0135-8

Wong, A. S., He, M. Y., & Chan, R. W. (2013). Effectiveness of computerized working memory training program in Chinese community settings for children with poor working memory. *Journal of Attention Disorders*. doi: 1087054712471427 [pii] 10.1177/1087054712471427

Xie, Y., Dixon, J. F., Yee, O. M., Zhang, J., Chen, Y. A., Deangelo, S., . . . Schweitzer, J. B. (2013). A study on the effectiveness of videoconferencing on teaching parent training skills to parents of children with ADHD. *Telemedicine Journal & E-Health, 19*, 192–199. doi: 10.1089/tmj.2012.0108

Zwi, M., Jones, H., Thorgaard, C., York, A., & Dennis, J. A. (2011). Parent training interventions for attention deficit hyperactivity disorder (ADHD) in children aged 5 to 18 years. *Cochrane Database System Reviews* (12), CD003018. doi: 10.1002/14651858.CD003018.pub3

CHAPTER 6
Targeted Treatments in Rett Syndrome

DANIEL C. TARQUINIO AND WALTER E. KAUFMANN

INTRODUCTION

Clinical Description and Standard Treatment

Rett syndrome (RTT) is a rare (approximately 1:10,000 females; Calfa, Percy, et al., 2011), sporadically transmitted, X-linked dominant neurodevelopmental disorder of females characterized by apparently normal early development; psychomotor regression involving loss of purposeful hand skills, language, and social interaction; and the emergence of gait abnormalities and stereotypical hand movements. Although Andreas Rett described this pattern in 1966, the medical community did not recognize RTT until Bengt Hagberg and colleagues reported 35 cases in 1983 (Hagberg, Aicardi, et al., 1983). Despite this initial gap of almost two decades, in the 30 years since then, researchers have clarified many clinical, neurobiological, and genetic aspects of RTT, including the identification of mutations in the methyl CpG binding protein 2 gene (*MECP2*) in the majority of RTT individuals (Amir, Van den Veyver, et al., 1999). Since the association with *MECP2*, research using mouse models of the disorder has provided insight into potential avenues for treatment and a foundation for clinical trials.

Clinical Presentation

The pattern of development in RTT is unique. Girls appear normal in early infancy, achieving appropriate developmental milestones, including sitting, walking, using single words or phrases, hand transfer, and pincer grasp. Although parents and physicians usually do not recognize abnormalities until a child is 6 to 18 months of age, parents later remark that the child was "too good" and relatively hypotonic from birth. A series of video reviews from early infancy have revealed abnormalities during the "apparently normal" period, including tongue protrusion, stiffness, asymmetrical eye opening, unusual finger movements, abnormal facies, a "bizarre" smile, abnormal spontaneous movements, limited gestural abilities, and atypical development of speech-language capacities (Einspieler, Kerr, et al., 2005; Marschik, Kaufmann, et al., 2013).

Signs and symptoms develop in a characteristic order. Growth failure, one of the earliest signs, begins with deceleration of fronto-occipital head circumference as early as one to two months of age, with microcephaly in 50–80% by age 5 (Tarquinio, Motil, et al., 2012) Therefore, deceleration of head growth is no longer a necessary criteria for diagnosis. Weight velocity decelerates at 6 months to 1 year, and linear growth follows at 15–17 months. The median weight and height both fall below the second percentile of normal children by age 12 (Tarquinio, Motil, et al., 2012).

Early symptoms include irritability and a plateau in the acquisition of motor and language skills. Regression begins between 6 months and 2.5 years with loss of fine motor skills. Communication can deteriorate abruptly or insidiously, and transiently decreased socialization gives the impression of autism spectrum disorder. As purposeful hand use deteriorates, stereotypical hand movements emerge (wringing, tapping, mouthing, clasping, squeezing, and finger rubbing), usually in the midline. Girls build an evolving repertoire of stereotypies and behaviors that include bruxism, air-swallowing, hyperventilation, and breath-holding (often alternating), and may include self-injury. While stress exacerbates these incessant behaviors, they cease during sleep. The diversity of these behaviors results in clinical phenotypes that are often dissimilar and may confound diagnosis.

After regression, development stabilizes and then gradually improves. Eighty percent learn to walk with a dyspraxic, wide-based gait, and although many lose this ability during regression, 60% remain ambulatory in adolescence. Stereotypies and breathing abnormalities may intensify throughout childhood, while autistic features are replaced by improved social interaction and decision-making. Communication is primarily nonverbal, and girls indicate desire through a characteristically intense, piercing eye gaze. After adolescence, hand stereotypies and breathing dysregulation decrease in intensity or disappear altogether.

Hagberg originally described four stages of progression: early onset stagnation, developmental regression, pseudostationary, and late motor degeneration (Hagberg & Witt-Engerstrom, 1986). The transition between stages is difficult to discern, and the length of each stage and age of transition are difficult to predict. Nonetheless, this system provides a rough temporal profile for anticipatory guidance.

Additional features of the disease present at different ages and with variable incidence. While EEG abnormalities are ubiquitous after age 2, seizures are rare prior to age 2, and seizure types vary from focal to generalized. Video EEG has confirmed that as many as two-thirds of paroxysmal events are non-epileptic, even in patients with an abnormal baseline EEG (Glaze, Percy, et al., 2010). Based on clinical assessment during a study of the natural history of RTT, 48% of 602 participants had seizures; however, prevalence estimates range from 30–80% in other studies. Other neurological abnormalities are common, and include dystonia and autonomic nervous system dysfunction (often resulting in small, cold feet). The majority have growth failure, frequently accompanied by osteopenia. Gastroesophageal reflux (GER) is common, and constipation is almost universal (Motil, Caeg, et al., 2012). Effective management exists for both of these conditions and can improve quality of life dramatically. Scoliosis is present in 53% overall, and can be severe, with up to 13% requiring surgery. However, certain *MECP2* mutations, R294X and R306C, have reduced risk for scoliosis (Ager, Fyfe, et al., 2006). Additional features include increased prevalence of prolonged QT syndrome (20%) and cholecystitis (Percy & Lane, 2005).

Although Andreas Rett initially described the syndrome as progressive and neurodegenerative, research on neurobiology and pathophysiology indicates that RTT is a stable neurodevelopmental condition. This notion is borne out by the longevity of patients with RTT. Survival is greater than 90% through age 10, and 75% of that of the unaffected population at age 35, dramatically superior to other disorders with profound cognitive impairment (Percy, 2002). While sudden death is more common in RTT, the etiology is unclear, and it may be a result of seizures, autonomic dysfunction, or cardiac conduction abnormality (Julu, Kerr, et al., 2001).

Diagnostic Criteria

Despite the discovery of a genetic etiology, 3–5% lack a mutation in *MECP2*, and diagnosis of RTT remains clinical (Neul, Kaufmann, et al., 2010). Because of the wide variability in phenotype within RTT and the nonspecific nature of certain RTT characteristics (e.g., stereotypies), to be diagnosed with classic RTT, patients must exhibit regression of previously acquired skills, fulfill four main diagnostic criteria (loss of hand skills, loss of spoken language, gait abnormalities, and hand stereotypies), and meet neither of the exclusion criteria (secondary brain injury or grossly abnormal psychomotor development prior to age 6 months) (Neul, Kaufmann, et al., 2010). Individuals can be diagnosed with atypical RTT if they exhibit regression of previously acquired skills, fulfill at least two of the four main diagnostic criteria, and five of eleven supportive criteria (breathing disturbances and/or bruxism when awake, impaired sleep, abnormal muscle tone, peripheral vasomotor disturbances, scoliosis/kyphosis, growth retardation, small cold hands and feet, inappropriate laughing/screaming, diminished pain response, intense eye gaze). Within the category of atypical RTT are three variants: the early onset seizure, or "Hanefeld" variant (typically associated with mutations in *CDKL5*); the congenital onset, or "Rolando" variant, lacking normal early development (typically associated with mutations in *FOXG1*); and the preserved speech, or "Zapella" variant (often associated with *MECP2* mutation). Of all individuals with RTT characteristics, over 80% have classic RTT, and 15–20% have atypical RTT. Although the diagnosis of RTT does not require *MECP2* testing, the role of *MECP2* mutations in RTT and other disorders is under investigation.

Management

No treatment targets defective methyl CpG binding protein 2 (MeCP2) production in RTT. Strategies for modifying protein production or inserting exogenous DNA have not reached the stage of clinical application. Therefore, management strategies are supportive, symptomatic, and preventive.

The degree of cognitive impairment in RTT is difficult to assess. Classical methods reveal a mental age of 8–10 months and a gross motor age of 12–18 months, though eye-gaze technology may offer a window for more detailed evaluation (Baptista, Mercadante, et al., 2006). Girls rarely acquire adaptive skills such as dressing and toileting. However, aggressive physical, occupational, and speech therapy, and augmentative communications are crucial to improve functional ability and prevent deterioration. Though time-consuming, behavioral therapy has long been recognized to increase function (Bat-Haee, 1994). Girls and women with RTT demonstrate universal appreciation of music, and music therapy can improve socialization and hand use (Yasuhara & Sugiyama, 2001).

Breathing irregularities can involve breath-holding in excess of one minute or severe abdominal distention from air swallowing. Behaviors cease during sleep, therefore severe snoring or apnea during sleep should prompt investigation for obstructive sleep apnea. Interrupted sleep patterns, including playing quietly or laughing for no reason (colloquially referred to as "Rett parties"), are common and may disrupt caregivers' sleep, but are otherwise harmless. Melatonin can help induce sleep, but will not prevent arousals. Antihistamines may restore sleeping patterns, but tachyphylaxis is common. Zolpidem and trazodone are effective sleep aids, and have been successful in RTT (Prater & Zylstra, 2006).

Seizures in RTT can be difficult to manage, and even more difficult to differentiate from non-epileptic events. If diagnosis is unclear, video EEG should be pursued. Routine EEG typically shows background slowing with recurrent spike or slow spike-and-wave activity. In the absence of clinical seizures, this pattern alone does not warrant anti-epileptic medication. Clinical seizures frequently respond to carbamazepine (or oxcarbazepine), sodium valproate, levetiracetam, or lamotrigine. Topiramate may produce anorexia, exacerbating growth failure. Levetiracetam often provokes or exacerbates behavioral abnormalities. In documented non-epileptic events, the cause is often anxiety, which has been treated effectively in RTT with selective serotonin reuptake inhibitors.

Pubertal onset occurs early in 12% of girls with RTT; however, the ages of menarche and completion of puberty are similar to the unaffected population (Garcia-Rudaz, Deng, et al., 2009). When early adrenarche or thelarche occurs, consultation with an endocrinologist is warranted. Menses are often accompanied by increased behaviors, anxiety, pain, and exacerbation of seizures, and consultation for hormonal control of menstruation can alleviate these symptoms.

Since the majority of girls with RTT develop scoliosis, screening should begin at an early age. Bracing is used for a curvature greater than 25 degrees, although its efficacy is unclear. Surgery is recommended if the curve progresses beyond 40 degrees. Once girls develop scoliosis, they should be followed by an orthopedic surgeon (Downs, Bergman, et al., 2009). Dual-energy X-ray absorptiometry scanning often reveals osteopenia or osteoporosis. Vitamin D deficiency is common in RTT, and not clearly related to nutritional status, use of anticonvulsants, degree of mobility, or MECP2 status (Motil, Barrish, et al., 2011). To support bone health, girls should receive adequate calcium and vitamin D, and should bear weight as much as possible.

Routine care should include consultation with a nutritionist who has experience with RTT. Girls with RTT have increased protein and calorie requirements. Feeding difficulties are common, resembling the difficulties in Parkinson disease, and occupational therapists can help achieve successful feeding through positioning and augmentative devices. Constipation is pervasive in RTT, and either magnesium hydroxide suspension (milk of magnesia) or polyethylene glycol powder (tasteless and odorless laxative) can be titrated into daily fluids to achieve normal bowel movements without the complications of enemas or mineral oil. Other gastrointestinal (GI) issues include GER, esophagitis, and gallbladder dysfunction. Severe GER is common, and frequently requires the assistance of a GI specialist. In severe growth failure, a gastrostomy tube allows caregivers to provide adequate calories and nutrition, administer medications easily and accurately, and relieve abdominal bloating due to air swallowing.

MOLECULAR, EPIGENETIC AND NEUROBIOLOGICAL ASPECTS

Neurobiology and Pathophysiology

Early autopsy studies in RTT patients revealed global abnormalities. Brain weight in RTT is reduced in all age groups to 60–70% of expected weight. The frontal cortex and deep nuclei have reduced volume, and melanin pigmentation is decreased in the substantia nigra. Although the overall appearance of the brain is normal in RTT, it is smaller and characterized by diffuse abnormalities. The neuropil is denser with smaller, more tightly packed neurons; short, primitive dendrites; and reduced arborizations, all features suggesting an immature pattern or a developmental arrest of synaptic connections (Kaufmann, Johnston, et al., 2005). Immunochemical profiling of dendritic proteins supports this hypothesis, demonstrating selective impairment in microtubule-associated protein 2, a key protein during dendritic expansion (Kaufmann, MacDonald, et al., 2000). Early neurochemical studies found low biogenic amine concentration in older patients; however, subsequent studies did not support this finding (Percy, 1992). Cerebrospinal fluid levels of monoamines, lactate, and pyruvate are generally normal, while β-endorphin immunoreactivity was elevated in several studies and unremarkable in others (Budden, Myer, et al., 1990). Choline acetyltransferase activity is reduced in several forebrain cortical and subcortical regions, and nerve growth factor fails to stimulate its production (Wenk & Hauss-Wegrzyniak, 1999). Imaging studies have revealed impaired binding of radioligand to benzodiazepine receptors, relative decreased frontal lobe blood flow, and decreasing N-acetyl aspartate:creatine ratio with age, suggesting progressive neuropil loss. However, normal neuronal migration, involvement of multiple neurotransmitter (NT) systems, and immature dendrites suggest developmental arrest late in the third trimester or early in infancy, rather than a progressive disorder (Armstrong, 2002; Kaufmann, Johnston, et al., 2005).

Experimental models of RTT display both immature synapses and deficient synaptic reorganization after development. The latter seems to reflect disruption of calcium-dependent activation of MeCP2 secondary to synaptic stimulation as well as loss of MeCP2's epigenetic function. Long-term potentiation (LTP), which is normal in pre-symptomatic Mecp2-deficient mice, becomes abnormal in symptomatic mice, which supports the concept that in RTT, a synaptopathy accounts for most clinical phenomena, including regression (Weng, McLeod, et al., 2011). Decreased Mecp2 levels are associated with reductions in the key post-synaptic protein PSD-95, as well as abnormal excitatory and inhibitory signaling (Chao, Zoghbi, et al., 2007). The abnormal excitatory-inhibitory balance in Mecp2 deficiency seems to reflect changes in multiple neurotransmitter (NT) systems, as suggested by the ontogeny of MeCP2 expression (Shahbazian, Young, et al., 2002), which lead to specific features of the disorder. For instance, abnormal GABA release may explain prevalent seizures (Medrihan, Tantalaki, et al., 2008), while abnormal excitatory NT release may be associated with motor and cardiorespiratory manifestations (Kron, Howell, et al., 2012). The brainstem of patients with RTT exhibits inappropriate serotonin transporter binding in the dorsal motor nucleus of the vagus compared to age-matched controls, which could explain poor autonomic control over gastrointestinal and cardiac functions (Paterson, Thompson, et al., 2005). Abnormal synaptic connections in the hippocampus are associated with abnormal socialization and motor apraxia (Moretti, Levenson, et al., 2006). Dysfunction in the hypothalamic-pituitary-adrenal (HPA) axis and enhanced corticotropin-releasing hormone expression may contribute to anxiety (McGill, Bundle, et al., 2006).

Although MeCP2 is expressed in all tissues, central nervous system expression predominates. Faulty or absent MeCP2 results in immature neurons through several mechanisms: abnormal gene repression, increased transcriptional noise, over-transcription of certain genes, and downstream effects on other processes (Kerr and Ravine 2003). Level of affinity of MeCP2 for methylated DNA is associated with phenotypical severity in the case of missense mutations. For example, an R106W mutation (associated with a severely affected phenotype) results in a 100-fold reduced affinity, while T158M (associated with a less severe phenotype) causes a moderate reduction in binding (Kudo, Nomura, et al., 2001). Affinity of R133C (the least affected phenotype) displays similar DNA binding to that of the wild-type protein (Ballestar, Yusufzai, et al., 2000; Kudo, Nomura, et al., 2001).

Regulation of brain-derived neurotrophic factor (BDNF) by MeCP2 and subsequent neurosecretory signaling is particularly critical to the phenotype (Wang, Chan, et al., 2006). In *Mecp2* knockout (KO) mice, a model that recapitulates features of RTT, BDNF levels are paradoxically low (Sun and Wu 2006), possibly due to global reductions in synaptic activity or to over-transcription of neuronal transcriptional repressors which subsequently downregulate BDNF. Specific to the clinical presentation, low BDNF levels in the nucleus tractus solitarius (nTS) of the brainstem in a RTT KO model are associated with abnormal neuronal gating, a phenomenon thought to be associated with the cardiorespiratory abnormalities in RTT (Kline, Ogier, et al., 2010). Abnormalities downstream to BDNF have also been implicated in hippocampal function. BDNF signaling affects membrane currents and dendritic calcium signals in the hippocampus through the transient receptor potential canonical (TRPC) channels TRPC3 and TRPC6. *Trpc3* is a target of *MeCP2* transcriptional regulation, and calcium signals are impaired in CA3 pyramidal neurons of symptomatic *Mecp2* mutant mice (Li, Calfa, et al., 2012).

While much remains to be learned about the roles of *Mecp2*, an encouraging experiment asked the question—could mature individuals with defective *Mecp2* benefit from presence of the normal protein? Researchers silenced *Mecp2* in mice with a genetic "switch" and activated the gene after the RTT phenotype was evident, resulting in restoration of function. This proof-of-principle experiment showed that neurological defects, including those in synaptic plasticity, can be reversed in the mouse model by the presence of a normal *Mecp2* gene (Guy, Gan, et al., 2007). Restoration of function is more pronounced when *Mecp2* is activated earlier in postnatal life, but still occurs in adult mice (Robinson, Guy, et al., 2012)

MECP2 Mutations

Given that RTT occurs almost exclusively in females, and is transmitted in an X-linked dominant fashion, early efforts at finding a genetic etiology focused on mutations in the X-chromosome. Although familial cases were scarce, linkage studies performed in these families helped narrow the search to Xq28 and ultimately identify mutations in *MECP2* as the etiology of RTT (Amir, Van den Veyver, et al., 1999). Most cases are the result of a *de novo* mutation, typically of paternal origin (Trappe, Laccone, et al., 2001). Numerous mutations in *MECP2* can cause RTT, and despite over 200 specific mutations associated with the RTT phenotype, 66% of affected individuals have one of eight common mutations. Soon after *MECP2* was identified as the gene responsible for RTT, researchers recognized that *MECP2* mutations are present in individuals with disorders other than RTT.

Approximately 95% with classic RTT and 50% with atypical RTT have a mutation in *MECP2*. However, known pathological mutations display remarkable phenotypic variability (Bebbington, Anderson, et al., 2008; Neul, Fang, et al., 2008). Affected individuals with an *MECP2* mutation without RTT range from asymptomatic, to mildly learning disabled, to autistic; some may fulfill diagnostic criteria for Angelman syndrome (AS) (Jedele, 2007). Phenotype in X-linked dominant disease may depend on the process of lionization, or X-chromosome inactivation (XCI), as well as other epigenetic factors (Hoffbuhr, Moses, et al., 2002). Because XCI occurs early in a female embryo's life, random silencing of one X-chromosome results in a mosaic pattern of cell lines distributed thereafter. Although XCI is random, unbalanced silencing can either mask or expose a mutation on one of the X-chromosomes. Family studies have shown that identical mutations with differing degrees of XCI can result in dramatically different phenotypes, including mothers who are "silent" carriers, or monozygotic twins of whom one girl with balanced XCI developed RTT and the other, with skewed XCI, was asymptomatic (Hoffbuhr, Moses, et al., 2002). Skewing of greater than 75% normal gene expression is present in such cases (Huppke, Maier, et al., 2006).

Remarkably, XCI can change over the lifespan of an individual, and in KO mice, *Mecp2* production in cortex increases from 50% to 70% with age (Metcalf, Mullaney, et al., 2006). Although the XCI ratio of peripheral tissue in humans is only weakly associated with phenotype, in KO mice, XCI testing of brain and spinal cord not only varies among different regions of one subject's central nervous system, it is also associated with specific behaviors (Wither, Lang, et al., 2013). Although the majority of individuals have balanced XCI, understanding and manipulating XCI is an area of active research interest.

The association between specific mutations and phenotypes is complicated and not thoroughly elucidated. Factors such as type of mutation and functional site on the protein can account for some of the variability in loss of function of the final protein product. In general, nonsense mutations are associated with a more severe phenotype than missense. Due to small sample sizes and inconsistent diagnosis and rating scales, most comparisons of genotype and clinical phenotype have found only weak trends. However, two studies using consistent criteria to assess larger populations found significant associations. Neul et al. found that ambulation, hand use, and language ability are more severely affected in those with the R168X mutation than in those with the R294X and late carboxy-terminal mutations (Neul, Fang, et al., 2008). Those with the R133C mutation are less severely affected than those with R168X or large deletions. Surprisingly, while those with the R306C mutation (thought to confer a less severe pheno-type) showed better scores for ambulation and hand use, their communication was severely affected (Neul, Fang, et al., 2008). Using similar criteria, Bebbington et al., found that R270X and R255X are the most severe, while R133C and R294X are the mildest (Bebbington, Anderson, et al., 2008). Other studies have examined genotype–phenotype associations pertaining to specific aspects of the disorder. Epilepsy is more common in T158M (74%) and R106W (78%) mutations, and less common in R255X and R306C (both 49%) (Glaze, Percy, et al., 2010). Regarding behavior, specific *MECP2* mutations demonstrate complex associations with autistic features from an early age (Marschik, Kaufmann, et al., 2013). Growth failure is most severe in large deletions, T158M, R168X, R255X, R270X, and other pre-C-terminal truncations (Tarquinio, Motil, et al., 2012).

Several males with *MECP2* mutations have been identified, and as many as 1.7% of males with intellectual disability (ID) have mutations in *MECP2* (Villard 2007). Males with *MECP2* mutations fall into three general categories. First, mutations resulting in RTT in females generally cause a severe early postnatal encephalopathy in males, resulting in death during infancy. However, males with a *MECP2* mutation and either Klinefelter syndrome (47 XXY) or somatic mosaicism of the X chromosome have a RTT phenotype "diluted" by the presence of a normal *MECP2* gene. Second, males with mutations that do not cause RTT in females can present with a variety of phenotypes, ranging from mild ID to severe cognitive impairment with or without motor abnormalities (e.g., A140V). Third, males with duplication of the entire *MECP2* gene, as well as other genes at the Xq28 locus, present with infantile hypotonia, recurrent respiratory infections, seizures, spasticity, absent speech, and severe ID (Gadalla, Bailey, et al., 2011).

Genetic Testing

MECP2 testing is expensive and should be approached in a stepwise fashion. While physicians are tempted to test all children with ID or autism spectrum disorder, testing should be reserved for specific scenarios. Children with clinical criteria of classic or atypical RTT should be tested. Females aged 6 to 24 months with features of RTT should be tested if they also display one of the following: low muscle tone, deceleration of head circumference, or unexplained developmental delay. Three other situations warrant *MECP2* testing: 1) females who fulfill clinical criteria for AS but have negative AS testing, 2) males with X-linked ID and normal fragile X syndrome (*FMR1*) testing, and 3) unexplained early postnatal encephalopathy.

Testing should begin by sequencing all four exons of *MECP2*; if no sequence variants are found, testing for large deletions is appropriate. In cases of familial, X-linked ID, or the third male phenotype listed above, testing for duplications should be pursued. Genes other than *MECP2* may be responsible for a minority of those with classic RTT, and screening for mutations in *CDKL5* or *FOXG1* without the variant phenotype described above is of questionable utility.

Epigenetics

Despite over 20 years of research on the function of MeCP2, knowledge of its epigenetic role and genes targeted during different stages of development is incomplete. Classically, MeCP2's primary function was thought to be binding methylated DNA and effecting transcriptional repression through two active sites, the methyl binding domain (MBD) and the transcriptional repression domain (TRD). Gene silencing results when MeCP2 binds to methylated CpG dinucleotides in gene promoter or other regulatory regions, then, along with the corepressor protein Sin3A, attracts histone deacetylases 1/2 to methylated DNA (Zachariah & Rastegar, 2012) (Figure 6.1). Several additional functions bolster MeCP2's profound role as an epigenetic regulator. Recently MeCP2 was found to cause activation of transcription in addition to repression. The TRD and C-terminal regions also interact directly with RNA, regulating the splicing of minigenes. Phosphorylation of ribosomal protein S6 is decreased in MeCP2-deficient neurons, resulting in downregulation of mTOR signaling (Ricciardi, Boggio, et al., 2011). MeCP2 also targets several microRNAs, some of which interact with the RNA-encoding BDNF (Wu, Tao, et al., 2010). Additionally, MeCP2 appears to share some of the characteristics of the core histone 1, and is involved in chromatin organization, in part through activity of the inter-domain region between the MBD and TRD (Zachariah & Rastegar, 2012). Through another mechanism, MeCP2 mediates formation of silent-chromatin loops during the process of imprinting, demonstrated through its regulation of the *DLX5* gene (Zachariah & Rastegar, 2012).

Epigenetic post-translational modifications to MeCP2 itself have been associated with both protein function and phenotype. Phosphorylation of MeCP2 at Serine 421 controls the ability of the protein to regulate dendritic morphology, BDNF transcription, and metabotropic glutamate receptor 5 transcription (Zhou, Hong, et al., 2006). Phosphorylation at Serine 80 appears to also regulate protein function; abnormal phosphorylation at

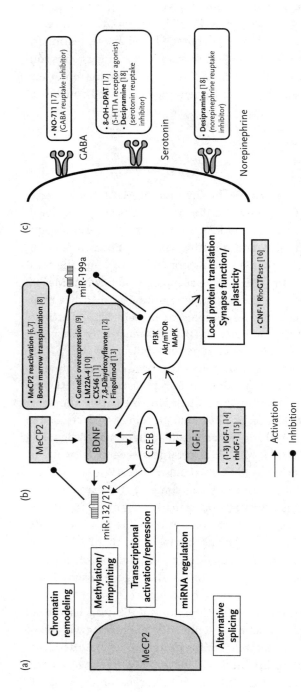

Figure 6.1:
Developmental Disorders

MeCP2-mediated molecular mechanisms that provide opportunities for therapeutics: (a) Schematic of different mechanisms by which MeCP2 can affect gene expression.

(b) Schematic showing how MeCP2 regulates protein-coding genes and miRNAs, so as to influence local translation and synaptic development, plasticity, and function. Also shown are attempted targets and molecules for therapeutic interventions. MeCP2 is known to increase the transcription of BDNF, which directly increases PI3K/Akt/MAPK signaling, or to affect plasticity-related miR-132, which in turn can target MeCP2 expression, thus forming a regulatory loop. In addition, BDNF can activate cyclic adenosine monophosphate Response Element-Binding protein (CREB), which can bind to the IGF-1 promoter and regulate transcription. IGF-1 is another positive regulator of the signaling pathways implicated in translation and synaptic plasticity. Akt/MAPK and mTOR are further involved in a double-negative inhibitory loop with miR-199a, a miRNA inhibited by MeCP2.

(c) Therapies aimed at restoring proper synaptic function by neurotransmitter rebalancing.

Key: BDNF, brain-derived neurotrophic factor; IGF-1, insulin-like growth factor 1; MeCP2, methyl CpG-binding protein 2; miRNA, microRNA.

Castro et al. Mechanisms and therapeutic challenges in ASDs. *Current Opinion in Neurology*, Volume 26, Number 2, April 2013. Copyright 2013 © Lippincott Williams & Wilkins, used with permission.

this site leads to locomotor deficits in mice (Tao, Hu, et al., 2009) Lastly, other epigenetic regulators also interact with MeCP2. For example, SIRT1, which plays a critical role in synaptic plasticity and memory, deacetylates MeCP2 and controls its binding activity to BDNF (Zocchi and Sassone-Corsi 2012) (Figure 6.1).

TARGETED TREATMENT INFORMATION

The age of neurobiologically targeted treatments for RTT is in its infancy. Yet, in the past 10 years, numerous mechanisms for treatment have been proposed, and several preclinical trials have shown promising results. A recent summary of preclinical investigations into targeted treatments identified 11 strategies, many of which are yet to be explored fully (Calfa, Percy, et al., 2011). To date, no clinical trials have yielded notable improvements in function; however, the equivocal or failed trials in the past are instructive, and summarized below.

Several challenges exist in designing a targeted treatment for RTT. Because MeCP2 is expressed variably in different cells in the brain and at different times in development, restoration of MeCP2 production may result in four scenarios: complete restoration of function, no restoration of function, decline in function due to overproduction of MeCP2, or restoration of function in certain cells but not those in which MeCP2 was critical at a certain period of development (Gadalla, Bailey, et al., 2011). Moreover, targeted treatments that restore function to processes regulated by MeCP2, without replacing MeCP2 itself, may only improve certain symptoms. Because MeCP2 production is prominent in early postnatal life, treatment may need to begin during the early stages of regression or even prior to regression to be effective, raising the issue of implementing neonatal screening. The fact that loss of previously normal *MECP2* function in adult mice leads to a severe phenotype (McGraw, Samaco, et al., 2011) supports the notion that MeCP2 is necessary for both developmental and mature brain synaptic plasticities ("double jeopardy") (Kaufmann, Johnston, et al., 2005), and that treatment would need to be administered throughout a patient's life.

The most attractive strategy from a mechanistic standpoint is insertion or activation of a normally functioning *MECP2* gene or MeCP2 protein. However, genetic manipulation is also the most challenging to implement. Alternately, targeting processes regulated by MeCP2 ("downstream") is a less complete but more realistic strategy. Genetic, neurosecretory, and other strategies will be examined below (Table 6.1).

Table 6.1 THERAPEUTIC STRATEGIES, AGENTS, AND IMPLEMENTATION

Category	Strategy	Compound	Target	Stage of Development
Genetic transcription/translation	Genetic transfection of *MECP2*	Transgene via viral vector	DNA	Preclinical
Genetic transcription/translation	Genetic Intervention	Satellite binding protein	Mutations affecting binding (R133C)	Preclinical
Genetic transcription/translation	Post-transcriptional modification	Synthetic aminoglycoside	Transcribed RNA coding MeCP2	Preclinical
Genetic transcription/translation	Chaperone	Investigational	Translated MeCP2 protein	Conceptual/Preclinical
Genetic binding	Enhanced binding of MeCP2	Folate and Betaine	DNA methylation	Phase II (completed—unsuccessful)
Neurotransmitter regulation	Increase DA, NE, 5-HT levels	Tyrosine/Tryptophan	NT precursors	Uncontrolled open label (completed—unsuccessful)
Neurotransmitter regulation	Stimulate DA receptors	Bromocriptine	DA receptors	Phase II (completed—selective improvement)
Neurotransmitter regulation	Inhibit NE reuptake	Desipramine	NE receptors	Phase II
Neurotransmitter regulation	Inhibit 5-HT reuptake	Fluoxetine	5-HT receptors	Uncontrolled open label (aborted prematurely—unsuccessful)
Neurotransmitter regulation	Increase ACh levels	Choline	ACh precursor	Preclinical
Neurotransmitter regulation	Antagonize glutamate receptors	Dextromethorphan	NMDA receptors	Phase II
Neurotransmitter regulation	Stimulate GABA receptors	Midazolam	GABA receptors	Preclinical
Neurotransmitter regulation	Block GABA reuptake/Stimulate 5-HT receptors	Investigational (NO-711/8-OH-DPAT)	GABA and 5-HT receptors	Preclinical

Genetic transcription/translation	Genetic Transfection of BDNF	Transgene via Viral Vector	DNA	
Neurotransmitter regulation	AMPA agonist to ↑ BDNF	Ampakines	AMPA receptor	Preclinical
Neurosecretory	↑ BDNF	Glatiramer acetate	BDNF transcription	Preclinical
Neurosecretory	↑BDNF	Fingolomod	BDNF transcription	Preclinical
Neurosecretory	Improve axonal transport to ↑ BDNF	Cysteamine	Huntingtin	Preclinical
Neurosecretory	TrkB agonist (BDNF target)	Investigational (LM22A-4)	TrkB receptor	Preclinical
Neurosecretory	Unclear (Huntingtin, TrkB)	Mecasermin	IGF-1R agonist	Phase II
Neurosecretory	Unclear (Huntingtin, TrkB)	Investigational (NNZ-2566)	IGF-1R agonist	Phase I
Neurotransmitter regulation	Improve astrocyte function	CNF1	Astrocytes	Preclinical
Neurotransmitter regulation	Decrease glial glutamate secretion, regulate glutamate clearance	Bone marrow transplant	Glia	Preclinical
Dietary/Metabolic	Induce ketosis	Ketogenic diet	CNS metabolism	Uncontrolled open label (selective improvement)
Dietary/Metabolic	Increase metabolic substrate	L-carnitine	CNS metabolism	Phase II (completed—inconsistent improvement)
Dietary/Metabolic	Increase metabolic substrate	Creatine	CNS metabolism	Phase II (completed—unsuccessful)
Neurotransmitter regulation	Opiate receptor antagonist	Naltrexone	Opioid receptors	Phase II (completed—unsuccessful)
Membrane potential	Sodium channel blockade to improve cardiac QT interval	Phenytoin	Sodium channels	Preclinical
Dietary/Metabolic	Improve mitochondrial efficiency	Investigational (EPI-743)	Mitochondria	Phase II

Key: dopamine (DA), norepinephrine (NE), serotonin (5-HT), neurotransmitter (NT), acetylcholine (ACh), insulin-like growth factor receptor (IGF-1R).

Preclinical and Clinical Studies

Pre-MECP2 *Era*

Prior to identification of *MECP2* mutations as causative of RTT, no specific animal models were available. Nonetheless, based on evidence from pathological specimens and imaging, clinical trials were conducted using tyrosine, tryptophan, bromocriptine, L-carnitine, the ketogenic diet, and the opiate agonist naltrexone (described below) (Percy, 2002).

Genetic and Molecular Strategies

Patients with RTT typically have random XCI, resulting in approximately 50% of cells expressing normal MeCP2 and 50% expressing either no protein or a mutated version. In the abnormal cells, a normal *MECP2* gene is present that was methylated early in embryonic life to inactivate its transcription. Reactivation of this normal gene is a strategy that could potentially cure the disease; however, the barriers to successful implementation are profound. Reactivation of an inactive X-chromosome is possible in theory, but it has never been accomplished. Moreover, if the entire silenced X-chromosome is reactivated, the "dose" of MeCP2 would approach normal levels in those cells; however, the dose of all other genes on the X-chromosome would be likely to reach pathological levels. Therefore a strategy for selective activation of silenced *MECP2* must also be developed.

Gene replacement is also an attractive strategy. A working copy of the *MECP2* gene could be transfected to specific cell types using a viral vector, and raise production of the normal protein in those cells. As in the reactivation strategy above, over-expression in normal cells is a concern. Strategies to overcome this include engineering feedback-inhibition of gene expression into the treatment, or silencing the *normal* endogenous gene in the hope that all normal neurons would only begin expressing the transfected gene (transgene) at a uniform dose. However, if more than one viral particle transfects a neuron, the dose of MeCP2 will be unpredictable. Additionally, technical barriers such as *in vivo* transfection of sufficient cells are not trivial. Many researchers have attempted transfection with a variety of vectors, with limited success and inconsistent functional improvement (Rastegar, Hotta, et al., 2009). Adeno-associated viruses (AAV) have been identified as the best vectors in RTT because of their ability to cross the blood–brain barrier and transfect globally. The Kaspar Laboratory (Ohio State University) is investigating transfection of mice using scAAV9, a vector that has proven successful in preclinical trials of spinal muscular atrophy. Additionally, the Crystal Laboratory (Weill Cornell Medical College) is investigating transfection of *MECP2* using AAVrh10.

One novel strategy addresses improving the function of mutated *MeCP2*. Recently, subregions of the MBD have been identified. A "pocket" responsible for 5-methyl cytosine binding (including the R133 amino acid) is bordered by two regions that are critical for chromatin rearrangement and aggregation. In the case of mutations that affect binding but not aggregation (e.g., R133C), targeted treatment with satellite binding proteins can restore both binding to heterochromatin and aggregation to normal levels in a mouse model (Casas-Delucchi, Becker, et al., 2012).

Considering that MeCP2 binds to methyl groups on DNA, increasing the number of methyl groups present using methyl donors could result in increased binding, even of dysfunctional MeCP2. To test this hypothesis, 68 participants with RTT were randomized in a double-blind randomized controlled trial (RCT) to receive placebo or 12 months of folate (a cofactor necessary for methyl donor pools) and betaine (a methyl group donor) (Glaze, Percy, et al., 2009). No objective improvements were noted; however, subjective improvement was reported in children less than 5 years old based on a parent questionnaire. Possible explanations for type II error included lack of controlling for genotype, and the authors cautioned that future studies should account for current knowledge about disease severity based on *MECP2* genotype.

Downstream Strategies

A strategy known as *post-transcriptional regulation* has been employed with varying success in disorders caused by a nonsense mutation. Aminoglycoside antibiotics (and other similar, less toxic molecules) can suppress premature stop codons producing a complete protein, probably by preventing stringent codon-anticodon pairing during translation. The caveat to this process is that amino acid substitution at the stop codon is random, and a protein with a missense mutation is the result.

Nonetheless, this strategy has met with limited success *in vivo* in other disorders (Sangkuhl, Schulz, et al., 2004). Approximately 35% of RTT is caused by nonsense mutations, and preclinical investigation in RTT is active. One synthetic aminoglycoside demonstrated 18–38% production of a full-length MeCP2 protein that was able to successfully translocate to the nucleus and was associated with increased levels of BDNF (Vecsler, Ben Zeev, et al., 2011).

After a mutated MeCP2 protein is translated, its function could be improved using molecular "chaperones." Such small molecules can address issues such as protein folding, a crucial step not only for protein function, but also for successful migration from the cytoplasm back to the nucleus where a protein like MeCP2 acts. Understanding protein conformation when MeCP2 is free in solution versus binding to DNA will instruct development of new molecules that target missense mutations (Hansen, Wexler, et al., 2011). Investigation into a chaperone to improve protein folding in the common T158M mutation is underway in the Bird Laboratory (University of Edinburgh).

Neurotransmitters

The understanding of NT function in models of RTT has expanded greatly with the ability to selectively decrease *MeCP2* expression in specific brain regions, specific cell types, or both in combination (Figure 6.1).

Monoamines

Dopamine: Many girls with RTT have low levels of CSF dopamine metabolites (19%) and serotonin metabolites (23%), especially those with severe mutations (Samaco, Mandel-Brehm, et al., 2009). Two decades ago, this early finding prompted treatment with tyrosine and tryptophan, which increased CSF monoamine metabolite levels but did not improve clinical outcomes over 10 weeks (Nielsen, Lou, et al., 1990); and bromocriptine (a dopamine agonist), which resulted in motor, communication, and cognitive improvements in some participants (Zappella, Genazzani, et al., 1990). When mouse models were developed, these exhibited low dopamine, serotonin, and norepinephrine (NE) levels, along with low levels of the enzymes responsible for production of these NTs (e.g., tyrosine hydroxylase [TH]). Region-specific KO models were able to demonstrate specific behavioral phenotypes associated with low levels of these NTs in various brainstem nuclei. Although no new clinical trials have been proposed, the prominent behavioral disruption and eventual onset of Parkinsonian features present in RTT suggest that dopamine regulation could improve function.

Norepinephrine: Respiratory abnormalities in *MECP2* deficient mice are associated with abnormalities in the medulla, and further brainstem and forebrain dysfunction can be associated with hyperexcitability in the locus ceruleus. Both regions exhibit a paucity of TH-expressing neurons, and low levels of NE (Taneja, Ogier, et al., 2009). *In vitro* administration of NE results in improvement in the rhythm of the respiratory network. Two follow-up studies demonstrated that MECP2-deficient mice treated with desipramine, which specifically inhibits NE reuptake, had improved respiratory rhythm and longer lifespan. Moreover, one study showed that desipramine treatment increases the number of TH-expressing neurons in the medulla to normal (Roux, Dura, et al., 2007), and the other study found that despite improved respiratory pattern, desipramine selectively *decreases* NE levels in the medulla (Zanella, Mebarek, et al., 2008). Based on the above animal studies, a phase II clinical trial is currently being conducted at six centers in France.

Serotonin: Based on direct assessment in postmortem tissue and case reports of improvement in respiratory function when girls with RTT were treated with serotonin agonists, serotonin receptors in the brainstem were implicated in cardiorespiratory dysregulation. To examine this hypothesis, researchers attempted to induce *Mecp2* expression by injecting male Wistar rats with fluoxetine, cocaine, a dopamine reuptake inhibitor, a norepinephrine reuptake inhibitor, or saline. The fluoxetine and cocaine groups showed increased expression of Mecp2 as well as another methyl-CpG binding domain protein, MBD1, suggesting that extracellular serotonin concentration is a regulator of *MeCP2* expression (Cassel, Carouge, et al., 2006). To target serotoninergic abnormalities, six patients were treated with fluoxetine in an open-label trial at Necker Enfants Malades University Hospital. None had a beneficial response at the end of the study, and three stopped the medication due to behavioral disturbances, sleep disorder, and/or anorexia. The study was ended prematurely by the French safety monitoring group.

Acetylcholine

Choline acetyltransferase (an enzyme involved in acetylcholine production) levels are low in the forebrain of girls with RTT (Wenk & Hauss-Wegrzyniak, 1999). Similarly, a knock-in mouse model demonstrated reduced choline levels in the striatum and increased levels in the hippocampus (Ricceri, De Filippis, et al., 2011). Researchers administered supplemental choline to these mice from birth to postnatal day 25 and found restoration of central choline levels and increased BDNF and nerve growth factor (NGF) expression. Although no major behavioral changes were observed, mice treated with choline maintained normal locomotion well beyond the period of choline supplementation, whereas control mice exhibited abnormal locomotor activity. Other studies have reported improvement in motor and behavioral function with choline treatment. RTT is almost never diagnosed in the perinatal period, and the impact of choline supplementation later in life has not been examined in a preclinical model.

Glutamate: Postmortem studies of patients with RTT have demonstrated age-related abnormalities in the glutamatergic system and NMDA receptors, characterized by early increase and late decrease in NMDA receptor levels, which have been reproduced in *Mecp2* KO mice (Blue, Kaufmann, et al., 2011). One possible mechanism is MeCP2's regulation of NMDA subunit NR1 splicing (Young, Hong, et al., 2005). Administration of the NMDA antagonist ketamine increased expression of the activity-dependent Fos protein in hypoactive regions such as the piriform and motor cortex of KO mice, as well as improved sensorimotor gating (a common index of cognitive function in neuropsychiatric disorders) (Kron, Howell, et al., 2012). The authors interpreted these findings as indicative of a network abnormality in the default mode network, also found in autism spectrum disorder, which can be partially rescued by administration of an NMDA antagonist. A study that administered memantine, another NMDA antagonist, transiently corrected LTP abnormalities in KO mice (Weng, McLeod, et al., 2011). Genetic deletion of the NMDA receptor subunit NR2A prevented the progressive visual loss exhibited by *Mecp2*-deficient mice (Durand, Patrizi, et al., 2012). Although the latter approach is not feasible in humans, it highlights the widespread effect that MeCP2 has on brain circuits and the key role that NMDA abnormalities play in synaptic dysfunction associated with RTT.

An open-label study of the NMDA antagonist dextromethorphan recruited 35 patients at the Hugo W. Moser Research Institute, and a double-blind RCT began in 2012. Researchers are collecting neuropsychological and behavioral data on children with RTT aged 2 to 10 years during a 3-month treatment period.

GABA: Cortical GABAergic neurons express 50% more MeCP2 than other neurons, and GABAergic cell-specific KO mice recapitulate the respiratory, compulsive, motor, and social symptoms in RTT (Voituron & Hilaire 2011). A cell- and region-specific KO model demonstrated that loss of MeCP2 in only forebrain GABAergic cells was sufficient to produce compulsive, motor, and social symptoms. Transcription of the genes responsible for intracellular GABA synthesis (*GAD1/GAD2*) is decreased, suggesting that the same mechanism resulting in decreased BDNF production in MeCP2-deficient cells is responsible. Although this KO model did not display seizures, this finding raises the possibility that GABA transaminase inhibitors, such as Vigabitrin, could target one of the mechanisms thought to generate epilepsy in RTT.

The GABA agonist midazolam transiently reversed the breathing dysfunction in KO mice (Voituron & Hilaire, 2011). Both GABA reuptake blockers and serotonin 1a agonists partially correct breathing dysfunction in a female KO model; however, both compounds in conjunction restore respiratory function to that seen in wild-type mice.

Growth Factors

Brain-derived neurotrophic factor: Several studies targeting BDNF have demonstrated both histological and functional improvements. Using a transgene in a mouse model of RTT, BDNF over-expression resulted in an extended lifespan and improved locomotion (Kline, Ogier, et al., 2010). Phosphorylation of MeCP2 releases the transcriptional repression of BDNF, leading to expansions in dendritic arborizations and synaptic maturation (Zhou, Hong, et al., 2006). Exogenous administration of BDNF successfully rescued the cardiorespiratory abnormalities present in KO mice; however, BDNF does not cross the blood–brain barrier (BBB). Administration of ampakines, compounds that facilitate activation of AMPA glutamate receptors and do cross the BBB, increased BDNF levels in a RTT mouse model and improved respiratory dysfunction (Kline, Ogier, et al., 2010). Glatiramer acetate, an immunomodulator used in multiple sclerosis (MS) increases BDNF levels in humans, and has been shown to increase BDNF expression to wild-type levels in KO mice; functional outcomes have not yet been assessed (Ben-Zeev, Aharoni, et al., 2011). Fingolimod, a sphingosine-1-phosphate receptor modulator also used to treat MS, increased BDNF levels, and improved lifespan, motor function, and size of the striatum in KO mice (Deogracias, Yazdani, et al., 2012). BDNF mimetics have also shown promise in reversing the phenotype of *Mecp2* KO mice.

A recent link between Huntington's disease (HD) and RTT suggested a therapeutic target to increase BDNF levels. Huntingtin and Huntingtin-associated protein are involved in axonal transport of BDNF, and decreased levels of BDNF in a model of HD are rescued by cysteamine treatment (Borrell-Pages, Canals, et al., 2006). In a KO model of RTT, the velocity of BDNF vesicle axonal trafficking was decreased, and treatment with cysteamine improved not only vesicular velocity and BDNF levels, but also lifespan and motor deficits (Roux, Zala, et al., 2012). Examining other targeted treatments being tested in HD may be indicated (e.g., calcineurin). Further downstream, tyrosine-related kinase B (TrkB), a target of BDNF, is critical for brainstem and hippocampal function and memory consolidation through LTP (Amaral, Chapleau, et al., 2007). Targeting this receptor with TrkB agonists improved respiratory function in heterozygous female *MECP2* mutant mice (Schmid, Yang, et al., 2012).

Insulin-like Growth Factor 1 (IGF-1): Insulin-like growth factor binding protein 3 (IGFBP3), a regulator of IGF-1, is modulated by MeCP2 (Itoh, Ide, et al., 2007). MeCP2 binds directly to the promoter of IGFBP3, and in the *Mecp2* KO mouse, IGFBP3 levels are elevated. The significance of this finding was underscored by the demonstration of increased IGFBP3 levels in RTT postmortem brain. The roles of hormones like IGF-1 in RTT are not completely understood. However, IGF-1 phosphorylates Huntingtin resulting in increased BDNF release (Zala, Colin, et al., 2008), and the IGF-1 receptor activates intracellular pathways also regulated by the TrkB receptor (Zheng & Quirion, 2004).

Treatment with an active peptide fragment of IGF-1 partially restored both functional and histological aspects of the disease in mice. Lifespan was extended by 50%, and locomotion, breathing abnormalities, and heart rate variability improved. Moreover, the treatment increased brain weight, dendritic spine density, synaptic amplitude, and PSD-95 (a marker of post-synaptic density) levels, and matured occipital cortex plasticity to wild-type levels (Tropea, Giacometti, et al., 2009).

Two phase I trials of recombinant full-length IGF-1 in girls with classic RTT were completed in 2012 and demonstrated safety and tolerability. In one, nine participants (ages 2–11) received the drug in escalating doses over a four-week period with good CSF penetration and without adverse events. In another, six patients (ages 4–11) received daily injections for six months without adverse events (Pini, Scusa, et al., 2012). A phase II crossover RCT began in March 2013 at Boston Children's Hospital and is collecting neurological, behavioral, neurophysiological, and autonomic outcome data.

A phase IIa RCT of NNZ-2566 (a tripeptide normally cleaved from IGF-1 in brain tissue) in RTT is underway at Baylor College of Medicine. The study is recruiting women 16 years and older and is collecting neurological, behavioral, and neurophysiological outcome data.

Miscellaneous Mechanisms

Glial function: Although classically conceived as a neuronal disorder, both *in vitro* and *in vivo* models of RTT have demonstrated that mutant *Mecp2* in astrocytes affects dendritic morphology and other phenotypical features. *In vitro,* dendrites of both mutant and wild type neurons were abnormal when neurons were co-cultured with mutant astrocytes (Ballas, Lioy, et al., 2009). Dendritic and synaptic abnormalities attributable to astrocytes are thought to be due to excessive secretion of glutamate; however, cultured KO astrocytes have an elevated glutamate clearance rate associated with impaired downregulation of excitatory amino acid transporters and excessive glutamate synthetase production (Okabe, Takahashi, et al., 2012). Dendritic abnormalities were reversed in Mecp2-deficient mice when Mecp2 function was selectively restored in astrocytes, and levels of the excitatory glutamate transporter VGLUT1 were increased. Moreover, these mice exhibited improved lifespan, locomotion, anxiety, and respiratory abnormalities, further supporting astrocytes as a therapeutic target (Lioy, Garg, et al., 2011). In a mouse model of RTT with atrophic and decreased numbers of astrocytes, targeting G-protein function with cytotoxic necrotizing factor 1 (CNF-1) improved both astrocyte number and morphology. Behavior also improved in these animals, as did levels of the cytokine IL-6 (associated with synaptic plasticity dysfunction when elevated) and astrocytic and neuronal metabolites (De Filippis, Fabbri, et al., 2012). Bone marrow transplant in *Mecp2* KO mice populated the brain with microglia with normal Mecp2 function (Derecki, Cronk, et al., 2012). Although this study corroborated previous *in vitro* evidence of microglial dysfunction in Mecp2 deficiency, the reported treatment required cranial irradiation to be effective, which limits its clinical application in patients with RTT. Moreover, if performed too late in development, the treatment resulted in little improvement.

Ketogenic diet: Apart from two case reports, only one uncontrolled trial has been conducted using ketogenic diet in RTT. Five of seven girls tolerated the diet and experienced reduction in seizures, but they experienced only "slight" improvements in behavior and motor function.

Naltrexone: Based on the observation of increased β-endorphin levels in girls with RTT, naltrexone was administered in a crossover RCT to 25 girls with RTT. The trial was complicated by an inadequate washout period; analysis of the first phase revealed improvement in respiratory parameters (potentially due to sedation), but no other behavioral or motor findings.

Carnitine: A crossover RCT examined L-carnitine supplementation in 35 girls with RTT, and found modest improvements in the "Patient Well-Being Index," as well as physician (but not parent) ratings of behavioral and orofacial/respiratory features. A follow-up six-month open-label study of 21 girls demonstrated "small but discernable improvements" in sleep efficiency, energy level, and communication skills (Ellaway, Peat, et al., 2001). Side effects included a fishy odor and diarrhea, necessitating dose adjustment in 9% of subjects. Despite the equivocal results of this clinical trial, a recent preclinical study examined carnitine supplementation in KO mice. The medication was administered from birth to death, and resulted in improved weight gain, activity, motor and cognitive features, as well as improved dendritic length and complexity. Neurotrophin levels were unaffected, despite being proposed as a mechanism for this treatment. Possible explanations for the discrepancy between this more recent preclinical trial and the older clinical trial are the model (male mice lack lionization characteristics) and age at start of treatment (equivalent to the human third trimester of pregnancy) (Schaevitz, Nicolai, et al., 2012).

Creatine: A crossover RCT of creatine supplementation enrolled 21 girls with RTT and was completed in 2009 (Freilinger, Dunkler, et al., 2011). Global DNA methylation, metabolic markers of methylation, motor and behavioral data were collected. Global DNA methylation increased significantly; however, neither metabolic markers nor functional variables changed with supplementation.

Cardiac conduction abnormalities: In addition to the several mechanisms described above, which contribute to cardiorespiratory dysfunction in RTT, abnormal sodium currents appear to play a role. In a KO mouse model in which only neurons carried the mutant allele, prolonged QT interval and ventricular tachycardia were present, and associated with increased persistent sodium current. Although β-blockade (the standard of care in human prolonged QT) failed to improve tachycardia, the sodium channel-blocking drug phenytoin improved QT interval, heart rate, and sodium current in these mice, introducing sodium channel blockade as a potentially novel treatment, specific for prolonged QT in RTT (McCauley, Wang, et al., 2011).

Mitochondria: In *Mecp2* KO mice, the nuclear gene for ubiquinol-cytochrome-c reductase core protein 1 (*UQCRC1*), which produces a component of mitochondrial complex III, is over-expressed due to lack of repression by Mecp2. Functionally, this results in an increased rate and decreased efficiency of mitochondrial respiration (Kriaucionis, Paterson, et al., 2006). An RCT is beginning shortly in Italy, using an orally absorbed small molecule that synchronizes energy generation in mitochondria.

SUMMARY

Successful treatments for RTT may emerge within the next several years. These treatments will be based on the neurobiology of the disorder, but will most likely target specific aspects of the disorder and will not be a panacea. However, treatments targeting symptoms of great distress to patients and families—seizures, anxiety, aggressive behavior, respiratory abnormalities, and communication impairment—would not only represent a great step forward in the management of RTT, but also a proof of principle for other disorders. Many other disorders, such as bipolar disorder with cognitive deficits, childhood-onset schizophrenia, and autism spectrum disorder, can be due to a mutation in *MECP2* and may benefit from identical treatments. Additionally, disorders caused by other genetic abnormalities, such as Down syndrome, fragile X syndrome, Angelman syndrome, and tuberous sclerosis, exhibit disruption of pathways also affected in RTT (e.g., mTOR), and may benefit from similar treatments. As treatments for the various NT and neurosecretory abnormalities resulting from deficient MeCP2 are identified, we anticipate a new, more neurobiologically based age of RTT management, with improved quality of life for both caregivers and children.

DISCLOSURES

Acknowledgments: Supported by grants from the International Rett Syndrome Foundation (IRSF), Autism Speaks, and NIH grants U54 RR019478 and P30 HD061222.

Conflict: Walter E. Kaufmann is a consultant of Genentech and receives research support from Ipsen and Novartis.

REFERENCES

Ager, S., Fyfe, S., et al. (2006). Predictors of scoliosis in Rett syndrome. *Journal of Child Neurology, 21*(9), 809–813.

Amaral, M. D., Chapleau, C. A., et al. (2007). Transient receptor potential channels as novel effectors of brain-derived neurotrophic factor signaling: potential implications for Rett syndrome. *Pharmacology Therapy, 113*(2), 394–409.

Amir, R. E., Van den Veyver, I. B., et al. (1999). Rett syndrome is caused by mutations in Xlinked MECP2, encoding methyl-CpG-binding protein 2. *Nature Genetics, 23*(2), 185–188.

Armstrong, D. D. (2002). Neuropathology of Rett syndrome. *Mental Retardation & Developmental Disability Research Review, 8*(2), 72–76.

Ballas, N., Lioy, D. T., et al. (2009). Non-cell autonomous influence of MeCP2-deficient glia on neuronal dendritic morphology. *Nature Neuroscience, 12*(3), 311–317.

Ballestar, E., Yusufzai, T. M., et al. (2000). Effects of Rett syndrome mutations of the methyl-CpG binding domain of the transcriptional repressor MeCP2 on selectivity for association with methylated DNA. *Biochemistry, 39*(24), 7100–7106.

Baptista, P. M., Mercadante, M. T., et al. (2006). Cognitive performance in Rett syndrome girls: a pilot study using eyetracking technology. *Journal of Intellectual Disability Research, 50*(Pt 9), 662–666.

Bat-Haee, M. A. (1994). Behavioral training of a young woman with Rett syndrome. *Perceptual & Motor Skills, 78*(1), 314.

Bebbington, A., Anderson, A., et al. (2008). Investigating genotype-phenotype relationships in Rett syndrome using an international data set. *Neurology, 70*(11), 868–875.

Ben-Zeev, B., Aharoni, R., et al. (2011). Glatiramer acetate (GA, Copolymer-1): a hypothetical treatment option for Rett syndrome. *Medical Hypotheses, 76*(2), 190–193.

Blue, M. E., Kaufmann, W. E., et al. (2011). Temporal and regional alterations in NMDA receptor expression in Mecp2-null mice. *Anatomical Record (Hoboken), 294*(10), 1624–1634.

Borrell-Pages, M., Canals, J. M., et al. (2006). Cystamine and cysteamine increase brain levels of BDNF in Huntington disease via HSJ1b and transglutaminase. *Journal of Clinical Investigation, 116*(5), 1410–1424.

Budden, S. S., Myer, E. C., et al. (1990). Cerebrospinal fluid studies in the Rett syndrome: biogenic amines and beta-endorphins. *Brain & Development, 12*(1), 81–84.

Calfa, G., Percy, A. K., et al. (2011). Experimental models of Rett syndrome based on Mecp2 dysfunction. *Experimental Biology & Medicine (Maywood), 236*(1), 3–19.

Casas-Delucchi, C. S., Becker, A., et al. (2012). Targeted manipulation of heterochromatin rescues MeCP2 Rett mutants and re-establishes higher order chromatin organization. *Nucleic Acids Research, 40*(22), E176.

Cassel, S., Carouge, D., et al. (2006). Fluoxetine and cocaine induce the epigenetic factors MeCP2 and MBD1 in adult rat brain. *Molecular Pharmacology, 70*(2), 487–492.

Chao, H. T., Zoghbi, H. Y., et al. (2007). MeCP2 controls excitatory synaptic strength by regulating glutamatergic synapse number. *Neuron, 56*(1), 58–65.

De Filippis, B., Fabbri, A., et al. (2012). Modulation of RhoGTPases improves the behavioral phenotype and reverses astrocytic deficits in a mouse model of Rett syndrome. *Neuropsychopharmacology, 37*(5), 1152–1163.

Deogracias, R., Yazdani, M., et al. (2012). Fingolimod, a sphingosine-1 phosphate receptor modulator, increases BDNF levels and improves symptoms of a mouse model of Rett syndrome. *Proceedings of the National Academy of Science, USA, 109*(35), 14230–14235.

Derecki, N. C., Cronk, J. C., et al. (2012). Wild-type microglia arrest pathology in a mouse model of Rett syndrome. *Nature, 484*(7392), 105–109.

Downs, J., Bergman, A., et al. (2009). Guidelines for management of scoliosis in Rett syndrome patients based on expert consensus and clinical evidence. *Spine, 34*(17), E607–E617.

Durand, S., Patrizi, A., et al. (2012). NMDA receptor regulation prevents regression of visual cortical function in the absence of Mecp2. *Neuron, 76*(6), 1078–1090.

Einspieler, C., Kerr, A. M., et al. (2005). Is the early development of girls with Rett disorder really normal? Pediatric Research, 57(5 Pt 1), 696–700.

Ellaway, C. J., Peat, J., et al. (2001). Medium-term open label trial of L-carnitine in Rett syndrome. *Brain & Development, 23*(Suppl 1), S85–S89.

Freilinger, M., Dunkler, D., et al. (2011). Effects of creatine supplementation in Rett syndrome: a randomized, placebo-controlled trial. *Journal of Developmental & Behavioral Pediatrics, 32*(6), 454–460.

Gadalla, K. K., Bailey, M. E., et al. (2011). MeCP2 and Rett syndrome: reversibility and potential avenues for therapy. *Biochemistry Journal, 439*(1), 1–14.

Garcia-Rudaz, C., Deng, V., et al. (2009). FXYD1, a modulator of Na,K-ATPase activity, facilitates female sexual development by maintaining gonadotrophin-releasing hormone neuronal excitability. *Journal of Neuroendocrinology, 21*(2), 108–122.

Glaze, D. G., Percy, A. K., et al. (2009). A study of the treatment of Rett syndrome with folate and betaine. *Journal of Child Neurology, 24*(5), 551–556.

Glaze, D. G., Percy, A. K., et al. (2010). Epilepsy and the natural history of Rett syndrome. *Neurology, 74*(11), 909–912.

Guy, J., Gan, J., et al. (2007). Reversal of neurological defects in a mouse model of Rett syndrome. *Science, 315*(5815), 1143–1147.

Hagberg, B., Aicardi, J., et al. (1983). A progressive syndrome of autism, dementia, ataxia, and loss of purposeful hand use in girls: Rett's syndrome: report of 35 cases. *Annals of Neurology, 14*(4), 471–479.

Hagberg, B., & Witt-Engerstrom, I. (1986). Rett syndrome: a suggested staging system for describing impairment profile with increasing age towards adolescence. *American Journal of Medical Genetics, 25*(Suppl 1), 47–59.

Hansen, J. C., Wexler, B. B., et al. (2011). DNA binding restricts the intrinsic conformational flexibility of methyl CpG binding protein 2 (MeCP2). *Journal of Biological Chemistry, 286*(21), 18938–18948.

Hoffbuhr, K. C., Moses, L. M., et al. (2002). Associations between MeCP2 mutations, X-chromosome inactivation, and phenotype. *Mental Retardation & Developmental Disability Research Review, 8*(2), 99–105.

Huppke, P., Maier, E. M., et al. (2006). Very mild cases of Rett syndrome with skewed X inactivation. *Journal of Medical Genetics, 43*(10), 814–816.

Itoh, M., Ide, S., et al. (2007). Methyl CpG-binding protein 2 (a mutation of which causes Rett syndrome) directly regulates insulin-like growth factor binding protein 3 in mouse and human brains. *Journal of Neuropathology & Experimental Neurology, 66*(2), 117–123.

Jedele, K. B. (2007). The overlapping spectrum of Rett and Angelman syndromes: a clinical review. *Seminars in Pediatric Neurology, 14*(3), 108–117.

Julu, P. O., Kerr, A. M., et al. (2001). Characterisation of breathing and associated central autonomic dysfunction in the Rett disorder. *Archives of Disease in Childhood, 85*(1), 29–37.

Kaufmann, W. E., Johnston, M. V., et al. (2005). MeCP2 expression and function during brain development: implications for Rett syndrome's pathogenesis and clinical evolution. *Brain & Development, 27*(Suppl 1), S77–S87.

Kaufmann, W. E., MacDonald, S. M., et al. (2000). Dendritic cytoskeletal protein expression in mental retardation: an immunohistochemical study of the neocortex in Rett syndrome. *Cerebral Cortex, 10*(10), 992–1004.

Kerr, A. M., & Ravine, D. (2003). Review article: breaking new ground with Rett syndrome. *Journal of Intellectual Disability Research, 47*(Pt 8), 580–587.

Kline, D. D., Ogier, M., et al. (2010). Exogenous brain-derived neurotrophic factor rescues synaptic dysfunction in Mecp2-null mice. *Journal of Neuroscience, 30*(15), 5303–5310.

Kriaucionis, S., Paterson, A., et al. (2006). Gene expression analysis exposes mitochondrial abnormalities in a mouse model of Rett syndrome. *Molecular & Cellular Biology, 26*(13), 5033–5042.

Kron, M., Howell, C. J., et al. (2012). Brain activity mapping in Mecp2 mutant mice reveals functional deficits in forebrain circuits, including key nodes in the default mode network, that are reversed with ketamine treatment. *Journal of Neuroscience, 32*(40), 13860–13872.

Kudo, S., Nomura, Y., et al. (2001). Functional analyses of MeCP2 mutations associated with Rett syndrome using transient expression systems. *Brain & Development, 23*(Suppl 1), S165–173.

Li, W., Calfa, G., et al. (2012). Activity-dependent BDNF release and TRPC signaling is impaired in hippocampal neurons of Mecp2 mutant mice. *Proceedings of the National Academy of Science, USA, 109*(42), 17087–17092.

Lioy, D. T., Garg, S. K., et al. (2011). A role for glia in the progression of Rett's syndrome. *Nature, 475*(7357), 497–500.

Marschik, P. B., Kaufmann, W. E., et al. (2013). Changing the perspective on early development of Rett syndrome. *Research in Developmental Disabilities, 34*(4), 1236–1239.

McCauley, M. D., Wang, T., et al. (2011). Pathogenesis of lethal cardiac arrhythmias in Mecp2 mutant mice: implication for therapy in Rett syndrome. *Science Translational Medicine, 3*(113), 113ra125.

McGill, B. E., Bundle, S. F., et al. (2006). Enhanced anxiety and stress-induced corticosterone release are associated with increased Crh expression in a mouse model of Rett syndrome. *Proceedings of the National Academy of Science, USA, 103*(48), 18267–18272.

McGraw, C. M., Samaco, R. C., et al. (2011). Adult neural function requires MeCP2. *Science, 333*(6039), 186.

Medrihan, L., Tantalaki, E., et al. (2008). Early defects of GABAergic synapses in the brain stem of a MeCP2 mouse model of Rett syndrome. *Journal of Neurophysiology, 99*(1), 112–121.

Metcalf, B. M., Mullaney, B. C., et al. (2006). Temporal shift in methyl-CpG binding protein 2 expression in a mouse model of Rett syndrome. *Neuroscience, 139*(4), 1449–1460.

Moretti, P., Levenson, J. M., et al. (2006). Learning and memory and synaptic plasticity are impaired in a mouse model of Rett syndrome. *Journal of Neuroscience, 26*(1), 319–327.

Motil, K. J., Barrish, J. O., et al. (2011). Vitamin D deficiency is prevalent in girls and women with Rett syndrome. *Journal of Pediatric Gastroenterology & Nutrition, 53*(5), 569–574.

Motil, K. J., Caeg, E., et al. (2012). Gastrointestinal and nutritional problems occur frequently throughout life in girls and women with Rett syndrome. *Journal of Pediatric Gastroenterology & Nutrition, 55*(3), 292–298.

Neul, J. L., Fang, P., et al. (2008). Specific mutations in methyl-CpG-binding protein 2 confer different severity in Rett syndrome. *Neurology, 70*(16), 1313–1321.

Neul, J. L., Kaufmann, W. E., et al. (2010). Rett syndrome: revised diagnostic criteria and nomenclature. *Annals of Neurology, 68*(6), 944–950.

Nielsen, J. B., Lou, H. C., et al. (1990). Biochemical and clinical effects of tyrosine and tryptophan in the Rett syndrome. *Brain & Development, 12*(1), 143–147.

Okabe, Y., Takahashi, T., et al. (2012). Alterations of gene expression and glutamate clearance in astrocytes derived from an MeCP2-null mouse model of Rett syndrome. *PLoS One, 7*(4), E35354.

Paterson, D. S., Thompson, E. G., et al. (2005). Serotonin transporter abnormality in the dorsal motor nucleus of the vagus in Rett syndrome: potential implications for clinical autonomic dysfunction. *Journal of Neuropathology & Experimental Neurology, 64*(11), 1018–1027.

Percy, A. K. (1992). Neurochemistry of the Rett syndrome. *Brain & Development, 14*(Suppl), S57–S62.

Percy, A. K. (2002). Clinical trials and treatment prospects. *Mental Retardation & Developmental Disability Research Review, 8*(2), 106–111.

Percy, A. K. (2002). Rett syndrome. Current status and new vistas. *Neurologic Clinics, 20*(4), 1125–1141.

Percy, A. K., & Lane, J. B. (2005). Rett syndrome: model of neurodevelopmental disorders. *Journal of Child Neurology, 20*(9), 718–721.

Pini, G., Scusa, M. F., et al. (2012). IGF1 as a potential treatment for Rett syndrome:Safety assessment in six Rett patients. *Autism Research & Treatments*, 679801.

Prater, C. D., & Zylstra, R. G. (2006). Medical care of adults with mental retardation. *American Family Physician, 73*(12), 2175–2183.

Rastegar, M., Hotta, A., et al. (2009). MECP2 isoform-specific vectors with regulated expression for Rett syndrome gene therapy. *PLoS One, 4*(8), E6810.

Ricceri, L., De Filippis, B., et al. (2011). Cholinergic hypofunction in MeCP2-308 mice: beneficial neurobehavioural effects of neonatal choline supplementation. *Behavioural Brain Research, 221*(2), 623–629.

Ricciardi, S., Boggio, E. M., et al. (2011). Reduced AKT/mTOR signaling and protein synthesis dysregulation in a Rett syndrome animal model. *Human Molecular Genetics, 20*(6), 1182–1196.

Robinson, L., Guy, J., et al. (2012). Morphological and functional reversal of phenotypes in a mouse model of Rett syndrome. *Brain, 135*(Pt 9), 2699–2710.

Roux, J. C., Dura, E., et al. (2007). Treatment with desipramine improves breathing and survival in a mouse model for Rett syndrome. *European Journal of Neuroscience, 25*(7), 1915–1922.

Roux, J. C., Zala, D., et al. (2012). Modification of Mecp2 dosage alters axonal transport through the Huntingtin/Hap1 pathway. *Neurobiology of Disease, 45*(2), 786–795.

Samaco, R. C., Mandel-Brehm, C., et al. (2009). Loss of MeCP2 in aminergic neurons causes cell-autonomous defects in neurotransmitter synthesis and specific behavioral abnormalities. *Proceedings of the National Academy of Science, USA, 106*(51), 21966–21971.

Sangkuhl, K., Schulz, A., et al. (2004). Aminoglycoside-mediated rescue of a disease-causing nonsense mutation in the V2 vasopressin receptor gene in vitro and in vivo. *Human Molecular Genetics, 13*(9), 893–903.

Schaevitz, L. R., Nicolai, R., et al. (2012). Acetyl-L-carnitine improves behavior and dendritic morphology in a mouse model of Rett syndrome. *PLoS One, 7*(12), E51586.

Schmid, D. A., Yang, T., et al. (2012). A TrkB small molecule partial agonist rescues TrkB phosphorylation deficits and improves respiratory function in a mouse model of Rett syndrome. *Journal of Neuroscience, 32*(5), 1803–1810.

Shahbazian, M., Young, J., et al. (2002). Mice with truncated MeCP2 recapitulate many Rett syndrome features and display hyperacetylation of histone H3. *Neuron, 35*(2), 243–254.

Sun, Y. E., & Wu, H. (2006). The ups and downs of BDNF in Rett syndrome. *Neuron, 49*(3), 321–323.

Taneja, P., Ogier, M., et al. (2009). Pathophysiology of locus ceruleus neurons in a mouse model of Rett syndrome. *Journal of Neuroscience, 29*(39), 12187–12195.

Tao, J., Hu, K., et al. (2009). Phosphorylation of MeCP2 at Serine 80 regulates its chromatin association and neurological function. *Proceedings of the National Academy of Science, USA, 106*(12), 4882–4887.

Tarquinio, D. C., Motil, K. J., et al. (2012). Growth failure and outcome in Rett syndrome: specific growth references. *Neurology, 79*(16), 1653–1661.

Trappe, R., Laccone, F., et al. (2001). MECP2 mutations in sporadic cases of Rett syndrome are almost exclusively of paternal origin. *American Journal of Human Genetics, 68*(5), 1093–1101.

Tropea, D., Giacometti, E., et al. (2009). Partial reversal of Rett Syndrome-like symptoms in MeCP2 mutant mice. *Proceedings of the National Academy of Science, USA, 106*(6), 2029–2034.

Vecsler, M., Ben Zeev, B., et al. (2011). Ex vivo treatment with a novel synthetic amino-glycoside NB54 in primary fibroblasts from Rett syndrome patients suppresses MECP2 nonsense mutations. *PLoS One, 6*(6), E20733.

Villard, L. (2007). MECP2 mutations in males. *Journal of Medical Genetics, 44*(7), 417–423.

Voituron, N., & Hilaire, G. (2011). The benzodiazepine Midazolam mitigates the breathing defects of Mecp2-deficient mice. *Respiratory Physiology & Neurobiology, 177*(1), 56–60.

Wang, H., Chan, S. A., et al. (2006). Dysregulation of brain-derived neurotrophic factor expression and neurosecretory function in Mecp2 null mice. *Journal of Neuroscience, 26*(42), 10911–10915.

Weng, S. M., McLeod, F., et al. (2011). Synaptic plasticity deficits in an experimental model of Rett syndrome: long-term potentiation saturation and its pharmaco-logical reversal. *Neuroscience, 180,* 314–321.

Wenk, G. L., & Hauss-Wegrzyniak, B. (1999). Altered cholinergic function in the basal forebrain of girls with Rett syndrome. *Neuropediatrics, 30*(3), 125–129.

Wither, R. G., Lang, M., et al. (2013). Regional MeCP2 expression levels in the female MeCP2-deficient mouse brain correlate with specific behavioral impairments. *Experimental Neurology, 239,* 49–59.

Wu, H., Tao, J., et al. (2010). Genome-wide analysis reveals methyl-CpG-binding pro-tein 2-dependent regulation of microRNAs in a mouse model of Rett syndrome. *Proceedings of the National Academy of Science, USA, 107*(42), 18161–18166.

Yasuhara, A., & Sugiyama, Y. (2001). Music therapy for children with Rett syndrome. *Brain & Development, 23*(Suppl 1), S82–S84.

Young, J. I., Hong, E. P., et al. (2005). Regulation of RNA splicing by the methylation-dependent transcriptional repressor methyl-CpG binding protein 2. *Proceedings of the National Academy of Science, USA, 102*(49), 17551–17558.

Zachariah, R. M., & Rastegar, M. (2012). Linking epigenetics to human disease and Rett syndrome: the emerging novel and challenging concepts in MeCP2 research. *Neural Plasticity,* 415825.

Zala, D., Colin, E., et al. (2008). Phosphorylation of mutant Huntingtin at S421 restores anterograde and retrograde transport in neurons. *Human Molecular Genetics, 17*(24), 3837–3846.

Zanella, S., Mebarek, S., et al. (2008). Oral treatment with desipramine improves breathing and life span in Rett syndrome mouse model. *Respiratory Physiology & Neurobiology, 160*(1), 116–121.

Zappella, M., Genazzani, A., et al. (1990). Bromocriptine in the Rett syndrome. *Brain & Development, 12*(2), 221–225.

Zheng, W. H., & Quirion, R. (2004). Comparative signaling pathways of insulin-like growth factor-1 and brain-derived neurotrophic factor in hippocampal neurons and the role of the PI3 kinase pathway in cell survival. *Journal of Neurochemistry, 89*(4), 844–852.

Zhou, Z., Hong, E. J., et al. (2006). Brain-specific phosphorylation of MeCP2 regulates activity-dependent BDNF transcription, dendritic growth, and spine matura-tion. *Neuron, 52*(2), 255–269.

Zocchi, L. and P. Sassone-Corsi (2012). SIRT1-mediated deacetylation of MeCP2 con-tributes to BDNF expression. *Epigenetics, 7*(7), 695–700.

CHAPTER 7

Cardio-Facio-Cutaneous Syndrome and Other RASopathies

Prospects for Treatment

WILLIAM E. TIDYMAN AND KATHERINE A. RAUEN

INTRODUCTION

Cardio-facio-cutaneous syndrome (CFC) was first described in a small cohort of three individuals who had unique craniofacial dysmorphology, ectodermal anomalies, and cardiac defects (Blumberg, Shapiro, et al., 1979). These three patients, along with five others, were subsequently reported as a new syndrome due to their common phenotypical features (Reynolds, Neri, et al., 1986). CFC is now known to be one in a group of syndromes known as *RASopathies* (Tidyman & Rauen, 2009). The RASopathies are a class of human genetic syndromes caused by germline mutations in genes that encode protein components of the Ras/mitogen-activated protein kinase (MAPK) pathway (Figure 7.1). The Ras/MAPK pathway is essential in the regulation of the cell cycle, differentiation, growth, and senescence, all of which are critical to normal mammalian development. The Ras/MAPK pathway has been extensively studied in the context of cancer since Ras was found to be somatically mutated in approximately 20% of malignancies (Bos, 1989), and hyperactivated extracellular signal-regulated kinase (ERK) is found in approximately 30% of human cancers due to activating mutations in either Ras or BRAF (Hoshino, Chatani, et al., 1999).

The Ras/MAPK pathway is an attractive target in the treatment of cancer, utilizing small molecule therapeutics that specifically inhibit the pathway. Many are in development and several are currently undergoing clinical trials, with some already FDA approved (Sebolt-Leopold, 2008). Because of

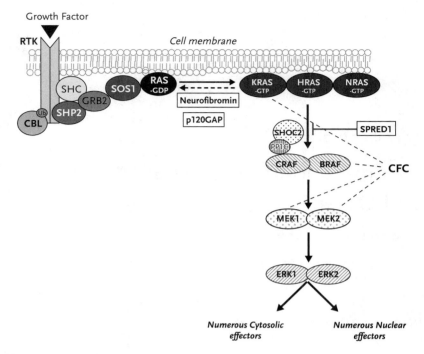

Figure 7.1:
The Ras/mitogen-activated protein kinase (MAPK) signaling pathway. The MAPK signaling pathway of protein kinases is highly conserved among eukaryotic organisms and is critically involved in cell proliferation, differentiation, survival, apoptosis, and senescence. The Ras/Raf/MEK/ERK signal transduction pathway is activated by multiple extracellular stimuli. Ras cycles between a GDP-bound, inactive state, and a GTP-bound active state. The transition between these two states is controlled by GTPase stimulating proteins (GAPs) and guanine exchange factors (GEFs). Activated Ras recruits Raf to the plasma membrane, which results in its activation. Active Raf, the first kinase of the cascade, phosphorylates MEK1 and/or MEK2, which then phosphorylates ERK1 and/or ERK2, the terminal effectors of the pathway. CFC is caused by activating germline mutations in *BRAF, MEK1/MAP2K1, MEK2/MAP2K2* and *KRAS*. CFC is one of the RASopathies, which also includes Noonan syndrome (NS) caused by activating mutations in *Shp2, SOS1, CRAF, KRAS, NRAS, SHOC2* and *CBL*; NS with multiple lentigines, caused by alteration of function of *Shp2*; capillary malformation-AV malformation, caused by haploinsufficiency of *RASA1*; neurofibromatosis type 1 (NF1), caused by inactivating mutations in the *NF1* gene; Costello syndrome, caused by activating mutations in *HRAS*; and Legius syndrome, caused by haploinsufficiency of SPRED1.

such intense focus on pathway inhibition, small molecular inhibitors such as RAF and MEK inhibitors may be of therapeutic use for syndromes in this pathway, especially for CFC. Thus, the same molecular inhibitors of the Ras/MAPK pathway for cancer may provide opportunities to therapeutically treat the developmental disorders caused by germline Ras/MAPK hyperactivation. Because many of the phenotypic signs and symptoms of the RASopathies are not static, the possible use of systemic therapies after birth to reduce MAPK activity holds the potential to ameliorate disease progression of some signs and symptoms.

CLINICAL PHENOTYPE

CFC syndrome is a rare, multiple congenital anomaly disorder character-ized by distinctive craniofacial features, congenital heart defects, psycho-motor delay, failure to thrive, and abnormalities of the skin and hair. CFC shares many overlapping phenotypical features with other RASopathies including Noonan and Costello syndromes (Rauen, 2006). Additionally, similar to Noonan and Costello syndromes, individuals with CFC display phenotypical variability and, therefore, each affected individual may not possess all characteristic features (Table 7.1). Craniofacial findings in CFC include macrocephaly, broad forehead, bitemporal narrowing, hypoplasia of the supraorbital ridges, down-slanting palpebral fissures with ptosis, short nose with depressed nasal bridge and anteverted nares, a high-arched palate, and low-set, posteriorly rotated, ears with prominent helices (Figure 7.2). Ectodermal findings typically consist of sparse, curly hair with sparse eyebrows and eyelashes, hyperkeratosis, keratosis pilaris, ulery-thema ophryogenes, hemangioma, progressive nevi formation, and ichthy-osis (Siegel, McKenzie, et al., 2011). Cardiac anomalies occur in about 80% of individuals, with pulmonic stenosis, septal defects and hypertrophic cardiomyopathy being the most prevalent. CFC individuals have a skeletal myopathy (Tidyman, Lee, et al., 2011) and are hypotonic with peripheral muscle weakness (Stevenson, Allen, et al., 2012). Musculoskeletal abnor-malities are common and include scoliosis, kyphosis, anterior chest wall anomalies, pes planus, and osteopenia (Stevenson and Yang, 2011). Ocular abnormalities, including strabismus, nystagmus, myopia, hyperopia, and astigmatism, are also common (Young, Ziylan, et al., 1993). Failure to thrive is typical in infancy, as is gastrointestinal dysfunction such as reflux, vomiting, oral aversion, and constipation (Sabatino, Verrotti, et al., 1997; Grebe & Clericuzio, 2000). Intestinal malrotation and renal anomalies are also common (Herman & McAlister, 2005). In addition, some instances of chylothoaces and lymphedema have been reported at birth (Chan, Chiu, et al., 2002).

Neurological abnormalities of some degree are universally present in CFC, which distinguishes it from Noonan syndrome. These include hypo-tonia, motor delay, speech delay, and learning disability (Yoon, Rosenberg, et al., 2007). Macrocephaly, ptosis, strabismus, and nystagmus are pres-ent in more than 50% of individuals, and corticospinal tract are findings

Table 7.1 GENERAL PHENOTYPICAL CHARACTERISTICS OF
CARDIO-FACIO-CUTANEOUS SYNDROME

Features	
Craniofacial Characteristics	High forehead, relative macrocephaly, bitemporal narrowing, hypoplasia of the supraorbital ridges, down-slanting palpebral fissures, epicanthal folds, ptosis, short nose with depressed bridge, anteverted nares, low-set and posteriorly rotated ears, ear lobe creases, deep philtrum, cupid's bow lip
Cardiac	Pulmonary valve stenosis, septal defects, valve dysplasia, hypertrophic cardiomyopathy, arrhythmias
Gastrointestinal	Gastroesophageal dysmotility and reflux, aspiration, vomiting, oral aversion, intestinal malrotation, constipation, splenomegaly, hepatomegaly
Growth	Failure to thrive, most with short stature, some with growth hormone deficiency
Neurological	Hypotonia, seizure disorders, ventriculomegaly, hydrocephalus, prominent Virchow-Robin spaces, abnormal myelination, Chiari malformation, structural anomalies
Cognition	Most with cognitive delay and/or learning disabilities, ranging from mild to severe
Ophthalmological Anomalies	Ocular hypertelorism, strabismus, nystagmus, astigmatism, myopia and/or hyperopia, optic nerve hypoplasia, cortical blindness, cataracts
Musculoskeletal Abnormality	Short neck, pterygium colli, pectus deformity, kyphosis and/or scoliosis, osteopenia, myopathy peripheral muscle weakness
Dermatologic—Skin	Xerosis, keratosis pilaris, ichthyosis, ulerythema oophorogenes, eczema, hemangiomas, café-au-lait macules, erythema, pigmented nevi, palmoplantar hyperkeratosis
Dermatologic—Hair	Sparse, curly, fine; or thick, woolly, or brittle; absent or normal eyelashes and eyebrows
Hematological and Lymphatic Abnormalities	Localized or generalized lymphedema, chylous pleural effusions

present in 32%. Ventriculomegaly or hydrocephalus are present in about 66% of CFC individuals, and seizures in about 38%. Additional neurological findings on MRI imaging include Virchow-Robin (perivascular) spaces, abnormal myelination, and brain structural anomalies.

It is unclear if individuals with CFC are at an increased risk for malignancies. Neoplasms, such as benign papillomas or malignancies observed in other RASopathies, have not been reported in CFC. Individuals with CFC may be at increased risk for acute lymphoblastic leukemia, although this has yet to be firmly established (Rauen, Tidyman, et al., 2010).

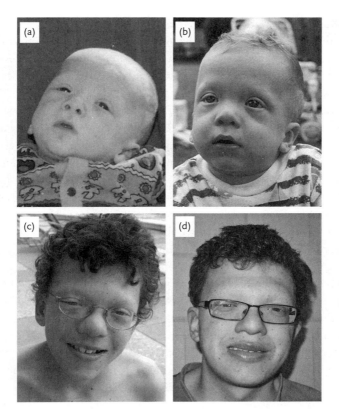

Figure 7.2:
Clinical images of an individual with cardio-facio-cutaneous syndrome (CFC) at different ages. (a) Newborn image of a male child who harbors a *MEK2* mutation. He has scant hair, lacks eyebrows, has down-slanting palpebral fissures with a short, upturned nose, and a cupid's bow upper lip. (b) By 10 months of age, his temporal alopecia persists. He still lacks eyebrows, and his low-set ears are more noticeable. (c) At 12 years old, his hair is very curly, and progressive mole formation becomes very noticeable. (d) At nearly 20 years old, his facial features are coarser, with numerous moles on his face.

MOLECULAR PATHOLOGY OF CFC SYNDROME

The Ras/MAPK pathway is one of several intracellular signaling cascades that exist in all eukaryotic cells and controls such fundamental cellular processes as proliferation, differentiation, survival, and apoptosis. The Ras/MAPK pathway is very complex, with multiple steps in the cascade allowing for both amplification of the input and branching of extracellular signaling to multiple pathways and effectors, but the pathway also allows for numerous regulatory inputs such that the strength, duration, and cell specificity of the pathway output is exquisitely controlled.

The Ras/MAPK pathway transduces extracellular input in the form of growth factors and small molecules to the intracellular environment (Figure 7.1). The pathway has been studied extensively in the context of oncogenesis, since its dysregulation is one of the primary causes of cancer. Ras proteins are small guanosine nucleotide-bound GTPases that comprise a critical signaling hub within the cell. Ras genes exist as a multigene family that includes HRAS, NRAS, and KRAS. They are activated through growth factors binding to receptor tyrosine kinases (RTK), G-protein-coupled receptors, cytokine receptors, and extracellular matrix receptors (for review, see Hancock, 2003). Ras proteins are capable of switching between an active conformation bound by GTP, and an inactive form bound by GDP. Activation through RTK occurs with the binding of a growth factor causing RTK auto-phosphorylation and interaction with the adaptor protein Grb2. Grb2 is bound to SOS, which is then recruited to the plasma membrane. SOS proteins are guanine nucleotide exchange factors (GEF) that increase the Ras nucleotide exchange rate of GDP for GTP, resulting in an increase in the active GTP-bound form of Ras. The MAPK pathway is one of several important downstream cascades of Ras. Activated Ras leads to the activation of Raf (ARAF, BRAF, and/or CRAF), the first MAPK kinase kinase of the cascade. Raf phosphorylates and activates MEK1 and/or MEK2 (MAPK kinase), which in turn phosphorylates and activates ERK1 and/or ERK2. ERK1 and ERK2 MAPKs are the ultimate effectors and exert their function on a large number of downstream molecules, both nuclear and cytosolic. ERK1/2 substrates include nuclear components, transcription factors, membrane proteins, and protein kinases (Yoon & Seger, 2006). Importantly, signaling through the pathway is terminated by the hydrolysis of Ras-bound GTP to GDP by a slow intrinsic Ras GTPase activity, or by Ras GTPase activity stimulated by GTPase activating proteins (GAPs) (Donovan, See, et al., 2002). The Ras/ MAPK pathway is downregulated by numerous phosphatases and specific pathway inhibitors such as SPRED1, which suppresses Ras activation of Raf, and MAP kinase phosphatase-1, which dephosphorylates ERK1/2 (Owens & Keyse, 2007).

At the present time, four known genes that encode proteins of the Ras/ MAPK pathway have been associated with CFC syndrome (Figure 7.1): BRAF (Niihori, Aoki, et al., 2006; Rodriguez-Viciana, Tetsu, et al., 2006), MEK1/ MAP2K1 and MEK2/MAP2K2 (Rodriguez-Viciana, Tetsu, et al., 2006), and KRAS (Niihori, Aoki, et al., 2006; Schubbert, Zenker, et al., 2006). The role of KRAS remains unclear in CFC, since KRAS mutations have also been identified in individuals clinically diagnosed with Noonan syndrome, as well as CFC.

BRAF Mutations

Heterozygous *BRAF* mutations are found in approximately 75% of mutation-positive CFC individuals (for review, see Tidyman and Rauen, 2009). BRAF is one member of the Raf family, along with CRAF and ARAF. *BRAF* is located on chromosome 7q34, contains 18 exons, and spans approximately 190 kb. BRAF is a serine/threonine protein kinase and is one of several direct downstream effectors of Ras (for review, see Wellbrock, Karasarides, et al., 2004). There are three conserved regions in BRAF. Conserved region 1 (CR1) is part of the regulatory amino-terminal region and contains the Ras binding domain and the cysteine-rich domain. Both of these domains are required for recruitment of BRAF to the cell membrane. CR2, also part of the N-terminal region, is the smallest of the conserved regions, but is serine- and threonine-rich and contains regulatory phosphorylation sites. CR3 encompasses the kinase domain and contains a glycine rich loop (exon 11) and the activation segment (exon 15) of the catalytic domain. BRAF is a known onco-protein, with somatic mutations reported in several different types of malignancies, including skin, thyroid, lung, ovarian, and colorectal cancer (Wan, Garnett, et al., 2004). Although the majority of *BRAF* mutations associated with CFC are novel, a small number are also found as somatic mutations in human cancer.

The most common CFC *BRAF* mutation is in exon 6, p.Q257R, followed by exon 12, p.E501 and exon 11, p.G469E. *In vitro* functional analyses of the BRAF mutant proteins have shown that the majority have increased kinase activity; however, a few mutant proteins are kinase-impaired (Niihori, Aoki, et al., 2006; Rodriguez-Viciana, Tetsu, et al., 2006). Interestingly, BRAF kinase impairment also causes increased MAPK pathway activity through CRAF activation (Heidorn, Milagre, et al., 2010). In addition, *in vivo* studies of CFC mutations in zebrafish demonstrated that both kinase-active and kinase-impaired mutations resulted in similar phenotypical activation of MAPK signaling (Anastasaki, Estep, et al., 2009).

MEK1/MAP2K1 and MEK2/MAP2K2 Mutations

Mutations in *MEK1/MAP2K1* and *MEK2/MAP2K2*, which encode the only known downstream effectors of BRAF, also cause CFC (Rodriguez-Viciana, Tetsu, et al., 2006). *MEK*, like the Raf genes, exists as a multigene family (Pearson, Robinson, et al., 2001). The *MEK1* gene is located on chromosome 15q22.31 and spans approximately 104 Kb. *MEK2* is located on chromosome 19p13.3 and spans approximately 34 Kb. Each *MEK* gene contains 11 exons with intervening sequences. The *MEK1* gene encodes the mitogen-activated protein kinase 1 (MEK1); likewise, *MEK2* encodes the protein MEK2. MEK1 and MEK2 are threonine/tyrosine kinases, with both isoforms having the ability to activate ERK1 and ERK2. The MEK1/2 proteins have about 85% amino acid identity (Wu, Harrison, et al., 1993) but do not serve redundant purposes (Brott, Alessandrini, et al., 1993; Alessandrini, Brott, et al., 1997). *MEK1* and *MEK2* mutations comprise approximately 25% of mutations in CFC individuals in which a gene mutation has been identified (for review, see Tidyman and Rauen, 2009). The vast majority of these are missense substitutions located in exons 2 and 3. The most common mutation is MEK1 p.Y130C, comprising approximately 40% of all the MEK mutations. Rare in-frame deletions have also been identified (Nava, Hanna, et al., 2007; Yoon, Rosenberg, et al., 2007). Functional studies on MEK mutant CFC proteins have shown that all are activating (Rodriguez-Viciana, Tetsu, et al., 2006; Estep, Palmer, et al., 2007).

DIAGNOSTIC METHODS

The initial diagnosis of CFC is based on clinical findings, typically involving characteristic craniofacial features, a heart anomaly, skin abnormalities, and developmental delay. A clinical diagnosis in the newborn period can be challenging, as many of the phenotypical features of CFC overlap with those of other RASopathies. Molecular genetic testing is exceptionally helpful to identify a mutation in one of the four genes known to be associated with CFC syndrome, *BRAF* (~75%), *MEK1* or *MEK2* (~25%), or *KRAS* (<2%). If a medical geneticist has a clinical suspicion of the gene that may be affected, single gene testing, by direct gene sequencing, may be done in a step-wise fashion beginning with the most commonly mutated gene, *BRAF* (exons 6, 11–17). If no causal mutation is identified, then one may move on to direct sequencing of specific exons of *MEK1/MAP2K1* (exons 2, 3, and 6) and *MEK2/MAP2K2* (exons 2, 3, and 7). If after this no causal mutation has been identified, then direct sequencing of *KRAS* may be performed where additional causal mutations have been demonstrated in individuals with a phenotype that overlaps with CFC. An alternative method for the molecular diagnosis of an individual suspected of having CFC is use of a multi-gene panel encompassing known causative RASopathy genes of the Ras/MAPK pathway. Such a molecular diagnostic test is now offered. The importance of determining the genetic etiology using molecular genetic testing is several-fold. Noonan syndrome and CFC have phenotypical overlap; thus, determining the genetic etiology by molecular testing is important to establish the correct diagnosis in an individual, as Noonan syndrome may be familial and thus inherited in an autosomal-dominant manner, whereas the majority of CFC individuals are singletons. Molecular information obtained through genetic testing is essential in the continuing effort to establish genotype/phenotype correlations for specific mutations. This will be of benefit in predicting the medical needs and directing the medical management of CFC patients. Additionally, the identification regarding which gene is mutated and the specific mutations will be critical in the context of clinical trials using small molecular inhibitors to treat CFC.

RELATED DISORDERS—OTHER RASOPATHIES

The RASopathies are a class of human genetic syndromes caused by germline mutations in genes that encode protein components of the Ras/mitogen-activated protein kinase (MAPK) pathway (Tidyman and Rauen, 2009, Fig. 2). Taken together, the RASopathies are one of the largest groups of malformation syndromes known, affecting approximately 1:1000 individuals. Mutations in these components all have a similar underling pathogenetic mechanism causing increased Ras/MAPK pathway activation. These syndromes include:

1. Noonan syndrome (NS) caused by activating mutations in *PTPN11* (Tartaglia, Mehler, et al., 2001), *SOS1* (Roberts, Araki, et al., 2007; Tartaglia, Pennacchio, et al., 2007), *RAF1* (Pandit, Sarkozy, et al., 2007; Razzaque, Nishizawa, et al., 2007), *KRAS* (Schubbert, Zenker, et al., 2006), *NRAS* (Cirstea, Kutsche, et al., 2010), *SHOC2* (Cordeddu, Di Schiavi, et al., 2009), and *CBL* (Martinelli, De Luca, et al., 2010; Niemeyer, Kang, et al., 2010);
2. NS with multiple lentigines caused by mutations in *PTPN11* (Digilio, Conti, et al., 2002) and *RAF1* (Pandit, Sarkozy, et al., 2007);
3. Capillary malformation-AV malformation (CM-AVN) caused by haploinsufficiency of the *RASA1* gene (Eerola, Boon, et al., 2003);
4. Costello syndrome (CS) caused by activating mutations in *HRAS* (Aoki, Niihori, et al., 2005);
5. Neurofibromatosis type 1 (NF1) caused by inactivating mutations in the *NF1* gene (Wallace, Marchuk, et al., 1990) and
6. Legius syndrome caused by inactivating mutations in the *SPRED1* gene (Brems, Chmara, et al., 2007).

The RASopathies each exhibit unique phenotypes; however, due to the common underlying mechanism of Ras/MAPK pathway dysregulation, they share numerous overlapping characteristics, including craniofacial dysmorphology; cardiac malformations; cutaneous, musculoskeletal, and ocular abnormalities; neurocognitive impairment; hypotonia; and an increased cancer risk.

CURRENT TREATMENT AND MANAGEMENT

CFC syndrome affects many organ systems, therefore, the vast majority of individuals require ongoing care by a multidisciplinary team of healthcare providers, preferable in a specialty genetics clinic. At present, there are no systemic therapies; because of this, deleterious phenotypical features caused by germline mutations in *BRAF, MEK1, MEK2,* or *KRAS* are treated as they would be in the general population. Cardiovascular management is dictated by the abnormality and usually managed by a pediatric cardiologist. Since many of the cardiovascular issues faced by patients with CFC also occur in the general pediatric population, standard medical treatments for these conditions are usually followed. If necessary, structural cardiac defects are treated surgically. Signs of hypertrophic cardiomyopathy are monitored by serial echocardiograms, whereas cardiac arrhythmias are medically managed in an aggressive manner. Severe feeding issues during the first years of life often require management by a pediatric gastroenterologist. Many children with CFC syndrome require nasogastric, or gastrostomy tube feeding because of failure to thrive. Increasing caloric intake may be of benefit to these patients. In addition, children with severe gastroesophageal reflux may require a Nissen fundoplication. Constipation affects the majority of individuals, so increased fiber in the diet, under the direction of a pediatrician, may be beneficial. Seizures are treated as in the general population. However, seizures may be refractory to single-agent therapy and may require polytherapy. Some individuals are growth-hormone deficient and may benefit from management by an endocrinologist. Ocular abnormalities such as myopia or hyperopia are corrected with lenses, and musculoskeletal abnormalities, such as scoliosis or pectus deformity, are managed as in the general population. Skin issues such as xerosis and pruritus may be relieved by increasing the ambient humidity or using hydrating lotions.

DEVELOPMENT OF RAS/MAPK PATHWAY TARGETED TREATMENT

The underlying molecular cause of the RASopathies is dysregulation of the Ras/MAPK pathway, which causes hyperactive ERK signaling. This makes pharmacological inhibition of the Ras/MAPK pathway signaling an attractive target for potential therapeutic treatment of these syndromes. Since the Ras/MAPK pathway is also frequently hyperactivated in cancer, numerous inhibitors of components of the pathway are under development as anti-cancer therapeutic agents. Ras pathway agents, such as farnesyl transferase inhibitors that prevent posttranslational modification of Ras, are being evaluated for cancer treatment and may be of therapeutic use for syndromes in this pathway. In addition, BRAF and MEK inhibitors offer the great potential in the possible treatment of the RASopathies, including CFC. Thus, the same molecular inhibitors developed for cancer treatment may provide opportunities to therapeutically treat the developmental disorders caused by germline mutations that hyperactivate the Ras/MAPK pathway. In addition, since many of the phenotypical features of the RASopathies progress throughout development and with aging, the use of systemic therapies after birth to normalize MAPK activity holds great potential to ameliorate the progression of deleterious phenotypes.

Studies utilizing RASopathy animal models have successfully demonstrated the effectiveness of Ras/MAPK pathway-specific inhibitors in reducing some of the phenotypical features associated with these syndromes. In particular, MEK1/2 specific inhibitors that block phosphorylation and activation ERK1/2 have shown great potential. The specific MEK1/2 inhibitor U0126 was shown to reduce the deleterious phenotype in a mouse model for Apert syndrome (Shukla, Coumoul, et al., 2007). Apert syndrome is caused by germline missense mutations in fibroblast growth factor receptor 2 (FGFR2), which results in constitutive activation of the Ras/MAPK pathway. It is characterized by a severe form of craniosynostosis that causes premature fusion of cranial sutures. This mouse model harbors an activating $Fgfr2^{S252W}$ mutation and mimics the abnormal cranial development characteristic of the syndrome. Mutant mice treated with U0126 restored normal Ras/MAPK signaling. In mice treated prenatally, abnormal cranial development was completely repressed, whereas with treatment postnatally it was significantly reduced.

Targeted treatment based on inhibition of the Ras/MAPK pathway has also been examined in several NF1 mouse models. NF1 is caused by heterozygous loss-of-function mutations in the NF1 gene that result in constitutive activation of Ras and hyperactivation of Ras/MAPK signaling. A significant portion of NF1 patients have neurocognitive impairment, with some having underlying structural brain abnormalities, including an enlarged corpus callosum. A mouse model for NF1 that has a conditional homozygous inactivation of Nf1 in neural progenitor cells mimics the brain abnormalities seen in NF1 patients. Mice treated postnatally, from P0.5 to P18 with the specific MEK inhibitor PD0325901, demonstrated normalization of fate determination of neural progenitor cells and a reduction in structural brain defects (Wang, Kim, et al., 2012). NF1 patients also develop benign neurofibromas, and some develop malignant peripheral nerve sheath tumors (MPNST) due to the hyperactivation of the Ras/MAPK pathway. The NF1 mouse model $Nf1^{fl/fl;DhhCre}$ conditionally ablates $Nf1$ in Schwann cell precursors and mimics the development of neurofibromas and MPNST seen in NF1 patients. Treatment of adult $Nf1^{fl/fl;Dhh-Cre}$ mice was shown to reduce aberrantly proliferating cells in neurofibromas and in MPNST, shrank neurofibromas in 80% of treated mice, and prolonged survival (Jessen, Miller, et al., 2013). Children with NF1 are predisposed to developing juvenile myelomonocyte leukemia (JMML). A NF1 mouse model $Nf1^{fl/fl;Mx1-Cre}$ that conditionally ablates $Nf1$ in hematopoetic cells produces a myeloproliferative neoplasm that accurately mimics JMML. Treatment of $Nf1^{fl/fl;Mx1-Cre}$ mutant adult mice with PD0325901 was shown to be effective in ameliorating the myeloproliferative disease and restoring normal erythropoiesis (Chang, Krisman, et al., 2013).

In addition, the use of the MEK inhibitor PD0325901 was successfully demonstrated in a mouse model for NS that carries a germline $Sos1^{E846K}$ activating mutation (Chen, Wakimoto, et al., 2010). This mutation results in increased Ras-GEF activity, causing sustained Ras activation. These mice exhibit several phenotypical features of NS such as facial dysmorphia, small size, reduced lifespan, and several cardiovascular defects, including ventricular septal defect, aortic valvular stenosis, and hypertrophic cardiomyopathy. Treatment with the MEK inhibitor PD032590 beginning prenatally, followed by postnatal treatment until day 28, normalized phosphorylation levels of ERK1/2. In addition, treated mice showed improved cranial dysmorphia and no signs of cardiac defects.

Using a zebrafish model for CFC that exhibits activation of the Ras/MAPK pathway and embryonic developmental defects associated with this activation, a large number of novel CFC mutations were screened and shown to be sensitive to MEK inhibitors (Anastasaki, Estep, et al., 2009). Moreover, it was shown that treatment with MEK inhibitors, including AZD6244, could normalize development (Anastasaki, Rauen, et al., 2012). The specific MEK inhibitor AZD6244 is a possible future therapeutic option for CFC, since this drug is currently in clinical trials for brain cancer. However, it was shown in the CFC zebrafish model that abrogating Ras/MAPK signaling can lead to severe developmental consequences. MEK inhibitors, including PD0325901, have also been reported to cause deleterious effects, such as visual disturbances, retinal vein occlusions, and neurological toxicities during clinical trials for cancer treatment (Rauen, Banerjee, et al., 2011). Because abrogating Ras/MAPK signaling has developmental consequences which can be easily observed in the CFC zebrafish, this model was used to assess whether low doses with MEK inhibitor could modulate Ras/MAPK signaling while avoiding detrimental effects on development. It was shown that low doses of MEK inhibition were sufficient to prevent the developmental defects in BRAF CFC zebrafish embryos and promote normal development (Anastasaki, Rauen, et al., 2012). Therefore, unlike treatment strategies for cancers that aim to inhibit MAPK signaling completely, suboptimal treatment strategies that partially modulate the signal intensity may be sufficient to prevent some of the developmental features caused by CFC mutations.

Currently there are two mouse models for CFC that should prove useful in further elucidating the molecular etiology of CFC and in the development of pharmacological intervention strategies targeting Ras/MAPK signaling in CFC. The first model consists of is a conditional knock-in mouse expressing a Cre-regulated *Braf* [L597V] mutation (Andreadi, Cheung, et al., 2012). The BRAF p.L597V mutation has been reported in both CFC and Noonan syndrome (Sarkozy, Carta, et al., 2009; Pierpont, Pierpont, et al., 2012) and results in an intermediate level of BRAF kinase activation typical of numerous other BRAF mutations shown to be causative for CFC (Rodriguez-Viciana, Tetsu, et al., 2006), as well as occurring somatically in some human cancers. The *Braf* [L597V] mouse phenocopies several of the hallmark characteristics of CFC, including reduced survival, small body size and weight, craniofacial dysmorphia, and cardiac abnormalities, including cardiac enlargement with thickening of the ventricular wall and septum caused by cardiomyocyte hypertrophy. Importantly, the *Braf* [L597V] mouse shows a significant increase in Ras/MAPK pathway activity, as indicated by increases in the phosphorylation of ERK. However, the mouse also demonstrated a predisposition towards the development of benign tumors with increased age, including skin papillomas and intestinal polyps, which are atypical in CFC.

The second CFC mouse model was generated by germline insertion of a hypomorphic *Braf* [V600E] allele which expresses at only 5–10% of the levels of wild-type BRAF (Urosevic, Sauzeau, et al., 2011). The level of kinase activation caused by the *Braf* [V600E] mutation is upwards of 50-fold higher than other mutations with CFC (Rodriguez-Viciana, Tetsu, et al., 2006) and is embryonically lethal (Mercer, Giblett, et al., 2005). The *Braf* [V600E] mutation is the most common somatic *BRAF* mutation found in human cancer, being found in 90% of cases (Davies, Bignell, et al., 2002).

Although 75% of individuals with CFC have *BRAF* mutations, the p.V600E mutation has never been identified as a causative mutation in CFC, probably because of its embryonic lethality (Rodriguez-Viciana, Tetsu, et al., 2006; Champion, Bunag, et al., 2011). This CFC mouse model expressing hypomorphic Braf p.V600E shows several phenotypical features characteristic of CFC, including decreased survival, reduced body size and weight, cardiac enlargement, and craniofacial dysmorphia. However, the cardiac enlargement present in this mouse model was associated with cardiomyocyte hyperplasia, not hypertrophy, which occurs in individuals with CFC. In addition, these mice showed neural defects, including an increased number of astrocytes, and developed abnormal behavioral characterized by hyperactivity and increased frequency of repetitive movements and seizures. The low levels of expression of the Braf p.V600E in the hypomorphic $Braf^{V600E}$ mouse was expected to approximate Ras/MAPK pathway hyperactivation typical of BRAF mutations causative of CFC. However, no increase was detected in the levels of phospho-ERK, which may limit the utility of this mouse model for investigating potential therapeutic agents that target inhibition of the Ras/MAPK pathway.

The data from animal models with an activated Ras pathway have supported the notion that phenotypes can be successfully normalized in both the prenatal and postnatal period by manipulating Ras/MAPK activity. Therefore, the possible use of systemic therapies after birth to reduce Ras/MAPK activity in CFC holds the potential to reduce the progression of the detrimental phenotype associated with CFC and provides support for moving towards clinical trials (Rauen, Banerjee, et al., 2011). Currently, there are approximately a dozen MEK inhibitors being evaluated in Phase I/II clinical trials for cancer treatment. The first clinical trial using a MEK inhibitor in a pediatric population is currently underway. The trial is a Phase I and pharmacokinetic study using the AstraZeneca compound AZD6244 for low-grade glioma. This trial will provide preliminary data about dose, safety, tolerability, and pharmacokinetics of a MEK inhibitor in a pediatric population and will serve as a starting point for further investigations of MEK inhibitors in non-cancer populations. It remains to be determined whether an efficacious dose for the treatment of CFC can be attained at levels sufficiently low to avoid possible side effects. Implementing clinical trials for CFC will require a step-wise approach: defining the best target population, choosing definitive endpoints, and selecting the appropriate small molecule inhibitor. Most importantly, clinical trials for the treatment of CFC, as well as the other RASopathies, will require close cooperation between basic and translational research, private industry, and advocacy organizations.

DISCLOSURES

Katherine A. Rauen and William E. Tidyman have no conflict of interest to disclose.

This work was supported in part by NIH/NIAMS R01AR062165.

Address correspondence to: Dr. Katherine A. Rauen, University of California, Davis Medical Center, Department of Pediatrics, Chief, Division of Genomic Medicine, UC Davis MIND Institute, 2825 50th Street, Room #2284, Sacramento, CA, 95817, Phone: (916) 703-0382, email: rauen@ucdavis.edu, and to Dr. William E. Tidyman, University of California Davis Medical Center, Department of Pediatrics, 2516 Stockton Blvd, Sacramento, CA, 95817, email: william.tidyman@ucdmc.ucdavis.edu.

REFERENCES

Alessandrini, A., Brott, B. K., et al. (1997). Differential expression of *MEK1* and *MEK2* during mouse development. *Cell Growth & Differentiation*, 8(5), 505–511.

Anastasaki, C., Estep, A. L., et al. (2009). Kinase-activating and kinase-impaired cardio-facio-cutaneous syndrome alleles have activity during zebrafish development and are sensitive to small molecule inhibitors. *Human Molecular Genetics*, 18(14), 2543–2554.

Anastasaki, C., Rauen, K. A., et al. (2012). Continual low-level MEK inhibition ameliorates cardio-facio-cutaneous phenotypes in zebrafish. *Disease Models & Mechanisms*, 5(4), 546–552.

Andreadi, C., Cheung, L. K., et al. (2012). The intermediate-activity (L597V)BRAF mutant acts as an epistatic modifier of oncogenic RAS by enhancing signaling through the RAF/MEK/ERK pathway. *Genes & Development*, 26(17), 1945–1958.

Aoki, Y., Niihori, T., et al. (2005). Germline mutations in HRAS proto-oncogene cause Costello syndrome. *Nature Genetics*, 37(10), 1038–1040.

Blumberg, B., Shapiro, L., et al. (1979). A New Mental Retardation Syndrome with Characterisitc Facies, Ichthyosis and Abnormal Hair. Report given at the March of Dimes Birth Defects Conference, Chicago, Il.

Bos, J. L. (1989). Ras oncogenes in human cancer: a review. *Cancer Research*, 49(17), 4682–4689.

Brems, H., Chmara, M., et al. (2007). Germline loss-of-function mutations in SPRED1 cause a neurofibromatosis 1-like phenotype. *Nature Genetics*, 39(9), 1120–1126.

Brott, B. K., Alessandrini, A., et al. (1993). MEK2 is a kinase related to MEK1 and is differentially expressed in murine tissues. *Cell Growth & Differentiation*, 4(11), 921–929.

Champion, K. J., Bunag, C., et al. (2011). Germline mutation in BRAF codon 600 is compatible with human development: de novo p.V600G mutation identified in a patient with CFC syndrome. *Clinical Genetics*, 79(5), 468–474.

Chan, P. C., Chiu, H. C., et al. (2002). Spontaneous chylothorax in a case of cardio-facio-cutaneous syndrome. *Clinical Dysmorphology*, 11(4), 297–298.

Chang, T., Krisman, K., et al. (2013). Sustained MEK inhibition abrogates myeloproliferative disease in Nf1 mutant mice. *Journal of Clinical Investigation*, 123(1), 335–339.

Chen, P. C., Wakimoto, H., et al. (2010). Activation of multiple signaling pathways causes developmental defects in mice with a Noonan syndrome-associated Sos1 mutation. *Journal of Clinical Investigation*, 120(12), 4353–4365.

Cirstea, I. C., Kutsche, K., et al. (2010). A restricted spectrum of NRAS mutations causes Noonan syndrome. *Nature Genetics, 42*(1), 27–29.

Cordeddu, V., Di Schiavi, E., et al. (2009). Mutation of SHOC2 promotes aberrant protein N-myristoylation and causes Noonan-like syndrome with loose anagen hair. *Nature Genetics, 41*(9), 1022–1026.

Davies, H., Bignell, G. R., et al. (2002). Mutations of the BRAF gene in human cancer. *Nature, 417*(6892), 949–954.

Digilio, M. C., Conti, E., et al. (2002). Grouping of multiple-lentigines/LEOPARD and Noonan syndromes on the PTPN11 gene. *American Journal of Human Genetics, 71*(2), 389–394.

Donovan, S., See, W., et al. (2002). Hyperactivation of protein kinase B and ERK have discrete effects on survival, proliferation, and cytokine expression in Nf1-deficient myeloid cells. *Cancer Cell, 2*(6), 507–514.

Eerola, I., Boon, L. M., et al. (2003). Capillary malformation-arteriovenous malformation, a new clinical and genetic disorder caused by RASA1 mutations. *American Journal of Human Genetics, 73*(6), 1240–1249.

Estep, A. L., Palmer, C., et al. (2007). Mutation analysis of BRAF, MEK1 and MEK2 in 15 ovarian cancer cell lines: Implications for therapy. *PLoS ONE, 2*(12), e1279.

Grebe, T. A., & Clericuzio, C. (2000). Neurologic and gastrointestinal dysfunction in cardio-facio-cutaneous syndrome: identification of a severe phenotype. *American Journal of Medical Genetics, 95*(2), 135–143.

Hancock, J. F. (2003). Ras proteins: different signals from different locations. *Nature Reviews Molecular Cellular Biology, 4*(5), 373–384.

Heidorn, S. J., Milagre, C., et al. (2010). Kinase-dead BRAF and oncogenic RAS cooperate to drive tumor progression through CRAF. *Cell, 140*(2), 209–221.

Herman, T. E., & McAlister, W. H. (2005). Gastrointestinal and renal abnormalities in cardio-facio-cutaneous syndrome. *Pediatric Radiology, 35*(2), 202–205.

Hoshino, R., Chatani, Y., et al. (1999). Constitutive activation of the 41-/43-kDa mitogen-activated protein kinase signaling pathway in human tumors. *Oncogene, 18*(3), 813–822.

Jessen, W. J., Miller, S. J., et al. (2013). MEK inhibition exhibits efficacy in human and mouse neurofibromatosis tumors. *Journal of Clinical Investigation, 123*(1), 340–347.

Martinelli, S., De Luca, A., et al. (2010). Heterozygous germline mutations in the CBL tumor-suppressor gene cause a Noonan syndrome-like phenotype. *American Journal of Human Genetics, 87*(2), 250–257.

Mercer, K., Giblett, S., et al. (2005). Expression of endogenous oncogenic V600EB-raf induces proliferation and developmental defects in mice and transformation of primary fibroblasts. *Cancer Research, 65*(24), 11493–11500.

Nava, C., Hanna, N., et al. (2007). CFC and Noonan syndromes due to mutations in RAS/MAPK signaling pathway: genotype/phenotype relationships and overlap with Costello syndrome. *Journal of Medical Genetics, 44*(12), 763–771.

Niemeyer, C. M., Kang, M. W., et al. (2010). Germline CBL mutations cause developmental abnormalities and predispose to juvenile myelomonocytic leukemia. *Nature Genetics, 42*(9), 794–800.

Niihori, T., Aoki, Y., et al. (2006). Germline KRAS and BRAF mutations in cardio-facio-cutaneous syndrome. *Nature Genetics, 38*(3), 294–296.

Owens, D. M., & Keyse, S. M. (2007). Differential regulation of MAP kinase signalling by dual-specificity protein phosphatases. *Oncogene, 26*(22), 3203–3213.

Pandit, B., Sarkozy, A., et al. (2007). Gain-of-function RAF1 mutations cause Noonan and LEOPARD syndromes with hypertrophic cardiomyopathy. *Nature Genetics*, *39*(8), 1007–1012.

Pearson, G., Robinson, F., et al. (2001). Mitogen-activated protein (MAP) kinase pathways: regulation and physiological functions. *Endocrine Reviews*, *22*(2), 153–183.

Pierpont, E. I., Pierpont, M. E., et al. (2012). Effects of germline mutations in the Ras/MAPK signaling pathway on adaptive behavior: cardiofaciocutaneous syndrome and Noonan syndrome. *American Journal of Medical Genetics A*, *152A*(3), 591–600.

Rauen, K. A. (2006). Distinguishing Costello versus cardio-facio-cutaneous syndrome: BRAF mutations in patients with a Costello phenotype. *American Journal of Medical Genetics A*, *140*(15), 1681–1683.

Rauen, K. A., Banerjee, A., et al. (2011). Costello and cardio-facio-cutaneous syndromes: Moving toward clinical trials in RASopathies. *American Journal of Medical Genetics. Part C, Seminars in Medical Genetics*, *157*(2), 136–146.

Rauen, K. A., Tidyman, W. E., et al. (2010). Molecular and functional analysis of a novel MEK2 mutation in cardio-facio-cutaneous syndrome: transmission through four generations. *American Journal of Medical Genetics. Part A*, *152A*(4), 807–814.

Razzaque, M. A., Nishizawa, T., et al. (2007). Germline gain-of-function mutations in RAF1 cause Noonan syndrome. *Nature Genetics*, *39*(8), 1013–1017.

Reynolds, J. F., Neri, G., et al. (1986). New multiple congenital anomalies/mental retardation syndrome with cardio-facio-cutaneous involvement—the CFC syndrome. *American Journal of Medical Genetics*, *25*(3), 413–427.

Roberts, A. E., Araki, T., et al. (2007). Germline gain-of-function mutations in SOS1 cause Noonan syndrome. *Nature Genetics*, *39*(1), 70–74.

Rodriguez-Viciana, P., Tetsu, O., et al. (2006). Germline mutations in genes within the MAPK pathway cause cardio-facio-cutaneous syndrome. *Science*, *311*(5765), 1287–1290.

Sabatino, G., Verrotti, A., et al. (1997). The cardio-facio-cutaneous syndrome: a long-term follow-up of two patients, with special reference to the neurological features. *Child's Nervous System*, *13*(4), 238–241.

Sarkozy, A., Carta, C., et al. (2009). Germline BRAF mutations in Noonan, LEOPARD, and cardiofaciocutaneous syndromes: molecular diversity and associated phenotypic spectrum. *Human Mutation*, *30*(4), 695–702.

Schubbert, S., Zenker, M., et al. (2006). Germline KRAS mutations cause Noonan syndrome. *Nature Genetics*, *38*(3), 331–336.

Sebolt-Leopold, J. S. (2008). Advances in the Development of Cancer Therapeutics Directed against the RAS-Mitogen-activated protein kinase pathway. *Clin Cancer Research*, *14*(12), 3651–3656.

Shukla, V., Coumoul, X., et al. (2007). RNA interference and inhibition of MEK-ERK signaling prevent abnormal skeletal phenotypes in a mouse model of craniosynostosis. *Nature Genetics*, *39*(9), 1145–1150.

Siegel, D. H., McKenzie, J., et al. (2011). Dermatological findings in 61 mutation-positive individuals with cardiofaciocutaneous syndrome. *The British Journal of Dermatology*, *164*(3), 521–529.

Stevenson, D. A., Allen, S., et al. (2012). Peripheral muscle weakness in RASopathies. *Muscle & Nerve*, *46*(3), 394–399.

Stevenson, D. A., & Yang, F. C. (2011). The musculoskeletal phenotype of the RASopathies. *American Journal of Medical Genetics. Part C, Seminars in Medical Genetics*, *157*(2), 90–103.

Tartaglia, M., Mehler, E. L., et al. (2001). Mutations in PTPN11, encoding the protein tyrosine phosphatase SHP-2, cause Noonan syndrome. *Nature Genetics, 29*(4), 465–468.

Tartaglia, M., Pennacchio, L. A., et al. (2007). Gain-of-function SOS1 mutations cause a distinctive form of Noonan syndrome. *Nature Genetics, 39*(1), 75–79.

Tidyman, W. E., Lee, H. S., et al. (2011). Skeletal muscle pathology in Costello and cardio-facio-cutaneous syndromes: developmental consequences of germline Ras/MAPK activation on myogenesis. *American Journal of Medical Genetics. Part C, Seminars in Medical Genetics, 157*(2), 104–114.

Tidyman, W. E., & Rauen, K. A. (2009). Molecular cause of cardio-facio-cutaneous syndrome. *Monographs in Human Genetics: Noonan Syndrome and Related Disorders—A Matter of Deregulated Ras Signaling.* Z.M. Bassel, Switzerland, Karger, Volume 17, 73–82.

Tidyman, W. E., & Rauen, K. A. (2009). The RASopathies: developmental syndromes of Ras/MAPK pathway dysregulation. *Current Opinion in Genetics & Development, 19*(3), 230–236.

Urosevic, J., Sauzeau, V., et al. (2011). Constitutive activation of B-Raf in the mouse germ line provides a model for human cardio-facio-cutaneous syndrome. *Proceedings of the National Academy of Sciences of the USA, 108*(12), 5015–5020.

Wallace, M. R., Marchuk, D. A., et al. (1990). Type 1 neurofibromatosis gene: identification of a large transcript disrupted in three NF1 patients. *Science, 249*(4965), 181–186.

Wan, P. T., Garnett, M. J., et al. (2004). Mechanism of activation of the RAF-ERK signaling pathway by oncogenic mutations of B-RAF. *Cell, 116*(6), 855–867.

Wang, Y., Kim, E., et al. (2012). ERK inhibition rescues defects in fate specification of Nf1-deficient neural progenitors and brain abnormalities. *Cell, 150*(4), 816–830.

Wellbrock, C., Karasarides, M., et al. (2004). The RAF proteins take centre stage. *Nature Reviews Molecular Cellular Biology, 5*(11), 875–885.

Wu, J., Harrison, J. K., et al. (1993). Identification and characterization of a new mammalian mitogen-activated protein kinase kinase, MKK2. *Molecular & Cellular Biology, 13*(8), 4539–4548.

Yoon, G., Rosenberg, J., et al. (2007). Neurological complications of cardio-facio-cutaneous syndrome. *Developmental Medicine & Child Neurology, 49*(12), 894–899.

Yoon, S., & Seger, R. (2006). The extracellular signal-regulated kinase: multiple substrates regulate diverse cellular functions. *Growth Factors, 24*(1), 21–44.

Young, T. L., Ziylan, S., et al. (1993). The ophthalmologic manifestations of the cardio-facio-cutaneous syndrome. *Journal of Pediatric Ophthalmology and Strabismus, 30*(1), 48–52.

CHAPTER 8

Targeted Treatments in Tuberous Sclerosis Complex (TSC)

PETRUS J. DE VRIES

INTRODUCTION

The term "tuberous sclerosis" was first coined by Bourneville, a French neurologist, in 1880. Bourneville described the case of a young girl at the La Salpêtrière Hospital in Paris who had severe intellectual disability and intractable epilepsy. After she died, postmortem examination of her brain showed that she had numerous white, hard, "potato-like" lesions on the surface of her brain, as well as multiple small subependymal nodules (Bourneville, 1880; Bourneville & Brissaud, 1881). There were earlier clinical case descriptions of similar phenomena documented by, for instance, Rayer (1835). The first description in English was published in 1890 by Pringle (1890), who described the case of a young woman who presented for consultation about her inability to have children. Pringle noted that she had a very unusual facial "rash" in a butterfly distribution over her nose and chin, sparing the upper lip. Bourneville had noted skin features in his cases, but attributed it to the bromide treatment used at the time to manage epilepsy. It was not until 1908 when Vogt recognized that the "cerebral tuberous sclerosis" described by Bourneville also included peripheral manifestations such as skin signs (Vogt, 1908). Moolten (1942) proposed the term "tuberous sclerosis complex" to refer to the multi-system nature of the disorder. The international consensus is to abbreviate the name to "TSC."

The century since first identification of the syndrome saw the emergence of detailed description of clinical features, the first set of diagnostic criteria by Manuel Gomez, a neurologist at the Mayo Clinic in the United States (see Gomez, 1988), and international revision of the Gomez criteria (Roach et al., 1998). Clinical case series and epidemiological studies confirmed the prevalence of TSC to be in the region of 1:10,000, with a birth incidence around 1:5,800 (Osborne et al., 1991). The disorder has an equal gender distribution, and individuals with TSC have been described worldwide. Prevalence rates suggest that there may therefore be 1–2 million people living with TSC across the globe.

Over the last two decades very significant progress has been made in understanding the pathophysiology of TSC. The *TSC2* gene was cloned in 1993, the *TSC1* gene in 1997 (Povey et al., 1994; European Chromosome 16 Tuberous Sclerosis Consortium, 1993; van Slegtenhorst et al., 1997). Both genes were recognized to be "tumor suppressors" of unknown function. Within the next five years, hamartin and tuberin, the protein products of *TSC1* and *TSC2*, respectively, were shown to act as a heterodimer intracellularly. Soon thereafter, the TSC1-TSC2 (hamartin-tuberin) complex was identified as a critical component of the mTOR (mammalian Target of Rapamycin) signaling pathway, and loss of either *TSC1* or *TSC2* (as seen in the clinical disorder) was shown to lead to mTOR overactivation (for a summary, see Crino et al., 2006; Curatolo et al., 2008; Huang & Manning, 2008). Through the good fortune of science, an FDA (U.S. Food and Drug Administration) approved mTOR inhibitor existed, and very rapidly the TSC basic and clinical scientific community were able to progress to animal and clinical trials of mTOR inhibitors for various features of TSC. In 2010–2012, everolimus, an mTOR inhibitor, was licensed by the FDA (www.fda.gov) and EMA (European Medicines Agency, www.ema.europa.eu) for the treatment of two TSC manifestations—subependymal giant cell astrocytomas (SEGAs) not amenable to curative surgery, and angiomyolipomas (AML) of the kidney larger than 3 cm. The first multi-center, international phase III randomized placebo-controlled trials were published in 2013 (Franz et al., 2013; Bissler et al., 2013). Various other clinical trials are underway to examine the safety and efficacy of mTOR inhibitors for the treatment of skin and lung features, epilepsy, and neuropsychiatric manifestations of TSC.

This chapter will outline some of the key features of this remarkable journey towards targeted treatments in tuberous sclerosis complex. We will first describe the clinical features of TSC, then summarize the molecular biology of the disorder, before proceeding to current management strategies and guidelines. In the final section, we will discuss pivotal findings in animal and human trials of mTOR inhibitors in TSC to date.

CLINICAL FEATURES OF TUBEROUS SCLEROSIS COMPLEX

TSC Is a Disorder with Variable Expression

Tuberous sclerosis complex is a multi-system disorder, and almost any organ can be affected. One of the key clinical challenges of TSC is the fact that clinical manifestations may have an extremely variable presentation (Crino et al., 2006; Curatolo et al., 2008; Kwiatkowski, Whittemore, & Thiele, 2010). Some individuals with TSC may have very mild and very few clinical features, while the severity and range of features in others may be profound. There are ongoing studies trying to understand this variability of expression at a molecular level, particularly with the aim of predicting likely manifestations and severity in individuals. To date there are no clear answers to this important question.

Genotype-phenotype studies have shown that, at a group-based level, *TSC2* mutations are associated with a more severe phenotype than *TSC1* (Jones et al., 1997; Dabora et al., 2001; Lewis et al., 2004; van Eeghen et al., 2012). However, variability of expression is large within both genotypes. At an individual level, knowing the mutation status or genotype of an individual does not yet have any robust predictive value.

TSC Has Age-Related Expression of Features

Many of the features of TSC have an age-related expression. Cortical tubers and subependymal nodules can be identified from about 16 weeks' gestation, and typically remain throughout the lifespan of an individual. Cardiac rhabdomyomas are typically present antenatally, and often spontaneously reduce in size or disappear during infancy or childhood (Curatolo et al., 2008; Kwiatkowski, Whittemore, & Thiele, 2010). Hypomelanotic macules (white patches) typically emerge in the first five years of life, while facial angiofibromata may become particularly pronounced towards adolescence. Angiomyolipoma of the kidney may be present from early childhood but may grow during and through adolescent years. SEGAs occur in 10–15% of individuals with TSC, and typically present in the first two decades of life. Lymphangiolyomyomatosis (LAM) of the lung typically develops in women with TSC in their 30s and 40s (Curatolo et al., 2008; Kwiatkowski, Whittemore, & Thiele, 2010).

The Physical Manifestations of TSC

Table 8.1 lists the main physical manifestations of TSC and the most likely ages of presentation (Curatolo et al., 2008; Kwiatkowski, Whittemore, &

Thiele, 2010). It is important to note that there have been very few longitudinal studies of the clinical features of TSC. There are international efforts to develop large-scale natural history studies, including an international study, TOSCA (TuberOus SClerosis registry to increase disease Awareness), which aims to identify and track 2,000 individuals with TSC over time (Jansen et al., 2013).

There are numerous other physical manifestations seen with TSC, and rare associations are described on a regular basis. Not all the features associated with TSC are regarded as diagnostic criteria. Table 8.1 also shows the physical characteristics that are part of the recently revised diagnostic criteria (marked with ** and *) (Northrup et al., 2013).

The Neuropsychiatric Manifestations of TSC

Tuberous sclerosis complex is associated with a vast range of neuropsychiatric manifestations across multiple levels of investigation. Similar to the physical phenotype of TSC, the neuropsychiatric features also have a wide range of variability, with about 10% of individuals very mildly affected, while about 30% are profoundly affected (de Vries & Prather, 2007; Joinson et al., 2003; de Vries, 2010a). The behavioral phenotype of TSC is therefore characterized by its variability. In spite of efforts to identify "subphenotypes," little progress has been made to date. Similarly, efforts to predict or understand the mechanisms underlying the phenotypical variability have not produced any robust findings. In particular, it has become clear that the number and location of cortical tubers are poor predictors of neuropsychiatric phenotype, as is the presence or type of epilepsy (de Vries & Howe, 2007; de Vries, 2010a). A few studies have investigated genotype–behavioral phenotype correlations in TSC (Lewis et al., 2004; van Eeghen et al., 2012). Similar to the physical phenotype, there is significant variability in the neuropsychiatric phenotype of both *TSC1* and *TSC2*. At present, clinicians are therefore advised not to use cortical tuber counts, presence or absence of epilepsy, or genotype as strong predictors of any neuropsychiatric phenotype in TSC. Below we will outline the different levels of investigation and manifestations typically seen in TSC. (For a more detailed account, please see de Vries, 2010a.)

Behavioral Manifestations

Here we use the term "behavioral" simply to refer to any observed behaviors causing concern to families or clinicians. There is evidence for a vast array

Table 8.1 PHYSICAL CHARACTERISTICS OF TUBEROUS
SCLEROSIS COMPLEX

Organ System Involved	Description	Typical Age at Onset
BRAIN		
Cortical dysplasias (Cortical Tuber (CT) and/or cerebral white matter radial migration lines)**	Potato-like white lesions in cerebral cortex or subcortical regions. Best detectable on FLAIR MRI images as hyperintense areas.	Prenatally
Subependymal Nodule (SEN)**	Small, hard growths in brain ventricles and adjacent subcortical matter. Typically appear in the thalamo-striatal region and close to Foramen of Munro. If calcified, detectable on CT scan of brain.	Presents prenatally. May calcify in childhood to adolescence.
Subependymal Giant Cell Astrocytoma (SEGA)**	SEN that show serial growth on MRI. Can become very large and lead to obstruction of cerebro-spinal fluid with resultant raised intracranial pressure (RICP), hydrocephalus, and papilloedema. SEGA may not show RICP until large in size.	Childhood to adolescence
Widespread Gray and White Matter Abnormalities		Prenatally. Becomes more pronounced into childhood as myelination progresses.
Epilepsy	Seen in at least 70% of individuals with TSC, often in complex combinations of seizure types that can be hard to treat.	Typically emerges in infancy and childhood, but can first present in adolescence or adulthood.
Infantile Spasms	Quick, sudden flexing movement of limbs, often referred to as "salaam spasms."	Typically emerge in first year of life.
SKIN		
Angiofibroma (≥3)**	Red, raised facial rash in butterfly distribution over nose and cheeks, sparing upper lip. May be confused with acne vulgaris.	Childhood to adulthood, often increases during adolescence
Ungual Fibroma (≥2)**	Growths in nail groove on hands and/or feet	Adolescence to adulthood
Shagreen Patch**	Coarse, thickened skin, typically in sacro-iliac region	Childhood

(continued)

Table 8.1 CONTINUED

Organ System Involved	Description	Typical Age at Onset
Hypomelanotic Macules (3 or more, at least 5 mm in diameter)**	White patches on skin, often only visible under Woods Lamp. Typically described as "ash-leaf" macules, but may often not have this typical appearance.	Infancy to childhood
"Confetti" Skin Lesions*	Groups of small, lightly pigmented spots	
EYES		
Multiple Retinal Hamartomas**	Hamartomatous growths in retina	Throughout life
Retinal Achromic Patch*		Throughout life
HEART		
Cardiac Rhabdomyoma**	Benign tumors in cardiac muscle, sometimes protruding into ventricles.	Prenatally. Typically reduces or disappears in childhood towards adolescence.
Wolff-Parkinson-White Syndrome	Supraventricular dysrhythmia sometimes seen in association with TSC.	Infancy to childhood
KIDNEYS		
Angiomyolipoma (two or more)**	Benign tumors of fat, smooth muscle, and blood vessels in kidneys. Can be single or multiple.	Childhood to adulthood. Typically increases during adolescence.
Multiple Renal Cysts*		
LUNG		
Lymphangioleio-myomatosis (LAM)**	Progressive cystic lesions of the lung. Lead to gradual deterioration in lung function; patient may become oxygen-dependent.	Adulthood. Almost exclusively seen in females.
OTHER MANIFESTATIONS		
Dental enamel pits (>3)*		
Intraoral fibromas (two or more)*		
Nonrenal hamartomas*		
Chordomas (rare)		
PNET (rare)		

**Major diagnostic criterion
*Minor diagnostic criterion
For a clinical diagnosis of "definite TSC," an individual needs to have two major criteria, or one major plus two or more minor criteria (Northrup et al., 2013).

of behavioral challenges, ranging from aggressive outbursts to self-injury, sleep problems, overactivity, restlessness, impulsivity, depressed and anxious mood, and social and communication problems (Hunt 1983, 1993; Prather & de Vries, 2004; de Vries et al., 2007; de Vries, 2010a). Some of these behaviors are correlated with the level of intellectual ability (de Vries et al., 2007; de Vries, 2010a). These include social and communication deficits, self-injury, and attention-related behaviors (overactivity, restlessness, impulsivity). In contrast, aggressive behaviors, temper tantrums, and mood features do not seem to correlate with the level of overall intellectual ability. Of clinical importance is the fact that all behavioral challenges are seen at high rates, even in children and adults with normal intellectual ability.

Psychiatric Manifestations

All behaviors causing concern require evaluation and consideration by clinicians and clinical teams, but not all cross thresholds to meet criteria for psychiatric disorders as defined in the *Diagnostic and Statistical Manual of Mental Disorders, 5th Edition* (DSM-5) or the *International Classification of Diseases, 10th Edition* (ICD-10) (APA, 2013; WHO, 1993). Tuberous sclerosis complex has a strong association with neurodevelopmental disorders, particularly autism spectrum disorder (ASD), attention-deficit hyperactivity disorder (ADHD), and intellectual disability (ID).

Autism spectrum disorders (ASD) are seen in about 50% of those with TSC (Bolton et al., 2002; de Vries et al., 2007; de Vries, 2010a). Even though there is a strong correlation between ASD and intellectual ability, with rates over 60% in those with ID, the rates of ASD in those with normal intellectual ability are still extremely high, at ~17% (de Vries et al., 2007). There is no clear evidence that the qualitative manifestations of ASD are distinct from those seen in individuals with ASD who do not have TSC. TSC has become a very interesting model in the study of mechanisms underlying the pathways to ASD, and is recognized as one of the medical conditions most commonly associated with ASD (Fombonne, 2003).

There have been fewer and less rigorous investigations of ADHD in TSC, but existing studies suggest that more than 50% of children with TSC may meet DSM criteria for ADHD (Gillberg et al., 1994; de Vries et al., 2007; de Vries, 2010a). Of clinical concern is the fact that, in one study, almost none of the children received a clinical workup for diagnosis and/or treatment for ADHD (de Vries, Gardiner, & Bolton, 2009). The study investigated the relationship between scores on the Connor Parent Rating Scale (CPRS), a widely used rating scale measure to suggest ADHD, and neuropsychological attention deficits, and showed that many children with TSC who did not have CPRS scores in the abnormal range had neuropsychological deficits. These results suggested that even children with TSC who do not present with features obviously suggestive of ADHD might have significant neuropsychological deficits in their attentional brain networks (de Vries, Gardiner, & Bolton, 2009) (Intellectual ability and disability will be discussed below).

Apart from the neurodevelopmental disorders, individuals with TSC are also at an increased risk of mood and anxiety disorders. There have been no systematic studies of bipolar mood disorder in TSC, but smaller-scale investigations have shown increased rates of depressive disorder and, in particular, anxiety disorder in adults with TSC. In a study performed by Lewis and colleagues, 60% of adults with TSC who had normal intellectual abilities met criteria for an anxiety disorder. Almost none of them had received a clinical diagnosis or treatment for their disorder (Lewis et al., 2004). To date, there is no clear evidence to suggest a raised rate of psychotic disorders in TSC. The reported rate of 1% is similar to the prevalence of schizophrenia in the general population (de Vries, 2010a). These data suggest that TSC may show a dissociation between neurodevelopmental and psychotic disorders, which may lend itself to interesting hypotheses regarding differential mechanisms of, for instance, ASD versus psychosis in the general population.

Intellectual Ability and Disability

Intellectual ability shows a bimodal distribution in TSC, in contrast to the majority of genetic disorders associated with neurodevelopmental disability that simply show a downward shift in the (unimodal) normal distribution of IQ. Approximately 70% of individuals with TSC fall on the typical normal distribution curve of IQ, but shifted downwards by 7–10 points (Joinson et al., 2003), while the remaining 30% fall in the profoundly impaired intellectual/developmental range with IQ/ Developmental Quotient score equivalents below 20. These results suggest two distinct intellectual phenotypes, referred to as the "normal distribution" (ND) phenotype and the "profound" (P) phenotype (de Vries & Prather, 2007). To date, there are no clear biomarkers to predict whether an individual will fall in the P or ND phenotype, or to predict where on the ND phenotype they are likely to fall. From a clinical perspective it is helpful to remind families that about 50% of those with TSC will have normal intellectual ability.

Clinicians and schools are often interested to know whether there is a specific intellectual profile of, for instance, stronger verbal versus performance/perceptual skills in TSC. Results by Prather and others (see de Vries, 2010a) showed that there is no predictable pattern of intellectual strengths and weaknesses, thus highlighting the need to perform an evaluation of each individual to determine their intellectual profile.

Scholastic/Academic Disorders

In spite of limited systematic data, the rates of specific disorders of learning (reading, writing, spelling, mathematics) appear to be high in TSC. A questionnaire-based approach suggested scholastic difficulties exist in at least 30% of school-aged children, including those with normal intellectual ability (de Vries, Gardiner, & Bolton, 2009; de Vries, 2010a).

Neuropsychological Profiles

There are no characteristic neuropsychological profiles or "signatures" in TSC. However, almost all individuals with TSC are at risk of having neuropsychological deficits in one or more domain of neuropsychological functioning (Prather & de Vries, 2004; de Vries, 2010a).

Executive and attention deficits appear to be the most commonly observed areas of weakness, with 50–75% of children and adults performing in the impaired range on one or more of these types of tasks (Ridler et al., 2007; de Vries, Gardiner, & Bolton, 2009; Tierney et al., 2011). Studies in children and adults with TSC revealed particular deficits in dual-tasking (divided attention), with deficits correlating with poor performance and feeling "overwhelmed easily" in daily life (Tierney et al., 2011). Many individuals have deficits in sustained auditory attention, but not typically in selective visual attention (de Vries, Gardiner, & Bolton, 2009; Tierney et al., 2011). Unilateral neglect (inability to attend to the left hemifield and preferentially attending to the right hemifield) has also been described in adults with TSC (McCartney, 2008; de Vries, 2010a). Executive deficits have been observed in attentional set-shifting, complex working memory, and planning in 40–60% of children and adults with TSC (Ridler et al., 2007; de Vries, 2010a).

Memory deficits have been described in about 30% of individuals, particularly in recall rather than recognition memory (Ridler et al., 2007; Davies et al., 2011). Visuospatial deficits are often seen in TSC, particularly where visuospatial constructional tasks are performed e.g. drawing a complex figure (Prather & de Vries, 2004; de Vries, 2010a).

Taking together all neuropsychological domains, a study of 21 adults with TSC who all had normal intellectual ability showed neuropsychological deficits (performance <5th percentile) in 20/21 participants. Eleven of the 21 had deficits in more than one domain (de Vries, 2010a). These and other results suggest that the majority of individuals with TSC have specific neuropsychological deficits.

THE MOLECULAR MECHANISMS OF TUBEROUS SCLEROSIS COMPLEX

Tuberous sclerosis complex is caused by a mutation in either the *TSC1* gene on chromosome 9q34 or the *TSC2* gene on chromosome 16p13.3 (van Slegtenhorst et al., 1997; European Chromosome 16 Tuberous Sclerosis Consortium, 1993). To date, mutational analysis can identify a disease-associated mutation in 85–90% of individuals with TSC (Kwiatkowski, Whittemore, & Thiele, 2010). A proportion of the missing mutations are attributable to low-level mosaicism. There are some research groups who are predicting that there might still be a third TSC gene, or related genes that might present with TSC-like phenotypes.

The protein products hamartin (TSC1) and tuberin (TSC2) are multifunctional proteins (Serfontein et al., 2011) and have domains to bind each other to form a heterodimer. More recent explorations of the quaternary structure of TSC1 and TSC2 have revealed that TSC1 and TSC2 interact to form large complexes containing multiple TSC1 and TSC2 subunits, rather than just heterodimers (Hoogeveen-Westerveld et al., 2012). This observation may have important implications for the functional consequences of different TSC mutations.

There is a wide range and location of mutations on *TSC1* and *TSC2*, including missense (rare in *TSC1*), nonsense, frame-shift, in-frame, and splice-site mutations. There are no obvious "hotspots" from mutations on any of the 21 *TSC1* coding exons or the 41 *TSC2* coding exons. Through the Leiden Open Variation Database (LOVD), a detailed TSC mutation database is curated by Professor Sue Povey and Dr. Rosemary Ekong (http://chromium.liacs.nl/LOVD2/TSC/home). To date, around 2,000 unique mutations have been submitted to the LOVD.

In contrast to earlier beliefs that all TSC mutations were null-mutations (that is, had a total loss of function), there is a growing body of evidence to show differential functional consequences of different *TSC1* and *TSC2* mutations. A recent examination of a range of *TSC2* mutations showed highly different profiles across mutations in relative levels of TSC2 and TSC1, as well as in the extent of phosphorylation of S6K at Threonine389 (Hoogeveen-Westerveld et al., 2013), supporting the notion of distinct functional consequences of different TSC mutations, implying distinct effects on TSC pathology (de Vries & Howe, 2007).

The TSC1-2 complex acts as a "molecular switchboard" and is a global regulator and integrator of a range of physiological processes (GRIPP) (de Vries & Howe, 2007; Crino et al., 2006; Curatolo et al., 2008; Huang & Manning, 2008; Kwiatkowski, Whittemore, & Thiele, 2010). Upstream, the TSC1-2 complex receives activating or inhibitory intracellular signals through the insulin signaling pathway (PI3K-AKT), through the mitogen-activated MAPK pathway (ERK1/2 and p38MAPK), and through the energy sensing AMPK pathway. Figure 8.1 shows a schematic representation of the TSC signaling pathway. For the primary evidence for intracellular signaling, see Huang and Manning, 2008; and Kwiatkowski, Whittemore, & Thiele, 2010.

The TSC1-2 complex directly inhibits Rheb (Ras homologue enriched in brain) by increasing the proportion of Rheb in its GDP state. Rheb in turn is an activator of mTOR (mammalian Target of Rapamycin). The mTOR

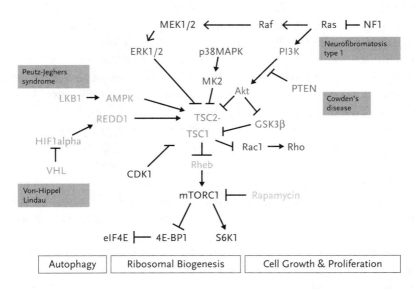

Figure 8.1:
Intracellular signaling in tuberous sclerosis complex
The TSC1-TSC2 complex acts as a molecular switchboard and integrates a range of upstream and downstream signals involved in core intracellular functions. The pathway is associated with a number of clinical conditions (shown in gray boxes). For further details, please see text.

protein complex has multiple, well-established roles in various aspects of intracellular signaling and functioning (Sarbassov, Ali, & Sabatini, 2005). It is present in two intracellular complexes, mTORC1 and mTORC2 (also referred to as TORC1 and TORC2). mTORC1 has roles in cell growth and proliferation, autophagy, ribosome biogenesis, and mRNA translation through activation of 4E-BP1 and S6K. mTORC2 appears to have roles in actin cytoskeletal function, metabolism, proliferation and cell survival through downstream outputs including Rho and PKCalpha.

The intracellular dynamics of TSC-mTOR proteins are clearly highly complicated, with new interacting proteins and intricacies discovered on an ongoing basis. At the most simplistic level, a mutation in the *TSC1* or *TSC2* gene leads to functional disturbance in the TSC1-2 complex, preventing its ability to receive and respond appropriately to upstream signals, and decreases the proportion of Rheb in its GDP state. Rheb-GTP leads to hyperphosphorylation of mTOR. As a result, a TSC mutation leads to mTOR overactivation. From a clinical perspective, TSC can therefore be conceptualized as an mTOR overactivation syndrome (de Vries & Howe, 2007; de Vries, 2010b; Kwiatkowski, Whittemore, & Thiele, 2010).

Given the role of mTOR in cell growth and proliferation, this mechanistic understanding has helped in understanding the basic pathophysiology of the disorder. (See, for instance, the description by Crino et al., 2006.) In cells and tissues with a TSC mutation, mTOR overactivation contributes to dysregulated growths, leading to skin, brain, and other tumors. In peripheral organs, it appears that loss of both TSC alleles is required (that is, loss of heterozygosity, LOH) to lead to the formation of tumors. In the brain, LOH is not required to lead to functional deficits (Crino et al., 2006). There is now ample evidence that heterozygous mutations are sufficient to lead to abnormalities in myelination, neuronal deficits, and so on.

The key observation of relevance to molecularly targeted treatments in TSC is the fact that the mTORC1 complex binds FKBP12-rapamycin and is inhibited by this interaction (Sarbassov, Ali, & Sabatini, 2005; de Vries, 2010b). In contrast, the mTORC2 complex is not rapamycin-sensitive under normal physiological conditions. Rapamycin (sirolimus) and other mTOR inhibitors such as everolimus therefore act as direct inhibitors of mTOR overactivation.

The evolutionary biology of the TSC proteins and related pathway proteins has revealed interesting results (Serfontein et al., 2010, 2011). Homologues of the TSC-TOR signaling pathway had been reported in animals, fungi, plants, and protozoa, and led to the impression that the proteins (and pathways) were evolutionarily conserved "throughout eukaryotes." Bioinformatic studies showed that the pathway was built up from a simpler one, probably to couple cell growth to energy signaling. Additional elements such as TSC1 and TSC2 were "bolted on" in particular eukaryotic lineages (Serfontein et al., 2010). Further exploration in different animal models (rat, mouse, zebrafish, fruit fly, and fission yeast) revealed that, while the structural and functional elements of the human TSC1 and TSC2 proteins showed high similarities to the rat and mouse sequences, this was not the case for *Danio rerio* (zebrafish), *Drosophila melanogaster* (fruit fly), *Schizosaccharomyces pombe* (fission yeast), or *Dictyostelium discoideum*. Findings therefore suggested caution in the interpretation of findings from these animal models of human TSC (Serfontein et al., 2011).

DIAGNOSING TUBEROUS SCLEROSIS COMPLEX

There are many possible routes to a diagnosis of TSC, but the most common is for an infant or child to present with seizures. MRI scan and physical workup may identify cortical tubers and other characteristics of the disorder. With improved prenatal ultrasound an increasing proportion of individuals are identified *in utero*, when cardiac rhabdomyomas are noted. Mildly affected parents are often only examined and diagnosed after a child has presented with clinical manifestations. While seizures are the most common reason for presentation, seizures themselves are not part of the diagnostic criteria for TSC. An International Consensus Panel was convened in 2012 to revise the diagnostic criteria for TSC. The revised criteria are not significantly different from the previously published criteria (Roach et al., 1998). The consensus panel did however make a few key changes which included adding genetic test results as a diagnostic criterion and reducing diagnostic classes from three (definite, probable, possible) to two (definite, possible) (Northrup et al., 2013).

Clinical Diagnostic Criteria

The clinical features typically associated with TSC are listed in Table 8.1. Major diagnostic criteria are indicated with a double asterisk (**) and so-called minor criteria are indicated with a single asterisk (*). For a clinical diagnosis of "definite TSC" an individual needs to have two major criteria or one major plus two or more minor criteria (Northrup et al., 2013). It has to be acknowledged that the diagnostic criteria have been developed based on clinical experience and expert opinion, rather than on careful analysis of diagnostic sensitivity and specificity using large datasets.

Given the variability of clinical manifestations, a strong emphasis is placed on doing a comprehensive workup of all newly diagnosed individuals. Given the age-related expression, it is also important to perform regular surveillance for the emergence of physical and neuropsychiatric features of TSC. General guidelines for initial evaluation and surveillance are presented below.

Initial Workup of Newly Diagnosed Individuals

Initial workup should be sufficiently comprehensive to identify all the diagnostic characteristics in every new individual with TSC (Roach et al., 1998; Roach et al., 1999; de Vries et al., 2005; Kwiatkowski, Whittemore, & Thiele, 2010; Krueger et al., 2013). Workup should start with a careful and detailed history, including a multigenerational genetic history and a careful history of all characteristics of TSC, including possible seizures, neurodevelopmental problems, and peripheral organ system involvement. Physical examination should consider all the diagnostic criteria, including dermatological examination, dental examination, eye examination, and screening for hypertension. Special investigations should include an MRI scan of the brain to look for cortical tubers (CT), subependymal nodules (SEN), and SEGAs; baseline routine EEG (wherever possible); MRI abdomen; ECG in the young; and pulmonary workup where required. Very importantly, comprehensive evaluation for all the TSC-associated neuropsychiatric disorders should be performed. Families should be offered genetic counseling, and, wherever possible, mutation analysis should be offered.

Surveillance Guidelines

In contrast to earlier views that further workup for individuals with TSC should be done as clinical symptoms emerge, there is now a significant body of evidence and strong consensus to suggest that a more pro-active approach to regular monitoring is required. All individuals with TSC are at high risk for a range of physical and neuropsychiatric manifestations, and should therefore have regular checks to screen for and identify problems as they emerge.

Consensus guidelines on surveillance of individuals with TSC were published in 2013 (Krueger et al., 2013). Recommendations outlined here are based on these guidelines.

For neurological manifestations, an MRI of the brain should be performed every one to three years in all individuals under the age of 25 to monitor for the development of SEGA. Individuals who already have SEGA should receive MRI monitoring significantly more frequently, and a multi-disciplinary team should discuss medical and surgical treatment options with individuals and their families.

Neuropsychiatric manifestations should be screened for at every clinic visit, and at least annually. The Neuropsychiatry Panel of the International Consensus Group undertook to develop a simple screening checklist to act as an *aide-mémoire* for clinicians to help in this task. This checklist, known as the TSC-Associated Neuropsychiatric Disorders Checklist (TAND Checklist) was under development and validation at the time of this writing (Leclezio et al., 2013). Apart from regular screening, individuals should also receive a comprehensive workup, as outlined in current assessment guidelines (de Vries et al., 2005; Krueger et al., 2013) at key stages. These include infancy, preschool years, early school years, middle school years, in adolescence, and—as required—in adulthood. The purposes of these evaluations are to ensure that a good baseline profile is established for each individual, and that problems are identified and managed as they emerge (Prather & de Vries, 2004; de Vries, 2010a).

Seizure disorders are very common in TSC, and individuals should therefore have regular monitoring for epilepsy, including routine (and more specialized) EEGs as required for known or suspected seizures.

Renal abnormalities also require ongoing monitoring. MRI abdomen is advised every one to three years. Renal function and blood pressure should be evaluated annually.

Skin and eye examination should be performed on an annual basis, dental examinations 6–12 monthly, and an ECG should be performed every one to three years in childhood until rhabdomyomas have disappeared.

RELATED DISORDERS

Disorders with Clinical Similarity to TSC

Whilst the diagnostic cluster of TSC features is unique, there are numerous differential possibilities when individuals may present with some of the characteristics suggestive of TSC. Here we outline a few possible areas of confusion.

Wolff-Parkinson-White syndrome (WPW) is a cardiac conduction disorder associated with a particular type of supraventricular tachycardia (O'Callaghan et al., 1998). There is an association between WPW and TSC. O'Callaghan and colleagues (1998) described a case series of 10 children with TSC who experienced WPW. WPW is also seen in association with other pathologies, including abnormalities in the *PRKAG2* gene (Gollob et al., 2001) and in association with Leber's hereditary optic neuropathy (LHON), a mitochondrial disorder (Mashima et al., 1996). Interestingly, it is also possible for WPW to confuse presentation in TSC—some of the clinical features of WPW include unexplained fainting or palpitations. These features have been attributed to anxiety disorders often seen in TSC, or to seizures commonly seen in TSC.

Hypomelanosis of Ito (HoI), also called *incontinentia pigmenti achromians*, is a rare disorder associated with areas of hypopigmented skin, typically in whorling patterns. HoI is often also associated with intellectual disability and seizures. The combination of these features may be confused with TSC. However, careful examination of the hypomelanosis should show a pattern quite distinct from that of TSC, in the absence of other diagnostic features of TSC. To date, only two cases of coexistence of TSC and HoI have been described (Muhammed & Mathew, 2007; Eussen et al., 2000).

Multiple neurological and neuropsychiatric disorders, including epilepsy, autism spectrum disorders, and intellectual disability, are commonly associated with TSC. As pointed out earlier, none of these is diagnostic of TSC. A diagnosis of infantile spasms should always raise suspicion of TSC, as should the combination of ASD, ID, and seizures.

Other mTOR Overactivation Syndromes

The mTOR signaling pathway is associated with a number of clinical syndromes. Figure 8.1 shows examples of some of these.

Neurofibromatosis Type 1 (NF1) is a neurocutaneous disorder associated with genetic abnormality in the *NF1* gene, on chromosome 17. The disorder has a prevalence of around 1:3,500 and is inherited in autosomal dominant fashion. The clinical characteristics include the presence of neurofibromas, skin abnormalities including café au lait spots, and axillary freckling. Individuals with NF1 are also at risk of a range of neuropsychiatric features, including increased rates of intellectual disability, ADHD, specific scholastic difficulties, and neuropsychological deficits. The NF1 protein, neurofibromin, is a RasGAP (Ras GTP-ase activating protein) and therefore acts as an intracellular inhibitor of Ras. Ras in turn activates both the PI3K pathway, ERK1/2, and potentially other MAPkinases (Johannessen et al., 2005; Krab, Goorden, & Elgersma, 2008). *NF1* mutations have been shown to lead to mTOR overactivation mediated through PI3K-AKT and ERK1/2, with TSC2 a central effector of this process. Some of the same targeted treatment strategies used in TSC, such as mTOR inhibitors, are therefore being explored in NF1.

Cowden's disease is an autosomal dominant disorder associated with mutations in the *PTEN* gene, located on chromosome 10 (Krab, Goorden and Elgersma, 2008). The PTEN protein functions as an inhibitor between PI3K and AKT, and therefore also has tumor suppressor function. Mutations in the gene lead to increased AKT phosphorylation, which in turn inhibits TSC2 signaling, ultimately leading to mTOR overactivation and to a multiple hamartoma syndrome. Characteristic features may include macrocephaly and various hamartomatous lesions, and Cowden's has been associated with autism and Lhermitte-Duclos disease (Kwon et al., 2006). Animal models with PTEN knock-out have shown autistic-like features, which can be reversed with mTOR inhibitors such as rapamycin (Kwon et al., 2006; Zhou et al., 2009).

Peutz-Jeghers syndrome, also referred to as *hereditary intestinal polyposis syndrome*, is also an autosomal dominant disorder characterized by the development of benign hamartomas in the GI tract, and areas of hyperpigmentation, typically in the oral mucosa, on hands and feet (Shackelford & Shaw, 2009). Mutations in the *LKB1* gene on chromosome 19 have been shown to lead to the syndrome. LKB1 is a direct activator of AMPK. Mutations in the *LKB1* gene lead to reduced AMPK phosphorylation, which in turn leads to reduced TSC2 phosphorylation, resulting in mTOR overactivation (Shaw et al., 2004).

Fragile X syndrome, a triplet repeat disorder, discussed in Chapter 9, also has upregulation of mTOR. Recent research has shown that mTOR and many of its downstream targets (S6K, 4E-BP1, EIF-4F) are overactivated in *Fmr1* knock-out animals through activation of PI3K and related proteins (Sharma et al., 2010).

It is therefore of significant interest that a number of disorders with physical and behavioral similarities may have shared molecular mechanisms, at least in part associated with mTOR overactivation. The TSC2 protein and the TSC1-2 complex appear to be pivotal in regulating input and output signals to mTOR for a range of genetic syndromes associated with clear-cut physical and neuropsychiatric disorders.

CURRENT MANAGEMENT OF TUBEROUS SCLEROSIS COMPLEX

It is clear from the outset that comprehensive management of TSC requires the involvement of a range of professionals across various health disciplines (e.g., pediatrician, neurologist, ophthalmologist, nephrologist, psychiatrist, psychologist) as well as other agencies/sectors (e.g., education, social care, voluntary sector). One of the key tasks in the management of individuals and families with TSC is therefore to aim for an integrated approach to assessment, monitoring, and treatment. There is a growing number of "comprehensive TSC centers" around the world where attempts are made to provide a seamless package of care across multiple disciplines, and incorporate a joined-up plan for monitoring, special investigations, and so on. Whilst this is clearly the strategy that will best serve families and individuals with TSC, there are numerous challenges involved for clinical and other service providers to develop and maintain such integrated care programs.

Management in TSC covers the broad range from initial assessment and regular screening/monitoring (both discussed above) to general and specific intervention strategies for specific problems. Given the multi-system nature of TSC, it is impossible to provide a comprehensive guide to intervention here. Below, we outline basic aspects of management for physical and neuropsychiatric problems in TSC.

Management of the Physical Manifestations of TSC

As outlined above, comprehensive assessment on first presentation is key to identifying the range and nature of manifestations for each individual with TSC. This helps the family and clinician determine a baseline from which to monitor individuals (as per monitoring guidelines) and to intervene as soon as required.

Cortical tubers in TSC do not tend to show change over time. However, SEN may transform into SEGA in at least 10–15% of children. Given that SEGA may grow rapidly and present with symptoms of raised intracranial pressure quite late (Franz, de Vries, & Crino, 2009), it is imperative to do regular monitoring with MRI scans every one to three years. Where a growing lesion is identified, more frequent scans are required, and a multidisciplinary team should discuss the possibilities for treatment with families. For asymptomatic SEGA, treatment may include ongoing monitoring, elective surgery, or an mTOR inhibitor (see section on targeted treatments, below). Where a SEGA presents as acutely symptomatic, surgical intervention (resection plus or minus shunting) is indicated.

Epilepsy can be complex and hard to treat in TSC. (For detailed discussions regarding epilepsy in TSC see Thiele and Weiner, 2010.) Vigabatrin is recommended as first-line treatment of infantile spasms in TSC. Adrenocorticotropin hormone (ACTH) is often tried where Vigabatrin treatment has been unsuccessful. Other types of seizures in TSC are typically treated using standard treatment guidelines as for seizures in individuals without TSC. A significant proportion of individuals have medically refractory seizures. Epilepsy surgery should be considered for such cases. Other modalities of seizure treatment include vagal nerve stimulation (VNS) and ketogenic (or modified ketogenic) diets (Thiele & Weiner, 2010). There are trials underway to explore the efficacy and safety of mTOR inhibitors to prevent or treat seizures such as the EXIST-3 trial (ClinicalTrials. gov NCT017139460).

Renal structure and function need to be monitored on a regular basis, as outlined above. Hypertension should be treated using standard treatment guidelines. Where angiomyolipoma have acute hemorrhage, embolization and post-embolization corticosteroids should be used. For asymptomatic angiomyolipoma larger than 3 cm in diameter, medical treatment with an mTOR inhibitor is recommended as first-line treatment (Krueger et al., 2013). Nephrectomy should be avoided (Bissler et al., 2013; Krueger et al., 2013).

Skin manifestations require regular monitoring. For rapidly changing or symptomatic lesions, there are options, including selective surgical resection or laser therapy. Great care should be taken and advice should be sought from clinicians who are expert in the treatment of TSC. (For a more detailed summary of skin treatment options, see Darling, Moss, & Mausner, 2010). There are currently trials exploring the potential utility of topical mTOR inhibitors for skin manifestations.

Lung manifestations require monitoring, and LAM may potentially be treated with mTOR inhibitors. A proportion of individuals with TSC and LAM receive a lung transplant (Krueger et al., 2013).

The core management task for all organ systems, including eyes, teeth, heart, and others not discussed above, is regular monitoring and appropriate intervention (Krueger et al., 2013). As can be seen above, molecularly targeted treatments have already made their way into treatment options for TSC. Some of the animal and clinical studies leading to these treatment recommendations will be outlined below.

Management of Neuropsychiatric Manifestations in TSC

The principles we have outlined of comprehensive assessment, regular monitoring, and appropriate intervention also apply to the management of the neuropsychiatric features of TSC. Comprehensive assessment on first presentation is key to identifying the range and nature of manifestations for each individual with TSC and to determining and documenting the profile of strengths and weaknesses of each individual. This helps the family and clinician establish a baseline from which to monitor individuals (as per monitoring guidelines) and to intervene as soon as required (de Vries et al., 2005; de Vries, 2010a; Krueger et al., 2013). (For a more detailed discussion of neuropsychiatric management in TSC, see de Vries, 2010a.)

Given the multilevel nature and variability of the neuropsychiatric presentation of TSC, individualized treatment plans are essential. There will be no individual professional or professional group who will be able to meet all the neuropsychiatric needs of a child or adult with TSC comprehensively. It is therefore crucial to aim for multidisciplinary and intersectorial working, with health, mental health, educational colleagues, and social care all important partners (de Vries, 2010a).

There are at present no "unique" treatments for the neuropsychiatric features of TSC, and almost no systematic intervention trials have been performed to determine the most efficacious treatments for the range of neuropsychiatric disorders seen in TSC. Clinicians are therefore advised to use the standards of care for the individual disorders to treat individuals with TSC. For instance, a child with TSC who presents with a possible autism spectrum disorder should receive evaluation, early interventions, and educational support in exactly the same way as any other child with possible ASD. Clinicians should guard against "diagnostic overshadowing," where the characteristics of a specific neuropsychiatric disorder such as ADHD, anxiety, and so on, are attributed simply to "being part of TSC." The treating clinician should use standard treatment strategies, but remain mindful of the multisystem involvement of TSC, which, in an individual patient, may include co-morbid seizures, renal impairment, other medications, or a cardiac rhythm disturbance.

Behavioral challenges should be explored in appropriate detail to determine whether they might be markers of a psychiatric disorder (de Vries, 2010a). Functional analysis of behaviors may be required, particularly where challenging behaviors such as aggression or self-injury are seen, in order to develop an understanding of the function of a particular behavior. Based on the understanding and "formulation" of the problem, treatments should be implemented. These may include behavior modification, environmental accommodations, and psycho-education of the family and school.

Psychiatric disorders, and in particular, neurodevelopmental disorders such as ASD and ADHD, are common in TSC. Clinicians should therefore have a very high index of suspicion and work with families to identify possible disorders as early as possible (de Vries et al., 2005). Early intervention programs for ASD should be accessed where indicated, and standard non-pharmacological and pharmacological treatment strategies for ADHD should be used as appropriate (Taylor et al., 2004).

Depressive and anxiety disorders should be treated using evidence-based treatments and may include cognitive-behavioral therapy (CBT), other talking treatments, and pharmacological treatment with, for instance, a selective serotonin reuptake inhibitor (SSRI). As pointed out above, there have been no systematic studies to date to indicate whether any particular psychopharmacological strategies are superior to others in TSC.

Psychotic disorders occur in TSC at the same rate as in the general population (de Vries, 2010a). When individuals present with possible psychotic phenomena, it is important first to explore the possibility of a seizure-related psychosis, for instance as associated with temporal lobe discharges.

Intellectual disability in TSC increases the likelihood of other mental health problems significantly (de Vries, Hunt and Bolton, 2007). Those with TSC and ID are therefore an even higher-risk group, and should be monitored and treated accordingly. Individuals with TSC and ID may require additional and special educational placements or support, and supported living in adulthood. Those with profound ID are likely to require lifelong support for most aspects of daily living.

The majority of children with TSC have some academic or scholastic challenges (de Vries, 2010a). Many will have specific learning disorders with reading, writing, spelling, or mathematics. Many others will struggle to remain in school because of anxiety or other mental health problems. All children with TSC should therefore be considered as having special educational needs and be considered for statutory support as provided through each country's educational system. In some countries, this process is referred to as an "IEP" (individual educational plan); in others it is referred to as a "statutory assessment of special educational needs."

As outlined above, various neuropsychological deficits are seen in TSC. Many of these have a direct impact on daily living, work, and quality of life (Prather & de Vries, 2004; Ridler et al., 2007; de Vries, Gardiner, & Bolton, 2009; Tierney et al., 2011). It is therefore important to be aware of each person's profile of strengths and weaknesses, and psycho-education should be provided to families and schools around each person's unique profile of what they are good at and what they are less good at. There are many educational, occupational therapy and "cognitive rehabilitation" strategies to help individuals develop specific areas of neuropsychological skills.

It is extremely important to remember that the presence of a multisystem disorder such as TSC has a significant impact on the psycho-social performance of an individual and their family. Parental stress, marital and relationship discord, poor self-esteem, and feelings of humiliation and shame are very high in families who live with TSC (de Vries, 2010a). Clinicians should therefore use appropriate strategies to discuss these challenges and to support families. This may sometimes be through counseling or formal family or other psychotherapies. Very often, support can be provided by being open, genuine, and warm with families, and by being willing to work in partnership with them. Some families find it extremely useful to link up with others who also have children or family members with TSC. There are now TSC parent/user organizations in many countries around the world, many of whom are members of TSCi (Tuberous Sclerosis Complex International; www.tscinternational.org). The U.S.-based TSAlliance (www.tsalliance.org) and the U.K. Tuberous Sclerosis Association (www.tuberous-sclerosis.org) have been established for many years and have supported numerous clinical, research, and organizational developments over the last few decades.

TARGETED TREATMENTS IN TUBEROUS SCLEROSIS COMPLEX

Discovery of Rapamycin

Rapamycin was discovered in 1965 in the soil of the Easter Island (known locally as *Rapa Nui*) (Benjamin et al., 2011). The substance was identified as a product of *Streptomyces hygroscopicus* and was later shown to have antifungal activity. It was not until the 1990s when the human protein FRAP and murine protein RAFT were shown to bind the rapamycin-FKBP12 complex, and that FRAP/RAFT were inhibited by the rapamycin-FKBP12 complex. FRAP/RAFT were renamed the mammalian Target of Rapamycin (mTOR). Rapamycin was approved by the FDA for prevention of organ rejection in 1999 (Benjamin et al., 2011).

Animal Models of Targeted Treatments in TSC

An increasing number of animal models of TSC have been developed over the last decade, and this chapter will not aim to provide a comprehensive summary. (For further details, see Kwiatkowski, Whittemore, & Thiele, 2010; Howe et al., 2014.)

With the discovery in *Drosophila* that the Tsc1-2 protein complex acted upstream to mTOR, and that *Tsc* mutations led to mTOR overactivation (e.g., Potter et al., 2001), there was a very rapid progression to test the hypothesis that rapamycin and other mTOR inhibitors rescue some of the phenotypes observed in $Tsc^{+/-}$ or $Tsc^{-/-}$ conditions.

Animal Models of Renal and Skin Manifestations

One of the first organ systems explored through animal models was the renal system. A small number of animal trials reported that rapamycin (sirolimus) or temsirolimus (a rapamycin derivative) were able to shrink renal cysts and reduce the volume of existing renal tumors, firstly in the Eker Rat, a naturally occurring $Tsc2^{+/-}$ animal, then in knock-out mice (Kennerson et al., 2005; Lee et al., 2005; Sampson, 2009). Given the fact that rapamycin was already FDA-approved, these preclinical studies were rapidly followed by early-phase clinical trials in humans with TSC and AML (see Clinical Trials of Targeted Treatments below). Using a nude mouse model, Rauktys and colleagues (2008) showed inhibition of skin tumor growth by topical rapamycin administration.

Animal Models of Neurocognition in TSC

For a number of years, basic neuroscientists were frustrated at not being able to develop animal models that recapitulated the typical brain lesions of humans with TSC such as cortical tubers, subependymal nodules, or SEGA (Wong, 2007). These researchers were keen to examine the role of mTOR dysregulation in the brain, but expressed concern that, without an animal model with tubers and seizures, experimental evidence would translate poorly to the human disorder. These views were based on the assumption in the 1990s that the neurocognitive and neurodevelopmental manifestations of TSC were attributable to the structural abnormalities (tuber number, location, load) and/or the electrophysiological profile (seizure type, onset, location, control), or combinations of these two variables (Goodman et al., 1997).

Christopher Howe and I challenged this "tuber and seizure causal assumption" and proposed that there is a direct molecular route from mutation to neuropsychiatric disorders in TSC, and that molecular dysregulation may be sufficient to cause the neurocognitive and other functional manifestations seen in the disorder (de Vries & Howe, 2007). The TSC1-TSC2 complex was therefore proposed by us to act as a "molecular switchboard," a term first used by us in 2007. Tubers and seizures were proposed to be neither necessary nor sufficient to lead to neuropsychiatric deficits. Two main hypotheses for testing stemmed from our GRIPP hypothesis—first, that a TSC mutation would be sufficient in animal models to lead to neurocognitive deficits; second, that rapamycin may reverse neurocognitive deficits by reducing mTOR dysregulation in the brain (de Vries & Howe, 2007).

Support for the first prediction came from two sources. A Dutch group published findings from a $Tsc1^{+/-}$ mouse (Goorden et al., 2007). The researchers confirmed that the mice had no structural abnormalities or seizures. On behavioral tasks, the mice showed significant spatial learning deficits, as well as socialization deficits, thus providing the first clear support for a direct molecular pathway from mutation to neurocognition in TSC not involving structural abnormalities or seizures. The second study was performed in the United States, where a $Tsc2^{+/-}$ knock-out mouse was shown also not to have any structural or seizure phenotypes, but clear deficits in spatial learning. Interestingly, the $Tsc2^{+/-}$ mice did not display any overt socialization deficits (Ehninger et al., 2008). Ehninger, Silva, and colleagues then administered rapamycin intraperitoneally for five days, and repeated the spatial memory tasks. They showed that the spatial learning deficits were reversed, and that the rapamycin-treated $Tsc2^{+/-}$ mice were indistinguishable from wild-type mice. Strikingly, the experimental mice were all of adult age, suggesting that some of these phenotypes may be reversible even in adult animals. In parallel with the above animal work, my colleagues and I started monitoring aspects of neurocognition as part of early-phase clinical trials (Ehninger, de Vries, & Silva, 2009; de Vries, 2010b) (see Clinical Trials of Targeted Treatments below).

Animal Models of Epilepsy in TSC

Seizures are a very significant burden in TSC and in the general population. Epilepsy affects about 1% of the general population. Many epilepsies do not respond well to medical treatment (Thiele & Weiner, 2010). There has been growing interest, not only in the identification of better treatments for seizures (so-called antiseizure drugs), but also in the prevention of epilepsy (so-called antiepileptogenic drugs) (Zeng et al., 2008; Wong, 2010). In a paradigm shift similar to that about neurocognition in TSC, it has become clear that epileptogenesis in TSC is driven by molecular aberration, and that mTOR signaling may be an important contributor to the pathogenesis of epilepsy. Wong and colleagues created a conditional $Tsc1$ knock-out in glial cells ($Tsc1^{GFAP}$CKO mice) (Zeng et al., 2008). The $Tsc1^{GFAP}$CKO mice developed glial proliferation, had progressive seizures, and died prematurely. Mice were administered rapamycin either "early" (postnatal day

14) or "late" (6 weeks of age). "Early" treatment prevented the onset of seizures and premature death. "Late" treatment suppressed seizures and prolonged survival. To confirm the mechanistic involvement in the observation, rapamycin reduced the mTOR overactivation in the brain, reduced neuronal disorganization, and increased brain size (Zeng et al., 2008). This and other subsequent studies have led the way for early-phase clinical trials of mTOR inhibitors for seizure disorders in TSC (see Clinical Trials of Targeted Treatments below).

Animal Models of Autism Spectrum Disorders in TSC

There is great interest in the pathophysiology of autism and ASD. TSC has become a very interesting model for examining the possible contributors, molecular mechanisms, early biomarkers, and treatments of ASD. Given that a number of disorders associated with ASD have mTOR overactivation as part of their molecular signature, there has been a growing interest in mTOR inhibitors as possible targeted treatments for ASD (de Vries, 2010b; Ehninger & Silva, 2011).

The first animal experiments of a targeted treatment for ASD-related phenomena in the mTOR pathway were described in a PTEN knockout mouse (Zhou et al., 2009). As described above, PTEN is an inhibitory protein between PI3K and AKT upstream of TSC1-2. Mutations in *PTEN* lead to mTOR overactivation and can be associated with Cowden's disease, autism, and intellectual disability. A conditional *Pten* knock-out mouse with PTEN loss in post-mitotic cortical and hippocampal neurons was created (Kwon et al., 2006). The knock-out mice developed neuronal hypertrophy, loss of neuronal polarity, and showed significant anxiety and social deficit behaviors. Treatment with rapamycin reversed structural deficits as well as anxiety and social deficits in the mice (Zhou et al., 2009). The PTEN findings led to increased interest in the likely rescue of ASD phenotypes in TSC and TSC animal models.

A handful of ASD-specific animal models of TSC have been described to date. An American group generated mice with *Tsc1* deleted in cerebellar Purkinje cells (Tsai et al., 2012). Behavioral experiments showed that both heterozygous and homozygous mice presented with autistic-like behaviors, including reduced social-approach behaviors, abnormal ultrasonic vocalizations, and inflexible behaviors during reversal on a water T-maze task. Treatment with rapamycin reversed the perseverative behavior on the T-maze and improved the social-approach behaviors in the mutant mice (but not in the heterozygotes) (Tsai et al., 2012).

Whilst these results were exciting, and experiments were conducted with particular care to show deficits across the "triad of impairments" in ASD (Tsai et al., 2012), highly specific knock-outs in highly specific tissues have some weaknesses in translation to the human condition. TSC in humans is essentially a heterozygous state, with (at least presumed) $TSC^{+/-}$ status in all tissue and cell types in the brain. Sato and colleagues published a study that reduced this concern to some extent (Sato et al., 2012). In their study, the researchers examined $Tsc1^{+/-}$ and $Tsc2^{+/-}$ mice across a set of behavioral paradigms and observed social deficits, including reduced performance on a social interaction task. Rapamycin administration to adult hetero-zygous $Tsc1$ and $Tsc2$ mice recovered the social interaction performance and reduced mTOR activation. Performance of the wild-type mice was not affected by rapamycin administration (Sato et al., 2012).

The Eker rat experiments conducted by Waltereit and colleagues (Waltereit et al., 2011) further illustrated the complexity of modeling human neurodevelopmental disorders in animals, and provided evidence to consider the role of gene–environment interaction. Waltereit used the Eker rat, a naturally occurring $Tsc2^{+/-}$ rat. These rats do not have any overt structural brain abnormalities or epilepsy. In order to study the impact of genotype and seizures on learning and social behavior in wild-type and Eker rats, seizures were induced at postnatal days 7 and 14. Following this, adult mice (aged 3–6 months) were assessed on a range of learning and social behavior tasks. No learning deficits were observed in the Eker rats at baseline, suggesting a very "able" group. Interestingly, seizures did not induce learning deficits in Tsc or wild-type animals. In contrast, $Tsc2^{+/-}$ sta-tus was sufficient to lead to some social deficit behaviors (social explora-tion, rearing, and novel-object exploration), while seizures induced anxiety and social evasion, and reduced social exploration and social contact behav-iors in wild-type and $Tsc2^{+/-}$ rats. These results therefore suggested that TSC haploinsufficiency may be sufficient to lead to some social deficit behaviors, and that seizures have a direct and additive effect to increase the likelihood and range of autistic-like behaviors (Waltereit et al., 2011). The Waltereit experiments did not introduce any mTOR inhibitors.

Taken together, there are various animal models of TSC that have pro-vided direct or indirect support for mTOR dysregulation as a molecular pathway to physical and neuropsychiatric disorders, and for the use of mTOR inhibitors as targeted treatments in TSC. Animal models across renal, skin, epilepsy, neurocognition, and autism-related behaviors have all contributed evidence towards the potential application of targeted treat-ments in humans with TSC. Needless to say, animal models are not free from limitations. In a recent review (Howe et al., 2014), we raised concern at three conceptual levels—*mutational equivalence* (the direct relevance of a particular animal mutation to actual mutations seen in humans), *structural/functional equivalence* (the fact that not all structural and functional domains of the TSC1 and TSC2 proteins are conserved in all animal models), and *behavioral/phenotypical equivalence* (the fact that some tumors are not seen in animal models and the challenge of modeling complex neuropsychiatric phenomena in simplistic animal models) (Howe et al., 2014). These concerns clearly will require careful consideration in further animal studies.

Clinical Trials of Targeted Treatments in TSC

Between 2003 and 2014, approximately 20 clinical trials of mTOR inhibitors in TSC were registered on the website ClinicalTrials.gov. These ranged from small-scale earlier-phase trials to relatively large international, randomized placebo-controlled trials. Trials have explored the efficacy and safety of mTOR inhibitors to treat renal AML, LAM (sporadic and TSC), SEGA, skin (facial angiofibromata), epilepsy, and neurocognition. Below we will outline some of the completed trials, and some of those still in progress.

Clinical Trials of SEGA, AML, and Facial Angiofibromata

Very swiftly after preclinical trials showed the efficacy of mTOR inhibitors for renal lesions, Bissler and colleagues initiated an open-label, non-randomized trial of the safety and efficacy of sirolimus in AML and LAM (Bissler et al., 2008). After 12 months of treatment, mean AML size was reduced by approximately 53%. After discontinuation of sirolimus, AML size increased to 86% of baseline diameter. Simultaneously, Sampson and colleagues in the United Kingdom conducted a very similar trial of 16 patients treated for two years on sirolimus. Results showed that half the subjects met (RECIST) criteria for partial response (Davies et al., 2008). Interestingly, results showed that some individuals had continued shrinkage of tumors even beyond the 12 months' study duration of the Bissler trial (Davies et al., 2008).

These open-label studies were sufficient to lead to a large-scale multicenter, randomized, placebo-controlled trial (EXIST-2), published early in 2013 (Bissler et al., 2013). In the study, 118 patients with TSC and angiomyolipoma (larger than 3 cm in diameter) from 24 centers in 11 countries were randomized 2:1 to everolimus or placebo. Response was defined as shrinkage of more than 50% of target angiomyolipoma volume from baseline. The response rate was 42% for the everolimus versus 0% for the placebo arm. The most common side effects in both groups were stomatitis (48% everolimus vs. 8% placebo), nasopharyngitis (24% everolimus vs. 31% placebo), and acne-like lesions (22% everolimus vs. 5% placebo). Results showed that everolimus reduced angiomyolipoma volumes with an acceptable safety profile and suggested that mTOR inhibitors such as everolimus could be a potential treatment for angiomyolipoma in TSC (Bissler et al., 2013). As mentioned earlier, the FDA and EMA approved the use of everolimus for the medical treatment of angiomyolipoma larger than 3 cm in individuals with TSC in 2012. At an international consensus conference in 2012, the Renal Expert Panel unanimously recommended everolimus as first-line treatment for asymptomatic angiomyolipoma >3 cm in TSC (Krueger et al., 2013).

In the absence of animal models of SEGA, Franz et al. (2006) performed a small open-label study of five individuals with SEGA and treated them with oral rapamycin from 2 to 20 months. All lesions showed regression, and in one case necrosis. Interruption of rapamycin treatment led to regrowth of the SEGA in one patient. Overall, treatment was well-tolerated and suggested that rapamycin may be a potential treatment for SEGA in TSC (Franz et al., 2006). The case series was followed by a larger open-label study of 28 patients with documented serial growth of SEGA (Krueger et al., 2010). Patients were treated on the mTOR inhibitor everolimus for 6 months. The primary efficacy endpoint was change in SEGA volume between baseline and 6 months. Thirty-two percent of patients showed a greater than 50% reduction, and 75% showed a greater than 30% reduction from baseline. Sixteen patients had 24-hour EEGs available. Nine of the 16 showed reductions in seizure frequency (Krueger et al., 2010). This open-label study was followed by a multicenter, randomized, placebo-controlled study of 117 patients across 24 centers in 10 countries (EXIST-1). The primary endpoint of the EXIST-1 trial was the proportion of patients with confirmed response, defined as a greater than 50% reduction in target volume from baseline. Thirty-five percent of patients on everolimus had a greater than 50% reduction in SEGA volume, versus 0% in the placebo arm. Seventy-eight percent of patients on everolimus had a greater than 30% reduction in SEGA size (Franz et al., 2013). The most common side effects were mouth ulceration (32% everolimus vs. 5% placebo), stomatitis (31% everolimus vs. 21% placebo), convulsion (23% everolimus vs. 26% placebo), and pyrexia (22% everolimus vs. 15% placebo). Results therefore supported the safety and efficacy of everolimus for SEGA in TSC. Based on the phase II data (Krueger et al., 2010) and confirmed by phase III data (Franz et al., 2013), FDA approval was granted in 2010 for the use of everolimus for the treatment of "patients with SEGA associated with TSC who require therapeutic intervention and are not candidates for curative surgery" (www.fda.gov). EMA approval was granted in 2011. At the international consensus conference held in 2012, the Brain Tumor Expert Panel did not reach a consensus to recommend everolimus as a first-line treatment of SEGA in TSC. The panel agreed to recommend everolimus as *one of the treatment options* for non-acute SEGA (Krueger et al., 2013).

Following reports of improvement in facial angiofibroma after systemic rapamycin administration (Hofbauer et al., 2008), clinical trials using topical rapamycin have started. There is now a handful of case reports indicating reduction in redness and raised aspects of facial angiofibromata. There are reports of shrinkage of shagreen patches and of reduction in ungual fibromas after systemic mTOR inhibitor drugs. One of the secondary outcomes in the EXIST-1 and EXIST-2 trials summarized above (Franz et al., 2013; Bissler et al., 2013) was clinician rating of the severity of skin lesions. In both studies, patients on everolimus showed a significantly greater improvement in skin signs than in the placebo group. There are ongoing trials of the efficacy and safety of everolimus for facial angiofibromas in TSC (ClinicalTrials.gov NCT01526356).

Clinical Trials of Neuropsychiatric Manifestations and Epilepsy

Results of the $Tsc2^{+/-}$ mouse study performed by Ehninger and colleagues (2008) led to great interest in mTOR inhibitors as targeted treatments of some aspects of the neuropsychiatric phenotype in TSC. As part of an open-label study, we introduced measures of immediate recall and recognition memory, as well as some measures of executive function (Davies et al., 2011). We predicted that, based on the animal literature, recall memory performance would be rapamycin-sensitive, while recognition memory would not be. Seven of the eight participants with TSC in the trial showed improvements in immediate recall memory, in contrast to none on the recognition memory tasks. Of the eight participants, four showed improvements in their immediate memory scores >1 standard deviation (SD) from baseline performance, suggesting clinically significant improvement (Davies, de Vries, et al., 2011; de Vries, 2010b). Based on the early animal and human data, there are currently three active phase II studies with neurocognition as primary endpoints, one in the United States (ClinicalTrials. gov NCT01289912; PIs Sahin, de Vries, & Krueger), one in the United

Kingdom (ISRCTN09739757; PIs Sampson & de Vries), and a third study in the Netherlands (ClinicalTrials.gov NCT01730209).

In spite of the great interest in neurocognitive trials in TSC and other genetic conditions, there are numerous challenges to acknowledge. Oncology trials have been conducted for years, and there is international consensus about criteria for treatment response, side effect monitoring, and so on. Neurocognitive trials using targeted treatments are relatively new, however, and there are no consensus agreements about measurement tools, quantifying endpoints, or guidelines on statistical management of complex, multilevel datasets. Neuropsychiatric measurement tools require knowledge of the age and developmental level of a participant; language and cultural factors need to be considered; and one of the grand challenges is therefore to identify measurement tools with good psychometric properties that have been standardized, validated, and normed across languages and cultures. A further challenge in clinical trials is the drive towards identification of a single primary outcome measure, which risks oversimplifying the complexity of, for instance, autism or intellectual disability, ADHD, or anxiety disorders. There will certainly never be a single tool that will summarize all of the dimensions of neuropsychiatric phenotypes.

At the time of this writing, a third large-scale multicenter, placebo-controlled trial had started (EXIST-3), with the primary purpose of examining the efficacy and safety of everolimus as an adjunctive treatment of focal seizures in TSC (ClinicalTrials.gov NCT01713946). The study was motivated by preclinical findings as outlined above (Zeng et al., 2008; Wong, 2010) and by reduction in seizure frequency observed in the phase II study by Krueger and colleagues (2010). A study of seizures brings some similar challenges in terms of primary endpoints and measurement tools, as discussed above.

Clinical Utility of mTOR Inhibitors in TSC

As listed above, the mTOR inhibitor everolimus (Afinitor®, Votubia®) has been licensed by the FDA and EMA for use in tuberous sclerosis complex. To our knowledge, this is the first-ever targeted treatment licensed for a named genetic condition associated with multisystem and neuropsychiatric manifestations. It is likely that approval for a skin preparation may be the next to emerge. There is clearly insufficient evidence to date to recommend clinical use or to pursue the licensing of mTOR inhibitors for epilepsy or aspects of neurocognition, in spite of positive preclinical and early-phase clinical studies.

One of the key challenges in the coming years will be to translate prescribing in the context of clinical trials into prescribing of mTOR inhibitors in "real-life" situations.

FUTURE PROSPECTS FOR TARGETED TREATMENTS IN TUBEROUS SCLEROSIS COMPLEX

There is a number of ongoing clinical trials of mTOR inhibitors in TSC (see ClinicalTrials.gov). Some are in extension phases, which will be very helpful in the collection of long-term safety data. Given that many patients may need to take an mTOR inhibitor as a lifelong treatment, it will be extremely important to collect information about the longer-term side-effect profiles of mTOR inhibitors. So far, it seems that longer-term mTOR inhibitor use is associated with an acceptable side-effect profile.

It will be with cautious optimism that the neurocognitive and epilepsy trials will be conducted. Given some of the measurement challenges, plus the challenging issue of "variable baselines" (the fact that individuals will enter studies at very different "baselines"), these studies will require careful monitoring and may require novel trial designs in a move away from the approaches borrowed from solid-tumor trials.

Given the interest in mTOR inhibitors as anti-epileptogenic drugs, there is an understandable interest in "pre-emptive" treatments. Some investigators have suggested mTOR inhibitor treatments to start *in utero*, or immediately postnatally (Jozwiak et al., 2007). While these are good and well-meaning sentiments, there are significant safety issues to clarify before any such trials should be supported. A recent study in an animal model showed neurological deficits in wild-type mice treated with mTOR inhibitors *in utero* (Tsai et al., 2013). Clearly, we need to learn much more in this regard in order to ensure that, above all, targeted treatments are safe.

There are already debates about the healthcare costs of new targeted treatments, and national insurance bodies, national health services, and service providers are starting to do simple economic health calculations. This will clearly be an area for further development and exploration. A particular challenge will be to do health economic modelling mindful that mTOR inhibitor treatment may have an impact on more than one organ system at a time and that the real-life impact of TSC happens in the context of multiple "systems" at any one time.

Finally, all discussions in this chapter have focused on mTOR inhibitors, specifically rapamycin and analogues, as targeted treatments in TSC. There are already laboratory-based investigations exploring other targets in the mTOR signaling pathway, and investigating feed-back and feed-forward mechanisms. There is no doubt that over time further potential molecular targets will be identified through basic science, molecular biological, or other exploratory routes. These will lead to new targets to explore, and new interactions or combinatorial treatments to consider. Our journey of targeted treatments in tuberous sclerosis complex and other genetic and neurodevelopmental disorders has clearly just begun.

DISCLOSURES

Dr. de Vries was a member of the Study Steering Committee for the EXIST-1, EXIST-2, and EXIST-3 multi-center, international phase III mTOR inhibitor trials sponsored by Novartis. He was also co-principal investigator on two investigator-initiated phase II clinical trials partly funded by Novartis. In addition, he has acted as an advisory board member to Novartis on the use of mTOR inhibitors in tuberous sclerosis complex. All payments received have been donated to the University of Cambridge, University of Cape Town, or the Society for the Study of Behavioural Phenotypes (SSBP).

Address for correspondence: Prof. Petrus J. de Vries, University of Cape Town, 46 Sawkins Road, Rondebosch, Cape Town, 7700, South Africa; email: petrus.devries@uct.ac.za or pd215@cam.ac.uk.

ABBREVIATIONS

4E-BP1:	Eukaryotic initiation factor 4E binding protein 1
AKT:	Protein kinase B
AMPK:	Adenosine monophosphate activated protein kinase
CDK1:	Cyclin dependent kinase 1
EIF4E:	Eukaryotic translation initiation factor 4E
ERK1/2:	Extracellular signal regulated kinase 1 and 2
GSK3β:	Glycogen synthase kinase 3 beta
HIF1α:	Hypoxia inducible factor-1 alpha
LKB1:	Serine/threonine kinase 1
MEK1/2:	MAPK/ERK kinase 1/2
MK2:	MAPK-activated protein kinase 2
mTORC1:	Mammalian target of rapamycin complex 1
NF1:	Neurofibromin, protein product of *NF1* gene
p38MAPK:	P38 mitogen-activated protein kinase
PI3K:	Phosphoinositide 3 kinase

PTEN:	Phosphatase and tensin homolog
Rac1:	Ras-related C3 botulinum toxin substrate 1
Raf:	MAP kinase kinase kinase (MAP3K)
Ras:	RAt Sarcoma, a small GTPase protein
REDD1:	REgulated in Development and DNA Damage responses 1
Rheb:	Ras homologue enriched in brain
Rho:	Ras homologue gene family, member A
S6K1:	Ribosomal p70 S6 kinase 1
TSC1:	Tuberous sclerosis complex 1 protein (hamartin)
TSC2:	Tuberous sclerosis complex 2 protein (tuberin)
VHL:	Von Hippel-Lindau tumour suppressor protein

REFERENCES

American Psychiatric Association. (2013). *Diagnostic and Statistical Manual of Mental Disorders*, 5th ed. Washington, DC: APA.

Benjamin, D., Colombi, M., Moroni, C., & Hall, M. N. (2011). Rapamycin passes the torch: a new generation of mTOR inhibitors. *Nature Reviews Drug Discovery, 10*, 868–880.

Bissler, J. J., Kingswood, J. C., Radzikowska, E., et al. (2013). Everolimus for angio-myolipoma associated with tuberous sclerosis complex or sporadic lymphan-gioleiomyomatosis (EXIST-2): a multi-centre, randomized, double-blind, placebo-controlled trial. *Lancet, 381*, 817–824.

Bissler, J. J., McCormack, F. X., Young, L. R., et al. (2008). Sirolimus for angiomyoli-poma in tuberous sclerosis complex or lymphangioleiomyomatosis. *New England Journal of Medicine, 258*, 140–151.

Bolton, P. F., Park, R. J., Higgins, J. N., et al. (2002). Neuro-epileptic determinants of autism spectrum disorders in tuberous sclerosis complex. *Brain, 125*, 1247–1255.

Bourneville, D. M. (1880). Sclerose tubereuse des circonvolutions cerebrales: idiotie et epilepsie hemiplegique [Tuberous sclerosis of the cerebral cortex: intellectual disability and hemiplegic epilepsy]. *Archives of Neurology (Paris), 1*, 81–91.

Bourneville, D. M., & Brissaud, E. (1881). Encephalite ou sclerose tubereuse de circon-volutions cerebrales [Encephalitis and tuberous sclerosis of the cerebral cortex]. *Archives of Neurology (Paris), 1*, 390–412.

Crino, P. B., Nathanson, K. L., & Henske, E. P. (2006). The tuberous sclerosis complex. *New England Journal of Medicine, 355*, 1345–1356.

Curatolo, P., Bombardieri, R., & Jozwiak, S. (2008). Tuberous sclerosis. *Lancet, 372*, 657–668.

Dabora, S. L., et al. (2001). Mutational analysis in a cohort of 224 tuberous sclerosis patients indicates increased severity of TSC2, compared with TSC1, disease in multiple organs. *American Journal of Human Genetics, 68*, 64–80.

Darling, T. N., Moss, J., & Mausner, M. (2010). Dermatologic manifestations of tuber-ous sclerosis complex (TSC). In D. J. Kwiatkowski, V. H. Whittemore, & E. A. Thiele (eds.), *Tuberous Sclerosis Complex: Genes, Clinical Features, and Therapeutics*. Weinheim, Germany: Wiley-Blackwell, 287–309.

Davies, D. M., de Vries, P. J., Johnson, S. R. et al. (2011). Sirolimus therapy for angiomyolipoma in tuberous sclerosis and sporadic lymphangioleiomyomato-sis: A phase 2 trial. *Clinical Cancer Research, 17*, 4071–4081.

Davies, D. M., Johnson, S. R., Tattersfield, A. E., et al. (2008). Sirolimus therapy in tuberous sclerosis or sporadic lymphangioleiomyomatosis. *New England Journal of Medicine, 358*, 200–203.

de Vries, P. J. (2010a). Neurodevelopmental, psychiatric and cognitive aspects of tuberous sclerosis complex. In D. J. Kwiatkowski, V. H. Whittemore, & E. A. Thiele (eds.), *Tuberous Sclerosis Complex: Genes, Clinical Features, and Therapeutics.* Weinheim, Germany: Wiley-Blackwell, 229–267.

de Vries, P. J. (2010b). Targeted treatments for cognitive and neurodevelopmental disorders in tuberous sclerosis complex. *Neurotherapeutics, 7*, 275–282.

de Vries, P. J., Gardiner, J., & Bolton, P. F. (2009). Neuropsychological attention deficits in tuberous sclerosis complex (TSC). *American Journal of Medical Genetics Part A. 149A*, 387–395.

de Vries, P. J., & Prather, P. (2007). The tuberous sclerosis complex. *New England Journal of Medicine, 356*(1), 92.

de Vries, P. J., & Howe, C. J. (2007). The tuberous sclerosis complex proteins—a GRIPP on cognition and neurodevelopment. *Trends in Molecular Medicine, 13*, 319–326.

de Vries, P. J., Hunt, A., & Bolton P. F. (2007). The psychopathologies of children and adolescents with tuberous sclerosis complex (TSC): a postal survey of UK families. *European Child and Adolescent Psychiatry, 16*, 16–24.

de Vries, P., Humphrey, A., McCartney, D., Prather, P., Bolton, P., Hunt, A., & the TSC Behaviour Consensus Panel (2005). Consensus clinical guidelines for the assessment of cognitive and behavioural problems in tuberous sclerosis. *European Child and Adolescent Psychiatry, 14*, 183–190.

Ehninger, D., & Silva A. J. (2011). Rapamycin for treating tuberous sclerosis and autism spectrum disorders. *Trends in Molecular Medicine, 17*, 78–87.

Ehninger, D., de Vries, P. J., & Silva, A. J. (2009). From mTOR to cognition: Molecular and cellular mechanisms of cognitive impairment in tuberous sclerosis. *Journal of Intellectual Disability Research, 53*, 838–851.

Ehninger, D., Han, S., Shilyansky, C., Shou, Y., Li, W., Kwiatkowski, D. J., Ramesh, V., & Silva, A. J. (2008). Reversal of learning deficits in a Tsc2$^{+/-}$ mouse model of tuberous sclerosis. *Nature Medicine, 14*, 843–848.

European Chromosome 16 Tuberous Sclerosis Consortium (1993). Identification and characterization of the tuberous sclerosis gene on chromosome 16. *Cell, 75*, 1305–1315.

Eussen, B. H. J., Bartalini, G., Bakker, L., et al. (2000). An unbalanced submicroscopic translocation t(8;16)(q24.3;p13.3)pat associated with tuberous sclerosis complex, adult polycystic kidney disease, and hypomelanosis of Ito. *Journal of Medical Genetics, 37*, 287–291.

Fombonne, E. (2003). Epidemiological surveys of autism and other pervasive developmental disorders: an update. *Journal of Autism and Developmental Disorders, 33*, 365–382.

Franz, D. N., Belousova, E., Sparagana, S., et al. (2013). Efficacy and safety of everolimus for subependymal giant cell astrocytomas associated with tuberous sclerosis complex (EXIST-1): a multicentre, randomized, placebo-controlled phase 3 trial. *Lancet, 381*, 125–132.

Franz, D. N., de Vries P. J., & Crino P. B. (2009). Giant cell astrocytomas in tuberous sclerosis complex. *Archives of Diseases in Childhood, 94*, 75–76.

Franz, D. N., Leonard, J., Tudor, C., Chuck, G., Care, M., Sethuraman, G., et al. (2006). Rapamycin causes regression of astrocytomas in tuberous sclerosis complex. *Annals of Neurology, 59*, 490–498.

Gillberg, I. C., Gillberg, C., & Ahlsen, G. (1994). Autistic behaviour and attention deficits in tuberous sclerosis: A population-based study. *Developmental Medicine Child Neurology, 36*, 50–56.

Gollob, M. H., Seger, J. J., Gollob, T. N., et al. (2001). Novel PRKAG2 mutation responsible for the genetic syndrome of ventricular preexcitation and conduction system disease with childhood onset and absence of cardiac hypertrophy. *Circulation, 104*, 3030–3033.

Gomez, M. R. (1988). Criteria for diagnosis. In M. R. Gomez (ed.), *Tuberous Sclerosis*, 2nd ed. New York: Raven Press.

Goodman, M., Lamm, S. H., Engel, A., Shepherd, C. W., Houser, O. W., & Gomez, M. R. (1997). Cortical tuber count: A biomarker indicating neurologic severity of tuberous sclerosis complex. *Journal of Child Neurology, 12*, 85–90.

Goorden, S. M., van Woerden, G. M., van der Weerd, L., Cheadle, J. P., & Elgersma, Y. (2007). Cognitive deficits in Tsc1$^{+/-}$ mice in the absence of cerebral lesions and seizures. *Annals of Neurology, 62*, 648–655.

Hofbauer, G. F., Marcollo-Pini, A., Corsenca, A., Kistler, A. D., French, L. E., Wuthrich, R. P., & Serra, A.L. (2008). The mTOR inhibitor rapamycin significantly improves facial angiofibroma lesions in a patient with tuberous sclerosis. *British Journal of Dermatology, 159*, 473–475.

Hoogeveen-Westerveld M., Ekong R., Povey S., et al. (2013). Functional assessment of TSC2 variants identified in individuals with tuberous sclerosis complex. *Human Mutation, 34*, 167–175.

Hoogeveen-Westerveld, M., van Unen, L, van den Ouweland, A., Halley, D., Hoogeveen, A., & Nellist, M. (2012). The TSC1-TSC2 complex consists of multiple TSC1 and TSC2 subunits. *BMC Biochemistry, 13*, 18.

Howe, C. J., Serfontein, J., Nisbet, R. E. R., & de Vries, P. J. (2014). Viewing animal models of tuberous sclerosis in the light of evolution. In P. Roubertoux (ed.), *Animal Models of Autism and Pervasive Neuro-Developmental Disorders*. Springer.

Huang J., & Manning B. D. (2008). The TSC1-TSC2 complex: A molecular switchboard controlling cell growth. *Biochemistry Journal, 412*, 179–190.

Hunt, A. (1983). Tuberous sclerosis: A survey of 97 cases. III. Family aspects. *Developmental Medicine Child Neurology, 25*, 353–357.

Hunt, A. (1993). Development, behaviour and seizures in 300 cases of tuberous sclerosis. *Journal of Intellectual Disability Research, 37*, 41–51.

Jansen, A.C., Kingswood, J.C. & TOSCA Consortium (2013). Tuberous Sclerosis Registry to Increase Disease Awareness (TOSCA). *Journal of Intellectual Disability Research, 57*, 799.

Johannessen, C. M., Reczek, E. E., James, M. F., Brems, H., Legius, E., & Cichowski, K. (2005). The NF1 tumor suppressor critically regulates TSC2 and mTOR. *Proceedings of the National Academy of Science USA, 102*, 8573–8578.

Joinson, C., O'Callaghan, F. J., Osborne, J. P., Martyn, C., Harris, T., & Bolton, P. F. (2003). Learning disability and epilepsy in an epidemiological sample of individuals with tuberous sclerosis complex. *Psychological Medicine, 33*, 335–344.

Jones, A. C., et al. (1997). Molecular genetic and phenotypic analysis reveals differences between *TSC1* and *TSC2* associated familial and sporadic tuberous sclerosis. *Human Molecular Genetics, 6*, 2155–2161.

Jozwiak, S., Domanska-Pakiela, D., Kotulska, K., & Kaczorowska, M. (2007). Treatment before seizures: New indications for antiepilepsy therapy in children with tuberous sclerosis complex. *Epilepsia, 48*(8), 1632.

Kenerson, H., Dundon, T. A., & Yeung, R. S. (2005). Effects of rapamycin in the Eker rat model of tuberous sclerosis complex. *Pediatric Research, 57,* 67–75.

Krab, L. C., Goorden, S. M. I., & Elgersma, Y. (2008). Oncogenes on my mind: ERK and mTOR signaling in cognitive diseases. *Trends in Genetics, 24,* 498–510.

Krueger, D. A., Care, M. M., Holland, K., et al. (2010). Everolimus for subependymal giant-cell astrocytomas in tuberous sclerosis. *New England Journal of Medicine, 363,* 1801–1811.

Krueger, D. A., Northrup, H., Roberds. S., Smith, K., Sampson J., Korf, B., et al. (2013). Tuberous sclerosis complex surveillance and management: recommendation of the 2012 International Tuberous Sclerosis Comsensus Conference. *Pediatric Neurology, 49,* 255–265.

Kwiatkowski, D. J., Whittemore, V. H., & Thiele, E. A. (2010). *Tuberous Sclerosis Complex: Genes, Clinical Features, and Therapeutics. Weinheim, Germany: Wiley-Blackwell.*

Kwon, C., Luikart, B. W., Powell, C. M., et al. (2006). Pten regulates neuronal arborization and social interaction in mice. *Neuron, 50,* 377–388.

Leclezio, L., Jansen, A. C., Whittemore, V. H., Wilmshurst J., Schlegel, B. & de Vries P. J. (2013). The Tuberous Sclerosis Complex Associated Nuropsychiatric Disorders (TAND) Checklist – pilot validation of a new screening tool for the neuropsychiatric manifestations in TSC. *Journal of Intellectual Disability Research.* 57, 800.

Lee, L., Sudentas, P., Donohue, B., et al. (2005). Efficacy of a rapamycin analog (CCI-779) and IFN-γ in tuberous sclerosis mouse models. *Genes Chromosomes Cancer, 42,* 213–227.

Lewis, J. C., Thomas, H. V., Murphy, K. C., & Sampson, J. R. (2004). Genotype and psychological phenotype in tuberous sclerosis. *Journal of Medical Genetics, 41,* 203–207.

Mashima, Y., Kigasawa, K., Hasegawa, H., et al. (1996). High incidence of preexcitation syndrome in Japanese families with Leber's hereditary optic neuropathy. *Clinical Genetics, 50,* 535–537.

McCartney, D. L. (2008). Spatial attention in tuberous sclerosis complex. PhD thesis, University of Cambridge, Cambridge, UK.

Moolten, S. E. (1942). Hamartial nature of the tuberous sclerosis complex and its bearing on the tumor problem. *Archives of Internal Medicine, 69,* 589–623.

Muhammed, K., & Mathew, J. (2007). Coexistence of two neurocutaneous syndromes: Tuberous sclerosis and hypomelanosis of Ito. *Indian Journal of Dermatology, Venereology & Leprology, 73,* 43–45.

Northrup, H., Krueger, D. A., Roberds. S., Smith, K., Sampson J., Korf, B., et al. (2013). Tuberous sclerosis complex diagnostic criteria update: recommendations of the 2012 international tuberous sclerosis complex consensus conference. *Pediatric Neurology, 49,* 243–254.

O'Callaghan, F. J. K., Clarke, A. C., Joffe, H., et al. (1998). Tuberous sclerosis complex and Wolff-Parkinson-White syndrome. *Archives of Diseases in Childhood, 78,* 159–162.

Osborne, J. O., Fryer, A., & Webb, D. (1991). Epidemiology of tuberous sclerosis. *Annals New York Academy of Sciences, 615,* 125–127.

Potter, C. J., Huang, H., & Xu, T. (2001). Drosophila Tsc1 functions with Tsc2 to antagonize insulin signalling in regulating cell growth, cell proliferation, and organ size. *Cell, 105,* 357–368.

Povey, S., Burley, M. W., Attwood, J., et al. (1994). Two loci for tuberous sclerosis: One on 9q34 and one on 16p13. *Annals of Human Genetics, 58,* 107–127.

Prather, P., & de Vries, P. J. (2004). Behavioral and cognitive aspects of tuberous sclerosis complex. *Journal of Child Neurology, 19,* 666–674.

Pringle, J. J. (1890). A case of congenital adenoma sebaceum. *British Journal of Dermatology*, 2, 1–14.

Rauktys, A., Lee, N., Lee, L., & Dabora, S. L. (2008). Topical rapamycin inhibits tuberous sclerosis tumor growth in a nude mouse model. *BMC Dermatology*, 8, 1.

Rayer, P. F. O. (1835). *Traite Theoretique et Practique des Maladies de la Peau*, 2nd ed. Paris: J. B. Bailliere.

Ridler, K., Suckling, J., Higgins, N. J., de Vries, P. J., Stephenson, C. M., Bolton, P. F., & Bullmore, E. T. (2007). Neuroanatomical correlates of memory deficits in tuberous sclerosis complex. *Cerebral Cortex*, 17, 261–271.

Roach, E. S., DiMario F. J., Kandt R. S., & Northrup, H. (1999). Tuberous Sclerosis Consensus Conference: Recommendations for diagnostic evaluation. *Journal of Child Neurology*, 14, 401–407.

Roach, E. S., Gomez, M. R., & Northrup, H. (1998). Tuberous Sclerosis Complex Consensus Conference: Revised clinical diagnostic criteria. *Journal of Child Neurology*, 13, 624–628.

Sampson, J. R. (2009). Therapeutic targeting of mTOR in tuberous sclerosis. *Biochemistry Society Transactions*, 37, 259–264.

Sarbassov, D. D., Ali, S. M., & Sabatini, D. M. (2005). Growing roles for the mTOR pathway. *Current Opinion in Cell Biology*, 17, 596–603.

Sato, A., Kasai, S., Kobayashi, T., et al. (2012). Rapamycin reverses impaired social interaction in mouse models of tuberous sclerosis complex. *Nature Communications*, 3, 1292.

Serfontein, J., Nisbet. R. E. R., Howe, C. J., & de Vries, P. J. (2011). Conservation of structural and functional elements of TSC1 and TSC2: A bioinformatic comparison across animal models. *Behavior Genetics*, 41, 349–356.

Serfontein, J., Nisbet, R. E. R., Howe, C. J., & de Vries, P. J. (2010). Evolution of the TSC1/TSC2-TOR signaling pathway. *Science Signaling*, 3, ra49.

Shackelford, D. B., & Shaw, R. J. (2009). The LKB1-AMPK pathway: Metabolism and growth control in tumour suppression. *Nature Reviews Cancer*, 9, 563–575.

Sharma, A., Hoeffer, C. A., Takayasu, Y., et al. (2010). Dysregulation of mTOR signaling in fragile X syndrome. *Journal of Neuroscience*, 13, 694–702.

Shaw, R. J., Bardeesy, N., Manning, B. D., et al. (2004). The LKB1 tumor suppressor negatively regulates mTOR signaling. *Cancer Cell*, 6, 91–99.

Taylor, E., Dopfner, M., Sergeant, J., et al. (2004). European clinical guidelines for hyperkinetic disorder—first upgrade. *European Child and Adolescent Psychiatry*, 13, 7–30.

Thiele, E. A., & Weiner, H. L. (2010). Epilepsy in TSC. In D. J. Kwiatkowski, V. H. Whittemore, & E. A. Thiele (eds.), *Tuberous Sclerosis Complex: Genes, Clinical Features, and Therapeutics*. Weinheim, Germany: Wiley-Blackwell, 187–210.

Tierney, K. M., McCartney, D. L., Serfontein, J. R., & de Vries, P. J. (2011). Neuropsychological attention skills and related behaviours in adults with tuberous sclerosis complex. *Behavior Genetics*, 41, 437–444.

Tsai, P. T., Greene-Collozzi, E., Goto, J., et al. (2013). Prenatal rapamycin results in early and late behavioural abnormalities in wild-type C57BL/6 mice. *Behavior Genetics*, 43, 51–59.

Tsai, P. T., Hull, C., Chu, Y., et al. (2012). Autistic-like behavior and cerebellar dysfunction in Purkinje cell *Tsc1* mutant mice. *Nature*, 488, 647–651.

Van Eeghen, A. M., Black, M. E., Pulsifer, M. B., Kwiatkowski, D. J., & Thiele, E. A. (2012). Genotype and cognitive phenotype of patients with tuberous sclerosis complex. *European Journal of Human Genetics*, 20, 510–515.

Van Slegtenhorst, M., de Hoogt, R., Hermans, C., et al. (1997). Identification of the tuberous sclerosis gene *TSC1* on chromosome 9q34. *Science, 277*, 805–808.

Vogt, H. (1908). Zur Pathologie und Patologischen Anatomie der Verschiedenen Idiotieform [Towards the pathology and pathological anatomy of different forms of intellectual disability]. *Monatschrift fur Psychiatrie und Neurologie, 24*, 106–150.

Waltereit, R., Japs, B., Schneider, M., et al. (2011). Epilepsy and *Tsc2* haploinsufficiency lead to autistic-like social deficit behaviors in rats. *Behavior Genetics, 41*, 364–372.

Wong, M. (2007). The utility of tuberless models of tuberous sclerosis. *Epilepsia, 48*, 1629–1630.

Wong, M. (2010). Mammalian target of rapamycin (mTOR) inhibition as a potential antiepileptogenic therapy: From tuberous sclerosis to common acquired epilepsies. *Epilepsia, 51*, 27–36.

World Health Organization (1993). *The ICD-10 Classification of Mental and Behavioural Disorders. Diagnostic Criteria for Research*. Geneva: WHO.

Zeng, L. H., Xu, L., Gutmann, D. H., & Wong, M. (2008). Rapamycin prevents epilepsy in a mouse model of tuberous sclerosis complex. *Annals of Neurology, 63*, 444–453.

Zhou, J., Blundell, J., Ogawa, S., et al. (2009). Pharmacological inhibition of mTORC1 suppresses anatomical, cellular, and behavioural abnormalities in neural-specific Pten knock-out mice. *Journal of Neuroscience, 29*, 1773–1783.

CHAPTER 9

Treatment of Fragile X Syndrome and Fragile X-associated Disorders

REYMUNDO LOZANO, EMMA B. HARE, AND
RANDI JENSSEN HAGERMAN

INTRODUCTION

Fragile X syndrome (FXS) and fragile X-associated disorders (FADs) are all related to mutations in the fragile X mental retardation 1 gene (*FMR1*) on the bottom end of the X chromosome at Xq27.3 position. In the normal range, there are 5 to 40 CGG repeats in the 5' untranslated region of *FMR1*. In carriers of the premutation, there are 55 to 200 CGG repeats, and in the full mutation there are more than 200 repeats that are usually methylated. In the full mutation, methylation shuts down transcription, and the lack or deficiency of the *FMR1* protein (FMRP) causes FXS. The premutation leads to the FADs because there is enhanced transcription leading to excessive *FMR1* mRNA and RNA toxicity (Tassone et al., 2000; Hagerman & Hagerman, 2013). The high end of the premutation can lead to lowered FMRP levels and mild symptoms that are typical in FXS (Goodlin-Jones et al., 2004). The RNA toxicity, however, can lead to emotional difficulties in childhood, including ADHD, autism spectrum disorders (ASD), shyness, and social anxiety (Farzin et al., 2006; Chonchiaya et al., 2012). These problems can persist into adulthood, although depression and anxiety are the most common difficulties of adults with the premutation and normal intellectual abilities (Bourgeois et al., 2011; Hagerman & Hagerman 2013).

The premutation is the most common genetic cause of primary ovarian insufficiency (FXPOI), meaning cessation of menses before age 40, and approximately 20% of carriers experience this problem (Sullivan et al., 2011). Approximately 54% of female and 27% of male premutation carriers experience migraine headaches (Au et al., 2013); the majority of carriers develop hypertension with age (Hamlin et al., 2012); and immune-mediated problems such as fibromyalgia and hypothyroidism are common in women who are carriers (Winarni et al., 2012a). Neurological problems are seen in aging premutation carriers, including neuropathy, tremor, ataxia, and cognitive decline, all symptoms of the fragile X-associated tremor ataxia syndrome (FXTAS). These neurological problems occur in approximately 40% of male carriers and 16% of female carriers, although the symptoms in females are less severe and dementia is rare (Hagerman & Hagerman, 2013).

This chapter will focus on targeted treatments developed for FXS, because recent progress in understanding the biological mechanisms of the disorder have led to the development of several medications that are leading the way for targeted treatments, not only in FXS, but also in related disorders, including autism and ASD. Some of the targeted treatments developed for FXS may also be helpful for premutation disorders (FAD), but additional research is needed before validating these treatments in carriers (Cao et al., 2012).

FXS is the most common inherited cause of intellectual disability (ID) and the most common single gene cause of autism known. The prevalence of the premutation in the general population is approximately 1 in 200 females and 1 in 450 males (Tassone et al., 2012), whereas the prevalence of the full mutation is approximately 1 in 4,000 males and females (Crawford et al., 2001).

CLINICAL FEATURES

Those with FXS usually do not have dysmorphic features, although the ears may be prominent with cupping in the upper aspect of the pinna, and the face may be long, but typically not until after adolescence (Figure 9.1). The skin is usually soft, and the finger joints may be hyperextensible in childhood because of loose connective tissue. The feet are generally flat with some degree of pronation, and the testicles become large in adolescence and then stabilize in size, such that they are two to three times larger than in normal males (Hagerman & Hagerman, 2002). A high arched palate is common, and this may influence the drainage of the Eustachian tubes. Ear infections are common in the first three to four years of life, and pressure equalizing (PE) tubes are often used to normalize hearing and improve

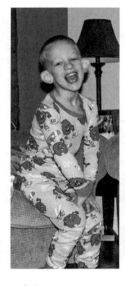
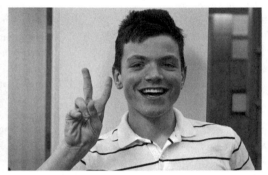

Figure 9.1:
Two boys with FXS. One displays typical fragile X features, specifically prominent ears, while the other does not.

language. Seizures occur in approximately 20% of children with FXS and up to 13% of children with the premutation, and anticonvulsants are an effective treatment (Hagerman & Hagerman 2002; Chonchiaya et al., 2012). The presence of seizures is associated with a higher risk for ASD, so treatment is essential (Chonchiaya et al., 2012).

Because most children with FXS look normal, the key to their diagnosis is in their behavior. By the second year of life, they develop increasing anxiety and hypersensitivity to sensory stimuli. Hyperactivity is seen in most boys and in up to 50% of girls with the full mutation, although attention and executive function deficits are common even when they are not hyperactive (Cornish et al., 2013). Infants are often hypotonic in the first and second year of life and delayed in language, typically not speaking at age two. Additional behavior problems include poor eye contact and hand-flapping with excitement, along with perseveration in behavior and tantrums. Autism is diagnosed in 30% of boys with FXS and an ASD is seen in up to 60% (Harris et al., 2008). The children with an ASD demonstrate significant social and language deficits beyond just poor eye contact or repetitive behaviors (Kaufmann et al., 2004) (Table 9.1).

Typically, children with FXS are diagnosed around three years of age with *FMR1* DNA testing (Bailey et al., 2009). High-functioning boys with an IQ greater than 70 and girls with FXS who typically present with learning

Table 9.1 CLINICAL CHARACTERISTICS OF FRAGILE X-ASSOCIATED DISORDERS

Premutation (55–200 CGG repeats)	Full Mutation (>200 CGG repeats)

Physical/Medical features (less frequent than in the full mutation):
 • Prominent ears
 • Hyperextensible finger joints
 • Seizures (8–13%)
 • Migraines
 • Immune mediated disorders
   • Fibromyalgia
   • Hypothyroidism
 • Primary ovarian insufficiency (FXPOI)
 • Aging: Fragile X-associated tremor/ataxia syndrome (FXTAS)
   • Neuropathy
   • Tremor
   • Ataxia
   • Cognitive decline
   • Executive function deficits
	Physical/Medical features:
	 • Prominent ears with cupping
	 • Elongated face after adolescence
	 • Hyperextensible joints
	 • Loose connective tissue
	 • Soft skin
	 • Flat feet with some pronation
	 • Macroorchidism after age 10
	 • High arched palate
	 • Seizures (20%)

Cognitive features: • Social anxiety • Depression • Anxiety • ADHD • Shyness • Autism spectrum disorders (ASD) • Executive function deficits	*Cognitive features:* • ADHD • Intellectual disability • Autism • Autism spectrum disorders (ASD) • Anxiety • Hypersensitivity to sensory stimuli • Executive function deficits • Social anxiety • Poor eye contact • Hand flapping • Perseveration • Tantrums • Social and language deficits • Learning disabilities
Prevalence: • 1 in 200 females • 1 in 450 males	*Prevalence:* • 1 in 4,000 males and females

disabilities, such as math problems, and anxiety, but without ID, are often not diagnosed until later in childhood or even adolescence. On occasion, a grandfather is diagnosed with FXTAS or a mother is diagnosed with FXPOI, which precipitates cascade testing of other family members, leading to diagnosis of a child with FXS or another family member with FAD.

The average IQ of an adult male with FXS is 40, but those with a lack or partial lack of methylation (methylation mosaicism) or those who have size mosaicism (some cells with the premutation and other cells with the full mutation) have an average IQ in the 60s (Hagerman & Hagerman, 2002). Approximately 15% of boys with FXS are high-functioning with an IQ greater than 70. Most girls with FXS, on the other hand, have an IQ above 70, although 25% have ID. The X-activation ratio, meaning the percentage of cells with the normal X as the active X, correlates with the overall IQ in girls with FXS (Loesch et al., 2004).

NEUROBIOLOGICAL MECHANISMS OF DISEASE

Over two decades of molecular research have led to significant advances in understanding the neurobiology of FXS and related disorders. FMRP is a selective RNA-binding protein, which regulates the translation of hundreds of mRNAs, usually through inhibition (Bagni et al., 2012; Darnell & Klann, 2013). FMRP contains three main RNA-binding domains; two hnRNP K-homology (KH) domains and one RGG box. In addition, a stem loop SoSLIP motif and U-rich sequences have been proposed to be RNA-binding sites. The I304N point mutation, which is located within the second KH domain, causes severe FXS and suggests that this domain plays an essential role in the FMRP function. FMRP is largely found in the cytoplasm; however, it contains a nuclear localization and nuclear export sequence. FMRP regulates RNA transportation, stabilization, and translation. *In vitro* FMRP is part of messenger ribonucleoparticles (structures that are involved in protein synthesis) and regulates dendritic transport of associated mRNAs, which result in the production of protein synthesis at the synapse (Bagni et al., 2012). FMRP interacts with several cytoplasmic and nuclear proteins, and it has been found in granules containing translationally silent preinitiation complexes. It is estimated that FMRP binds about 4% of total brain RNA and interacts with many other proteins, including approximately 30% of the proteins associated with autism (Bagni et al., 2012; Darnell et al., 2011, 2013; Iossifov et al., 2012).

In the brain, protein synthesis in the soma, axons, dendrites, and post-synaptic sites is required for long-term forms of synaptic plasticity, which form and consolidate long-term memories. Protein synthesis promotes synaptic plasticity activation, as well as the activation of different synaptic plasticity states, and it is coordinated by the action of the metabotrobic glutamate receptors (mGluRs) (Massey & Bashir 2007). Specifically, the activation of mGluR induces a synaptic plasticity state called "long-term depression" (LTD) (Massey & Bashir 2007), which triggers synaptic plasticity by regulating mRNA and the synthesis, degradation and recycling of somatic and axonic proteins. In the *Fmr1*-KO mice, LTD is significantly increased (Bagni et al., 2012). This effect on LTD is probably due to dysregulated local protein synthesis and has established the basis of the "mGluR theory" (Bear et al., 2004). The mGluR theory of FXS suggests that the psychiatric, cognitive, and neurological aspects of the syndrome are due to exaggerated downstream consequences of mGluR5 upregulation. This theory was validated by genetic mouse studies where rescue of several symptoms occurred when the mGluR5 heterozygous mouse was crossed with the *Fmr1*-KO mouse (Dolen et al., 2010). The *Fmr1*-KO shows an excess of protein translation, protein synthesis, and synaptic proteins (Berry-Kravis et al., 2011; Bagni et al., 2012). Additionally, FMRP binds and represses the catalytic subunit of PI3K, a signaling molecule downstream of the activation of mGluR5 (Gross et al., 2010). In summary, the absence of FMRP leads to dysregulation and usually over-expression of a number of its target genes, which causes abnormal synthesis of proteins involved in neurotransmission, dendritic morphology, and synaptic plasticity. Several approaches, including the use of mGluR5 antagonists, have led to positive outcomes for anatomical, electrophysiological, and behavioral measures in the animal model, leading to subsequent human trials (Hagerman et al., 2012) (Figure 9.2). Targeted treatments show promising results in mitigating or even reversing the neurobiological abnormalities caused by loss of FMRP. Furthermore, targeted treatments for FXS are leading the way for treatment of other neurodevelopmental disorders, including autism and ASD.

DIAGNOSTIC METHODS

The diagnosis of FXS or the premutation is made with molecular testing for the cytosine, guanine, guanine (CGG) expansion in *FMR1* (order the *FMR1* DNA test) that includes polymerase chain reaction (PCR) and Southern Blotting. The latter is most important to see if a large expansion in the full mutation range is present and to document the methylation status. PCR demonstrates the size of the premutation and the genetic report should

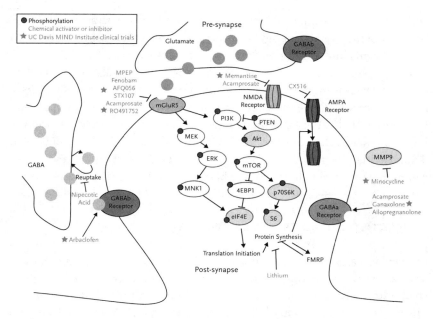

Figure 9.2:
Diagram of mechanism implicated in FXS altered synaptic plasticity and targeted treatments. Two signaling pathways downstream of mGluR5 affect translation, the MEK-ERK-Mnk1 and the PI3K-mTOR pathway. Also depicted are medications that affect the GABA receptors, MMP9 level, NMDA, and AMPA receptors. The stars represent clinical trials at the MIND Institute. Picture adapted from Levenga et al., 2010, and artistic input from Carolyn Yrigollen and Dr. Flora Tassone.

document the size of the CGG repeat. All children or adults diagnosed with ASD or ID of unknown etiology should be tested for FXS with the *FMR1* DNA testing. Those with neurological problems, including tremor or ataxia and women with POI, should also have *FMR1* DNA testing, and this can be ordered by any physician, usually the primary health care provider.

RELATED DISORDERS

There is a close association between ASD and FXS because FMRP regulates hundreds of genes at the synapse that are important for synaptic plasticity, and many of these genes are also associated with autism, including neuroligins, neurexins, *PSD 95, Shank 3, Arc*, etc. (Iossifov et al., 2012; Darnell & Klann, 2013). Therefore the lack of FMRP in FXS will lead to dysfunction of these other genes associated with autism. Low levels of FMRP in the CNS are also seen in autism without an *FMR1* mutation (Fatimi et al., 2011) and in other psychiatric conditions including schizophrenia, bipolar disorder, and depression (Fatimi et al., 2010). Recent studies have shown that FMRP levels in blood are associated with the age of onset and IQ in those with schizophrenia but without an *FMR1* mutation (Kovacs et al., 2013).

The gray zone includes those with 40 to 54 CGG repeats and it is called gray because it is unclear if disease is associated with this allele size. There is twice the rate of FXPOI in the gray zone than in the general population (Bretherick et al., 2005) and this is likely to be related to a mild elevation of *FMR1* mRNA levels (Loesch et al., 2007). In addition, FXTAS has now been diagnosed in the gray zone (Hall et al., 2011), and this is perhaps more common when others in the family have FXTAS (Liu et al., 2012).

CURRENT STANDARD TREATMENT OF FXS

Currently, early intervention with both speech and language therapy and occupational therapy with sensory integration techniques are given to children with FXS, most optimally beginning in the first year of life, but more typically obtained after diagnosis is made. Most children benefit significantly from special education support, but whenever possible, mainstreaming them into the regular classroom with the support of an aide is helpful (Hagerman & Hagerman, 2002). Enrichment of the environment is essential for an optimal outcome, and home intervention for early language development and motor development should start in the first year. For those with autism, the Early Start Denver Model (ESDM) developed by Sally Rogers and Geri Dawson is recommended (Dawson et al., 2010).

Many medications can be helpful in children with FXS, and the use of sertraline, a selective serotonin reuptake inhibitor (SSRI), may enhance language development at low doses beginning at age two (Winarni et al., 2012 a and b). However, hyperarousal can be seen in 20% of those treated with sertraline, and if activation or an increase in aggression occurs with sertraline, the dose should be lowered or discontinued. Typically sertraline or another SSRI can also decrease anxiety, and this may improve behavior and social interactions, which anxiety can worsen. The use of aripiprazole (Abilify) or risperidone (Risperdal) can help to stabilize mood, decrease aggression, and improve anxiety (Hagerman et al., 2009; Erickson et al., 2011). Clonidine or guanfacine can also have a calming effect in children with FXS and reduce hyperarousal, aggression, or hyperactivity. Clonidine can also help with sleep, although melatonin should be the first treatment for the sleep disturbances that are seen in the majority of young children with FXS (Wirojanan et al., 2009). Stimulants are helpful to treat ADHD symptoms in children with FXS who are five or older and can also be helpful throughout adolescence (Hagerman et al., 2009).

Currently, many of the targeted treatments outlined below are often mixed with standard treatments outlined above for an optimal effect for the child or adult with FXS.

TARGETED TREATMENTS

mGluR5 Antagonists

Since upregulation of the mGluR5 system leads to LTD, pharmaceutical interventions to downregulate mGluR5 activity have been shown to correct aspects of the FXS phenotype (Hagerman et al., 2012). There is a heightened focus on the development of mGluR5 negative allosteric modulators, resulting in the study of multiple compounds, including MPEP (2-methyl-6-phenylethynyl pyridine hydrochloride), fenobam (Neuropharm Ltd.), AFQ056 (Mavoglurant; Novartis Pharmaceuticals), RO4917523 (Hoffman-La Roche), and STX107 (Seaside Therapeutics).

Studies addressing MPEP treatment in *Fmr1*-KO mice have rescued an array of phenotypes typical of FXS, including correction of increased pre-pulse inhibition, audiogenic seizures, enhanced locomotor activity in the open field, increased density, and weak or immature synaptic architecture (reviewed in Hagerman et al., 2012). *In vitro* MPEP additionally rescued excessive AMPA receptor internalization in FMRP-deficient cultured neurons (Nakamoto et al., 2007). Of consideration, however, is the timing of mGluR5 antagonist treatment. When studying the effects of mGluR5 blockade on excitatory synaptic activity, normalization to wild-type values was only evident in hippocampal slices after two weeks of development, but not at one week or eight to ten weeks (Meredith et al., 2011). Chronic treatment with CTEP, another mGluR5 antagonist, corrected elevated hippocampal LTD, enhanced protein synthesis, audiogenic seizures, auditory hypersensitivity, irregular dendritic spine density, overactive ERK, and mTOR signaling, and partially corrected macroorchidism in young adult KO mice (Michalon et al., 2012). This study showed that pharmacological treatment after mature development can reverse many aspects of the FXS phenotype, and this has given hope to many families that have an adult with FXS.

Two genetic investigations of mGluR5 regulation in *Fmr1*-KO mice that reduced FMRP levels by 50% presented contradicting results of decreasing susceptibility to audiogenic seizures. While both studies presented the rescue of numerous phenotypes, reduced susceptibility to audiogenic seizures was only found in one study (Dolen et al., 2007), while the other reported no significant rescue of susceptibility to seizures (Thomas et al., 2012). This contradicting result demonstrates need for continued study and reinforces the consideration of factors such as background genetic effects or environmental factors that may contribute to the impact of treatment. Given the overall rescue of numerous phenotypical features of FXS in animal models, multiple mGluR5 antagonists are now under study in humans, with promising outcomes.

Human Studies

In a single-dose trial with fenobam administered to 12 adults with FXS, subjects showed a 20% improvement in prepulse inhibition (PPI), which involves sensorimotor gating and inhibition (Berry-Kravis et al., 2009). Due to financial constraints, however, Neuropharm was unable to pursue further development despite encouraging results.

The second clinical study with an mGluR5 antagonist was a randomized, double-blind, two-treatment, two-period, crossover study of AFQ056 in 30 males (18–35 years) (Jacquemont et al., 2011). While the primary outcome measure, the Aberrant Behavior Checklist–Community Edition (ABC-C), did not demonstrate significant treatment effects, an exploratory analysis showed seven patients with full *FMR1* methylation and no detectable *FMR1* messenger RNA improved significantly on the ABC-C compared to placebo. Eighteen patients with partial methylation showed a variable response, but overall there was no significant improvement on the medication. AFQ056 was well tolerated, with mild to moderate fatigue and headache the most commonly reported side effects (Jacquemont et al., 2011). Novartis is pursuing global, randomized, double-blind, placebo-controlled studies to evaluate the safety and efficacy of AFQ056 in children, adolescents, and adults with FXS (see the website clinicaltrials.gov for further information). In addition, open-label continuation studies are ongoing for adults and adolescents with FXS. Because there has been a mixed response to this medication, testing for biomarkers that could identify the responders, such as complete methylation of *FMR1*, is taking place.

Studies assessing efficacy of the mGluR5 antagonist RO4917523 (Hoffman-La Roche) are currently underway in children beginning at age five and into adulthood with FXS. These studies are at multiple centers internationally and are controlled trials, although open-label longitudinal studies have not yet been organized. If efficacy is seen in these studies, then phase 3 trials will be organized. Seaside Therapeutics, which recently partnered with Hoffman-La Roche, has developed another mGluR5 antagonist, STX107, which has been successful in animal studies and will be studied in patients with FXS in the future (Figure 9.2).

TARGETING GABA$_A$ RECEPTORS

In FXS, collective results show an imbalance between neuronal inhibition and excitation with overall excitation; therefore, changing the balance from excitation to inhibition has been considered through a GABAergic approach. The gamma amino-butyric acid (GABA) pathways are the main inhibitory system in the human brain and play a role in regulating neuronal excitability throughout the nervous system. There are two classes of GABA receptors: GABA$_A$ and GABA$_B$. GABA$_A$ receptors are ligand-gated ion channels, whereas GABA$_B$ receptors are G protein-coupled receptors. GABA$_A$ receptors allow the flow of chloride ions across the membrane, which hyperpolarizes the neuron's membrane and minimizes the effect of any coincident synaptic input. FMRP targets the mRNAs encoding eight different GABA$_A$ receptor subunits (α1, α3, α4, β1, β2, γ1, γ2, and χ), which were significantly reduced in the cortex of *Fmr1*-KO mice, particularly the γ subunit, which is believed to represent extrasynaptic (perisynaptic) GABA$_A$ receptors (D'Hulst et al., 2006). In addition, the *Fmr1*-KO mouse exhibits reduced inhibitory postsynaptic currents in the amygdala (Olmos-Serrano et al., 2010) and subicular neurons (Curia et al., 2009). Fly models of FXS also show lower levels of GABA receptors (Chang et al., 2008). GABA$_A$ agonists act to directly compensate for the GABA$_A$ subunit deficiencies by enhancing the function of the existing receptors.

A brief report of three patients with FXS and autism treated with acamprosate showed improvement in language and behavior in all the patients (Erickson et al., 2010). Acamprosate is a drug approved for treatment of alcohol withdrawal; it is thought to stabilize the excitatory/inhibition balance in the brain mainly by enhancing the function of GABA$_A$ receptors and possibly inhibitory effects at group I mGluRs (Erickson et al., 2010).

Ganaxolone (3a-hydroxy-3B-methyl analogue of allopregnanolone) is a GABA$_A$ receptor agonist through allosteric modulation; it is orally active and lacks hormonal side effects (Pin & Prézeau, 2007). In the *Fmr1*-KO, ganaxolone has been shown to decrease audiogenic seizures (Heulens et al., 2012). Similarly, studies in the *dfmr* mutant fly show that GABA$_A$ agonists ameliorate the lethality phenotype from glutamate-containing food, neuropathology, excessive protein translation, and abnormal courtship behavior (Chang et al., 2008). The chronic activation of GABA$_A$ receptors may have beneficial effects in ameliorating the learning deficits characteristic of the FXS (El Idrissi et al., 2009). Currently we are conducting a randomized, phase 2, double-blind, placebo-controlled crossover trial to investigate the efficacy of ganaxolone for the treatment of anxiety and attention deficits in children with FXS ages 6 to 17 (www.clinicaltrials.org).

TARGETING GABA$_B$ RECEPTORS

Arbaclofen (STX209, R-baclofen) is a γ-aminobutyric acid type B (GABA$_B$) receptor agonist and the active enantiomer of racemic baclofen, which acts presynaptically to block glutamate release. The resulting decreased glutamatergic drive indirectly reduces mGluR5 activation (Figure 9.2). In addition to exaggerated mGluR1/5 activation in FXS explained above is the deficiency of GABA-mediated inhibitory neurotransmission. Fmr1-KO mice show reduced GABAergic inhibition in the hippocampus, striatum, somatosensory cortex, and amygdala (Olmos-Serrano et al., 2010). Humans with FXS are shown to have excessive amgydala activation, as is evident during face-processing tasks (Watson et al., 2009). However, another recent study suggested the opposite; lower FMRP levels in fragile X spectrum involvement (FXSI) from the premutation to the full mutation were associated with lowered activation of the amygdala on fMRI studies (Kim et al., 2014). Dysregulation of the GABA pathways in the limbic system are hypothesized to be the basis of social anxiety and avoidance, characteristic of FXS (Cordiero et al., 2011). In the Fmr1-KO mice, arbaclofen reduced protein synthesis and translation to wild-type levels, corrected AMPAR trafficking in neurons, corrected the increased spine density, and rescued susceptibility to audiogenic seizures (Henderson et al., 2012). Therefore arbaclofen is considered a disease-modifying drug or targeted treatment for FXS.

Human Studies

A randomized, double-blind, placebo-controlled crossover study with arbaclofen evaluating improvements in behavioral symptoms of 63 subjects with FXS (55 males) aged 6–40 years showed significant treatment effects on numerous outcome measures (Berry-Kravis et al., 2012). While the primary outcome measure, the ABC-Irritability subscale, did not show significance, parent-nominated problem behaviors on the Visual Analog Scale (VAS) and the Clinical Global Improvement scale (CGI-I) showed positive trends with treatment of arbaclofen. Additional post hoc analysis demonstrated full study population improvement on the ABC-Social Avoidance (SA) subscale validated for FXS (Sansone et al., 2012), which is currently being used as an efficacy assessment in multiple clinical trials for FXS. Furthermore, a subset of patients who met diagnostic criteria for autism or had significant social deficits on the ABC (27 subjects) demonstrated additional improvements in the Vineland-Socialization subscale and all global measures. Overall, arbaclofen is a well-tolerated medication with few side effects, the most common being sedation and headache in only 8% (Berry-Kravis et al., 2012). Many of the subjects continued to extension studies. However, further controlled studies in those with ASD and in those with FXS did not show significant efficacy, leading to the collapse of the company and the termination of all studies.

LOVASTATIN

Lovastatin was originally isolated from the mold Aspergillus and it is also naturally found in the culinary oyster mushroom. It was the first statin utilized clinically, and it has the greatest transcellular permeability coefficient; therefore, it reaches the highest central nervous system (CNS) levels when compared to other statins. Lovastatin is a specific inhibitor of the rate-limiting enzyme in cholesterol biosynthesis (3-hydroxy-3-methylglutaryl coenzyme A [3HMG-CoA] reductase), and it is widely used for treatment of hyperlipidemia in children and adults (Figure 9.2). Although lovastatin is FDA-approved for use in children 10 years and older for treatment of familial hypercholesterolemia, it has been used in younger children for other conditions, such as cholesterol ester storage disease and nephrotic syndrome (Prata et al., 1994). Most recently, lovastatin has been used successfully in infants to treat hypoxia and ischemic encephalopathy (Buonocore et al., 2012). Lovastatin is also a targeted treatment for neurofibromatosis type 1 (NF1) because it can inhibit small GTPases (including Ras) (Li et al., 2007). In mice with $Nf1+/-$ mutation, lovastatin improved memory and long-term deficits in potentiation without significant side effects (Acosta et al., 2011).

Pertinent to FXS, lovastatin reduces the activation of the small guanosine triphosphatase (GTPase) Ras and subsequently the activation of the extracellular signal regulated kinase (ERK1/2), a signaling molecule downstream to the activation of mGluRs (Gross et al., 2010). Specifically, lovastatin interferes with recruitment of Ras to the membrane, a process required to transition from inactive GDP to active GTP. The interaction of Ras with the membrane requires the post-translational addition of a farnesyl group to the C terminus of Ras. Lovastatin inhibits Ras farnesylation by targeting the upstream mevalonate pathway (Osterweil et al., 2010).

In the *Fmr1*-KO, lovastatin decreased the excessive protein production (Osterweil et al., 2010) by inhibition of the Ras-ERK1/2 signaling in the hippocampal neurons (Li et al., 2007). In addition, the use of lovastatin blocked the induction of mGluR-mediated epileptiform activity in hippocampal slices, lowered seizures, and corrected hyperexcitability in visual cortex in the *Fmr1*-KO (Osterweil et al., 2013).

We have utilized lovastatin clinically in five children with FXS, and we have seen a response in enhanced language. For instance, the mother of an 11-year-old old boy with autism and FXS who was started on lovastatin (20 mg a day) stated that he "came out of the fog"; he started verbalizing more with the utilization of phrases for the first time and "using more combinations of new words." His eye contact improved, as did his overall behavior. Although his mother states that he is still "spinning things," she adds that "he is now using pretend play, which is new for him." There were no side effects, and his cholesterol and other laboratory studies remain normal. However, these are anecdotal reports and there is a need for a controlled trial of lovastatin to assess its safety and efficacy in children with FXS.

MINOCYCLINE

Animal Studies

When Bilousova et al. (2009) published the first *fmr1*-KO mouse studies utilizing minocycline, the fragile X field was surprised that one month of minocycline after birth could rescue the dendritic spine defects seen in FXS. The long, thin and immature spines converted to normal mature spines on minocycline, and there were improvements in anxiety on the elevated plus maze along with improvements on a cognitive task (Bilousova et al., 2009). These researchers found elevated matrix metalloproteinase 9 (MMP9) levels in the *fmr1*-KO mouse compared to wild type and minocycline lowered the MMP9 levels to normal (Figure 9.2).

MMP9 is an endopeptidase that is extracellular, but it also appears to be an important protein for the development of synaptic connections and plasticity, particularly in the hippocampus (Michaluk et al., 2011). In the *Drosophila* model of fragile X (*dfmr1* mutants), Kendall Broadie's laboratory demonstrated that over-expression of the only tissue inhibitor of MMPs, tissue inhibitor of metalloproteinase (TIMP), prevented the synaptic defects seen in the *dfmr1* mutants (Siller & Broadie, 2011). Minocycline treatment of the *dfmr1* mutants normalized synaptic structure and brain morphology (Siller & Broadie 2011). Subsequently, Rotschafer et al. (2011) have demonstrated decreased ultrasonic calling vocalizations during mating in the *fmr1*-KO mouse compared to wild type, and treatment for four weeks after birth with minocycline normalized the deficient vocalizations. These animal studies have paved the way for clinical trials with minocycline in patients with FXS.

Human Studies

Minocycline is a semisynthetic tetracycline-derivative antibiotic that has been available since the 1960s and is a common treatment for multiple conditions, including Rocky Mountain spotted fever and acne vulgaris. The initial human studies in FXS involved a survey of the families whose children with FXS were treated clinically with minocycline after the Bilousova study was published. Utari et al. (2010) utilized a Likert scale to survey the parents of 50 children treated for at least two weeks and up to a year and found that 70% of families noted improvement in language, attention, and/or social interactions, although side effects occurred in over one-third of patients. Paribello et al. (2010) carried out an open-label add-on-study of minocycline in 20 males with FXS who were 13 to 32 years of age and found improvement in a variety of measures, including the Vineland and the ABC scale. They found minocycline to be well tolerated, but 2 of the 20 patients treated developed a positive antinuclear antibody (ANA) test.

Due to these initial positive responses, Leigh et al. initiated a randomized, double-blind, placebo-controlled, crossover trial in individuals with FXS, ages 3.5–16 years (*n* = 55, mean age 9.2, SD 3.6 years) (Leigh et al., 2013). Participants were first randomized to three months of minocycline or placebo, and then switched to the other treatment arm for an additional three months. Primary outcome measures were the Clinical Global Impressions Scale–Improvement (CGI-I) and the Visual Analogue Scale (VAS) for behavior difficulties. Sixty-nine subjects were screened and 66 were randomized. Fifty-five subjects (83.3%) completed at least the first period, and 48 (72.7%) completed the full trial. The results demonstrated, in an intention-to-treat analysis, significantly greater improvement (lower score) in the primary outcome, CGI-I, after minocycline compared to placebo (least squares means ± standard error: 2.49 ± 0.13, 2.97 ± 0.13, respectively, p 0.0173) and greater improvement (higher number) in an ad hoc analysis of anxiety and mood-related behaviors on the VAS (minocycline 5.26 cm ± 0.46 cm, placebo 4.05 cm ± 0.46 cm; p 0.0488). The secondary outcome measures, including the ABC, the Vineland Adaptive Behavior

Scales (2nd edition), and the Expressive Vocabulary Test (EVT), had no significant improvement on minocycline. Side effects were not significantly different during the minocycline and placebo treatment periods. No serious adverse events occurred during minocycline treatment even in the young children at 3.5 years (Leigh et al., 2013).

The benefit of minocycline is that it is available by prescription currently and it can be used clinically, whereas the mGluR5 antagonists and the GABA$_A$ and GABA$_B$ agonists described above are not currently available clinically, although this may change in 2015. Minocycline is usually well tolerated, although it can cause GI upset, loose stools, skin sensitivity to the sun, and darkening of the skin, gums, or nails with prolonged use (Smith & Leyden 2005; Utari et al., 2010). Graying of the permanent teeth can also occur when used by children under age eight before the permanent teeth have emerged, so it is not FDA-approved for children under eight. Parents must decide whether the use of minocycline that can improve synaptic connections is worth the chance of gray teeth, although the latter problem can be fixed cosmetically with dental plating. In rare cases a lupus-like syndrome can develop, with a rash, swollen joints, or an autoimmune hepatitis, but this is reversible once the minocycline is stopped. Rarely, increased intracranial pressure can develop, leading to a severe headache called *pseudotumor cerebri*, so parents should be warned that if a rash, swollen joints, or persistent headache occur, the minocycline should be stopped.

Because minocycline is an antibiotic, it will change the flora in the GI tract, so it is recommended that a probiotic be utilized during treatment with minocycline. Minocycline and milk or milk products can chelate together, so milk should be avoided ½ to 1 hour before and after minocycline is given orally (Utari et al., 2010). We also recommend checking an ANA level every six months during minocycline treatment. Our preliminary data show that approximately 26% of children with FXS develop a positive antinuclear antibody (ANA) titer; however, 20% have a baseline positive titer (Rafika et al., unpublished data), similar to the autism population (20%, Mostafa & Kitchener, 2009) but higher than the 5% to 15% positive ANA in children in the general population (Wananukul et al., 2005).

Minocycline has been studied as a neuroprotective agent in diseases such as Huntington's disease and multiple sclerosis (Plane et al., 2010). There are several mechanisms by which minocycline has been theorized to exert its neuroprotective effects and anti-inflammatory effects, including inhibiting microglial activation, decreasing caspase activity, and through anti-apoptotic properties (Plane et al., 2010; Figure 9.3). It is unclear whether these neurobiological effects may be beneficial for those with FXS and perhaps also for those with premutation developmental problems. For some

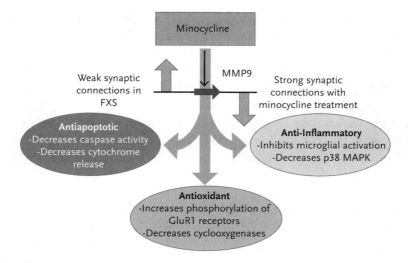

Figure 9.3:
Roles played by minocycline in neuroprotection and in lowering MMP9 levels to strengthen synaptic connections in those with FXS. Figure art developed by Dr. Paul Hagerman and Paul Doucet.

children with the premutation, there is a lowering of FMRP levels, particularly in the upper premutation range, which in turn would increase MMP9 levels. Therefore, those with the premutation and developmental problems related to lowered FMRP levels are predicted to improve on minocycline. This has been seen on a clinical basis in a handful of children, but controlled studies have not been carried out in premutation carriers. It is also possible that the immune-mediated problems that are experienced by some adult premutation carriers, such as fibromyalgia or multiple sclerosis, may also improve with minocycline. The neuroprotective and antiapoptotic effects of minocycline may also be beneficial for FXTAS, but so far these studies have not been carried out.

ADDITIONAL CONSIDERATIONS FOR TREATMENT

While the medications listed above are the focus of currently available targeted treatments, additional compounds have promising mechanisms for treatment in FXS. A recent open-label study of lithium in patients with FXS showed improvements in social behavior according to the ABC-C total score, VAS, Vineland-II maladaptive behavior subscale, and Repeatable Battery for the Assessment of Neuropsychological Status (RBANS) list learning (Berry-Kravis et al., 2008) (Figure 9.2). Only mild side effects were seen, although seven subjects experienced polyuria/polydipsia (Berry-Kravis et al., 2008). P21-activated kinase (PAK) inhibitors are another targeted treatment under development for FXS. Hayashi et al. (2007) demonstrated biological and behavioral phenotypical rescue in the *fmr1*-KO mouse, including partial restoration of irregular spine density and shape in the forebrain as well as partial and full amelioration of locomotor activity, stereotypy, anxiety, and trace fear conditioning with the *dnPAK* transgene. PI3K inhibitors are also targeted treatments in the *fmr1*-KO mouse and will probably be helpful in human studies when they are initiated (Gross et al., 2010).

The most robust treatment plan should be multifaceted, including non-pharmaceutical interventions such as speech, language, and/or occupational sensory integration therapy; educational/behavioral interventions such as the use of Early Start Denver Model for ASD (Dawson et al., 2010) ; the use of digital technology such as the iPAD learning programs to enhance academic, language, and socialization skills; in combination with targeted treatments, symptom-focused medications, and a healthy diet including antioxidants. There is strong evidence for oxidative stress in neurons with either the premutation (Chen et al., 2010; Cao et al., 2012) or the full mutation (de Diego-Otero et al., 2008), and the use of antioxidants such as NAC (N-acetylcysteine), alpha tocopherol (vitamin E), or melatonin (Romero-Zerbo & Decara, 2009) has been shown to normalize synaptic connections in the *fmr1*-KO mouse (de Diego-Otero et al., 2008). We therefore recommend antioxidants in the diet of children or adults with the premutation or the full mutation.

This is an exciting time for the use of targeted treatments in those with FXS because of the possibility of reversing the ID and behavioral problems associated with this and other related disorders with similar neurobiological changes. The future looks bright if the funding can be marshaled to carry out the studies that will demonstrate efficacy in individuals with FXS.

DISCLOSURES

This work was supported by grant R40 MC 22641 from the Maternal and Child Health Research Program, Maternal and Child Health Bureau (Combating Autism Act of 2006, as amended by the Combating Autism Reauthorization Act of 2011); Health Resources and Services Administration, Department of Health and Human Services, National Institutes of Health grants HD036071, HD02274, AG032119, and AG032115; DOD PR101054; support from the Health and Human Services

Administration on Developmental Disabilities grant 90DD05969; and the National Center for Advancing Translational Research UL1 TR000002.

Corresponding author—Dr. Randi J. Hagerman, MIND Institute, UC Davis Health System, 2825 50th Street, Sacramento, CA 95817; email: randi.hagerman@ucdmc.ucdavis.edu; telephone: (916) 703-0247.

REFERENCES

Acosta, M. T., Kardel, P. G., Walsh, K. S., Rosenbaum, K. N., Gioia, G. A., & Packer, R. J. (2011). Lovastatin as treatment for neurocognitive deficits in neurofibromatosis type 1: Phase I study. *Pediatric neurology*, *45*(4), 241–245.

Au, J., Akins, R., Berkowitz-Sutherland, L., Tang, H., Chen, Y., Boyd, A., et al. (2013). Prevalence and risk of migraine headaches in adult fragile X premutation carriers. *Clinical genetics*, *84*(6), 846–551. doi: 10.1111/cge.12109

Bailey, D. B. Jr, Raspa, M., Bishop, E., & Holliday, D. (2009). No change in the age of diagnosis for FXS: Findings from a national parent survey. *Pediatrics*, *142*, 527–533.

Bagni, C., Tassone, F., Neri, G., & Hagerman, R. (2012). Fragile X syndrome: Causes, diagnosis, mechanisms, and therapeutics. *Journal of clinical investigation*, *122*(12), 4314.

Bear, M. F., Huber, K. M., & Warren, S. T. (2004). The mGluR theory of fragile X mental retardation. *Trends in neurosciences*, *27*, 370–377.

Berry-Kravis, E., Sumis, A., Hervey, C., Nelson, M., Porges, S. W., Weng, N., et al. (2008). Open-label treatment trial of lithium to target the underlying defect in fragile X syndrome. *Journal of developmental & behavioral pediatrics*, *29*(4), 293–302

Berry-Kravis, E., Hessl, D., Coffey, S., Hervey, C., Schneider, A., Yuhas, J., et al. (2009). A pilot open label, single dose trial of fenobam in adults with fragile X syndrome. *Journal of medical genetics*, *46*(4), 266–271.

Berry-Kravis, E., Knox, A. & Hervey, C. (2011). Targeted treatments for fragile X syndrome. *Journal of neurodevelopmental Disorders*, *3*, 193–210.

Berry-Kravis, E. M., Hessl, D., Rathmell, B., Zarevics, P., Cherubini, M., Walton-Bowen, K., et al. (2012). Effects of STX209 (arbaclofen) on neurobehavioral function in children and adults with fragile X syndrome: a randomized, controlled, phase 2 trial. *Science and translational medicine*, *4*, 152ra127.

Bilousova, T. V., Dansie, L., Ngo, M., Aye, J., Charles, J. R., Ethell, D. W., & Ethell, I. M. (2009). Minocycline promotes dendritic spine maturation and improves behavioural performance in the fragile X mouse model. *Journal of medical genetics*, *46*(2), 94–102.

Bourgeois, J. A., Seritan, A. L., Melina Casillas, E., Hessl, D., Schneider, A., Yang, Y., et al. (2011). Lifetime prevalence of mood and anxiety disorders in fragile X premutation carriers. *Journal of clinical psychiatry*, *72*(2), 175.

Bretherick, K. L., Fluker, M. R., & Robinson, W. P. (2005). FMR1 repeat sizes in the gray zone and high end of the normal range are associated with premature ovarian failure. *Human genetics*, *117*(4), 376–382.

Buonocore, G., Perrone, S., Turrisi, G., Kramer, B. W., & Balduini, W. (2012). New pharmacological approaches in infants with hypoxic-ischemic encephalopathy. *Current pharmaceutical design*, *18*(21), 3086–3100.

Cao, Z., Hulsizer, S., Tassone, F., Tang, H. T., Hagerman, R. J., Rogawski, M. A., et al. (2012). Clustered burst firing in *FMR1* premutation hippocampal neurons: Amelioration with allopregnanolone. *Human Molecular Genetics*, *21*, 2923–2935.

Chang, S. Bray, S. M., Li, Z., Zarnescu, D. C., He, C., Jin, P., Warren, S. T. (2008). Identification of small molecules rescuing fragile X syndrome phenotypes in Drosophila. *Nature chemical biology, 4*, 256–263.

Chen, Y., Tassone, F., Berman, R. F., Hagerman, P. J., Hagerman, R. J., Willemsen, R., & Pessah, I. N. (2010). Murine hippocampal neurons expressing Fmr1 gene premutations show early developmental deficits and late degeneration. *Human molecular genetics, 19*(1), 196–208.

Chonchaiya, W., Au, J., Schneider A., et al. (2012). Increased prevalence of seizures in boys who were probands with the *FMR1* premutation and co-morbid autism spectrum disorder. *Human genetics, 131*(4), 581–589.

Cornish, K., Cole, V., Longhi, E., Karmiloff-Smith, A., & Scerif, G. (2013). Mapping developmental trajectories of attention and working memory in fragile X syndrome: Developmental freeze or developmental change? *Development and psychopathology, 25*(02), 365–376.

Cordeiro, L., Ballinger, E., Hagerman, R., & Hessl, D. (2011). Clinical assessment of DSM-IV anxiety disorders in fragile X syndrome: prevalence and characterization. *Journal of neurodevelopmental disorders, 3*(1), 57–67.

Crawford, D. C., Acuña, J. M., & Sherman, S. L. (2001). *FMR1* and the fragile X syndrome: human genome epidemiology review. *Genetics in medicine, 3*(5), 359–371.

Curia, G., Papouin, T., Séguéla, P., & Avoli, M. (2009). Down-regulation of tonic GABAergic inhibition in a mouse model of fragile X syndrome. *Cerebral cortex, 19*(7), 1515–1520.

D'Hulst, C., De Geest, N. et al. (2006). Decreased expression of the GABAA receptor in fragile X syndrome. *Brain research, 1121*, 238–245.

Darnell, J. C., Van Driesche, S. J., Zhang, C., Hung, K. Y. S., Mele, A., Fraser, C. E., et al. (2011). FMRP stalls ribosomal translocation on mRNAs linked to synaptic function and autism. *Cell, 146*(2), 247–261.

Darnell, J. C., & Klann, E. (2013). The translation of translational control by FMRP: therapeutic targets for FXS. *Nature neuroscience, 16*(11), 1530–1536. doi: 10.1038/nn.3379

Dawson, G., Rogers, S., Munson, J., Smith, M., Winter, J., Greenson, J., et al. (2010). Randomized, controlled trial of an intervention for toddlers with autism: the Early Start Denver Model. *Pediatrics, 125*(1), e17–e23.

de Diego-Otero, Y., Romero-Zerbo, Y., el Bekay, R., Decara, J., Sanchez, L., Rodriguez-de Fonseca, F., & del Arco-Herrera, I. (2008). α-tocopherol protects against oxidative stress in the fragile X knockout mouse: An experimental therapeutic approach for the Fmr1 deficiency. *Neuropsychopharmacology, 34*(4), 1011–1026.

Dolen, G., Osterweil, E., Rao, B. S., Smith, G. B., Auerbach, B. D., Chattarji, S., Bear, M. F. (2007). Correction of fragile X syndrome in mice. *Neuron, 56*, 955–962.

Dölen, G., Carpenter, R. L., Ocain, T. D., & Bear, M. F. (2010). Mechanism-based approaches to treating fragile X. *Pharmacology & therapeutics, 127*(1), 78–93.

Erickson, C. A., Mullett, J. E., & McDougle, C. J. (2010). Brief report: acamprosate in fragile X syndrome. *Journal of autism and developmental disorders, 40*(11), 1412–1416.

Erickson, C. A., Stigler, K. A., Wink, L. K., Mullett, J. E., Kohn, A., Posey, D. J., & McDougle, C. J. (2011). A prospective open-label study of aripiprazole in fragile X syndrome. *Psychopharmacology, 216*(1), 85–90.

El Idrissi, A., Boukarrou, L., Dokin, C., & Brown, W. T. (2009). Taurine improves congestive functions in a mouse model of fragile X syndrome. *Taurine 7*, 191–198.

Farzin, F., Perry, H., Hessl, D., Loesch, D., Cohen, J., Bacalman, S., et al. (2006). Autism spectrum disorders and attention-deficit/hyperactivity disorder in boys with the fragile X premutation. *Journal of developmental & behavioral pediatrics, 27*(2), S137–S144.

Fatemi, S. H., Kneeland, R. E., Liesch, S. B., & Folsom, T. D. (2010). Fragile X mental retardation protein levels are decreased in major psychiatric disorders. *Schizophrenia research, 124*(1–3), 246.

Fatemi, S. H., Folsom, T. D., Kneeland, R. E., & Liesch, S. B. (2011). Metabotropic glutamate receptor 5 upregulation in children with autism is associated with underexpression of both fragile X mental retardation protein and GABAA receptor beta 3 in adults with autism. *The Anatomical record: advances in integrative anatomy and evolutionary biology, 294*(10), 1635–1645.

Goodlin-Jones, B. L., Tassone, F., Gane, L. W., & Hagerman, R. J. (2004). Autistic spectrum disorder and the fragile X premutation. *Journal of developmental & behavioral pediatrics, 25*(6), 392.

Gross, C., Nakamoto, M., Yao, X., Chan, C. B., Yim, S. Y., Ye, K., Warren, S. T., & Bassell, G. J. (2010). Excess phosphoinositide 3-kinase subunit synthesis and activity as a novel therapeutic target in fragile X syndrome. *Journal of neuroscience, 30,* 10624–10638.

Hamlin, A. A., Sukharev, D., Campos, L., Mu, Y., Tassone, F., Hessl, D., et al. (2012). Hypertension in *FMR1* premutation males with and without fragile X-associated tremor/ataxia syndrome (FXTAS). *American journal of medical genetics part a, 158A,* 1304–1309.

Hagerman, R. J., & Hagerman, P. J. (Eds.). (2002). *Fragile X syndrome: Diagnosis, treatment, and research.* Baltimore, MD: Johns Hopkins University Press.

Hagerman, R. J., Berry-Kravis, E., Kaufmann, W. E., Ono, M. Y., Tartaglia, N., Lachiewicz, A., & Tranfaglia, M. (2009). Advances in the treatment of fragile X syndrome. *Pediatrics, 123*(1), 378–390.

Hagerman, R. J., Lauterborn, J., Au, J., & Berry-Kravis, E. (2012). Fragile X syndrome and targeted treatment trials. *Results and problems in cell differentiation, 54,* 297–335.

Hagerman, R. J. & Hagerman, P. (2013). Advances in the clinical and molecular research regarding the premutation including FXTAS: The other side of fragile X. *Lancet neurology, 12,* 786–798.

Hall, D. A., Berry-Kravis, E., Zhang, W., Tassone, F., Spector, E., Zerbe, G., et al. (2011). *FMR1* gray zone alleles: Association with Parkinson's disease in women. *Movement disorders, 26*(10), 1900–1906.

Harris, S. W., Hessl, D., Goodlin-Jones, B., Ferranti, J., Bacalman, S., Barbato, I., et al. (2008). Autism profiles of males with fragile X syndrome. *American journal on mental retardation, 113,* 427–438.

Hayashi, M. L., Rao, B. S., Seo, J. S., Choi, H. S., Dolan, B. M., Choi, S. Y., et al. (2007). Inhibition of p21-activated kinase rescues symptoms of fragile X syndrome in mice. *Proceedings of the national academy of sciences, 104*(27), 11489–11494.

Henderson, C., Wijetunge, L., Kinoshita, M. N., Shumway, M., Hammond, R. S., Postma, F. R., et al. (2012). Reversal of disease-related pathologies in the fragile X mouse model by selective activation of GABAB receptors with arbaclofen. *Science and translational medicine, 4,* 152ra128.

Heulens, I., D'Hulst, C., Van Dam, D., De Deyn, P. P., & Kooy, R. F. (2012). Pharmacological treatment of fragile X syndrome with GABAergic drugs in a knockout mouse model. *Behavioural brain research, 229*(1), 244–249.

Iossifov, I., Ronemus, M., Levy, D., Wang, Z., Hakker, I., Rosenbaum, J., et al. (2012). De novo gene disruptions in children on the autistic spectrum. *Neuron, 74*(2), 285–299.

Jacquemont, S., Curie, A., Des Portes, V., Torrioli, M. G., Berry-Kravis, E., Hagerman, R. J., et al. (2011). Epigenetic modification of the FMR1 gene in fragile X syndrome is associated with differential response to the mGluR5 antagonist AFQ056. *Science translational medicine, 3*(64), 64ra1–64ra1.

Kaufmann, W. E., Cortell, R., Kau, A., Bukelis, I., Tierney, E., Gray, R., et al. (2004). Autism spectrum disorder in FXS: communication, social interaction, and specific behaviors. *American journal of medical Genetics part a, 129A,* 225–234.

Kim, S. Y., Burris, J., Bassal, F., Koldewyn, K., Chattarji, S., Tassone, F., et al. (2014). Fear-specific amygdala function in children and adolescents on the fragile X spectrum: a dosage response of the *FMR1* gene. *Cerebral cortex, 24*(3), 600–613. doi: 10.1093/cercor/bhs341

Kovács, T., Kelemen, O., & Kéri, S. (2013). Decreased fragile X mental retardation protein (FMRP) is associated with lower IQ and earlier illness onset in patients with schizophrenia. *Psychiatry research, 210*(3), 690–693. doi: 10.1016/j.psychres.2012.12.022

Leigh, M. J. S., Nguyen, D. V., Mu, Y., Winarni, T. I., Schneider, A., Chechi, T., et al. (2013). A randomized double-blind, placebo-controlled trial of minocycline in children and adolescents with fragile X syndrome. *Journal of developmental & behavioral pediatrics, 34*(3), 147–155.

Li, M., & Losordo, D. W. (2007). Statins and the endothelium. *Vascular pharmacology, 46*(1), 1–9.

Liu, Y., Winarni, T. I., Zhang, L., Tassone, F., & Hagerman, R. J. (2012). Fragile X-associated tremor/ataxia syndrome (FXTAS) in grey zone carriers. *Clinical genetics, 84*(1), 74–77. doi: 10.1111/cge.12026.

Loesch, D. Z., Huggins, R. M., & Hagerman, R. J. (2004). Phenotypic variation and FMRP levels in fragile X. *Mental retardation and developmental disabilities research reviews, 10*(1), 31–41.

Loesch, D. Z., Bui, Q. M., Huggins, R. M., Mitchell, R. J., Hagerman, R. J., & Tassone, F. (2007). Transcript levels of the intermediate size or grey zone fragile X mental retardation 1 alleles are raised, and correlate with the number of CGG repeats. *Journal of medical genetics, 44*(3), 200–204.

Massey, P. V., & Bashir, Z. I. (2007). Long-term depression: Multiple forms and implications for brain function. *Trends in neurosciences, 30,* 176–184.

Meredith, R. M., De Jong, R., Mansvelder, H. D. (2011). Functional rescue of excitatory synaptic transmission in the developing hippocampus in Fmr1-KO mouse. *Neurobiology of disease, 41,* 104e110.

Michalon, A., Sidorov, M., Ballard, T. M., Ozmen, L., Spooren, W., Wettstein, J. G., et al. (2012). Chronic pharmacological mGlu5 inhibition corrects fragile X in adult mice. *Neuron, 74,* 49e56.

Michaluk, P., Wawrzyniak, M., Alot, P., Szczot, M., Wyrembek, P., Mercik, K., et al. (2011). Influence of matrix metalloproteinase MMP-9 on dendritic spine morphology. *Journal of cell science, 124*(19), 3369–3380.

Mostafa, G. A., & Kitchener, N. (2009). Serum anti-nuclear antibodies as a marker of autoimmunity in Egyptian autistic children. *Pediatric neurology, 40*(2), 107–112.

Nakamoto, M., Nalavadi, V., Epstein, M. P., Narayanan, U., Bassell, G. J., Warren, S. T. (2007). Fragile X mental retardation protein deficiency leads to excessive mGluR5-dependent internalization of AMPA receptors. *Proceedings of the national academy of sciences USA, 104*, 15537–15542.

Olmos-Serrano, J. L., Paluszkiewicz, S. M., Martin, B. S., Kaufmann, W. E., Corbin, J. G., & Huntsman, M. M. (2010). Defective GABAergic neurotransmission and pharmacological rescue of neuronal hyperexcitability in the amygdala in a mouse model of fragile X syndrome. *Journal of neuroscience, 30*, 9929–9938.

Osterweil, E. K., Krueger, D. D., Reinhold, K., & Bear, M. F. (2010). Hypersensitivity to mGluR5 and ERK1/2 leads to excessive protein synthesis in the hippocampus of a mouse model of fragile X syndrome. *Journal of neuroscience, 30*(46), 15616–15627.

Osterweil, E. K., Chuang, S.-C., Chubykin, A. A., Sidorov, M., Bianchi, R., Wong, R. K., & Bear, M. F. (2013). Lovastatin corrects excess protein synthesis and prevents epileptogenesis in a mouse model of fragile X syndrome. *Neuron, 77*(2), 243–250.

Paribello, C., Tao, L., Folino, A., Berry-Kravis, E., Tranfaglia, M., Ethell, I., & Ethell, D. (2010). Open-label add-on treatment trial of minocycline in fragile X syndrome. *BMC Neurology, 10*(1), 91.

Plane, J. M., Shen, Y., Pleasure, D. E., & Deng, W. (2010). Prospects for minocycline neuroprotection. *Archives of neurology, 67*(12), 1442.

Pin, J. P., & Prézeau, L. (2007). Allosteric modulators of GABAB receptors: mechanism of action and therapeutic perspective. *Current neuropharmacology, 5*(3), 195.

Prata, M. M., Nogueira, A. C., Pinto, J. R., Correia, A. M., Vicente, O., Rodrigues, M. C., & Miguel, M. J. (1994). Long-term effect of lovastatin on lipoprotein profile in patients with primary nephrotic syndrome. *Clinical nephrology, 41*(5), 277.

Romero-Zerbo, Y., Decara, J., et al. (2009). Protective effects of melatonin against oxidative stress in Fmr1 knockout mice: a therapeutic research model for the fragile X syndrome. *Journal of pineal research, 46*(2), 224–234.

Rotschafer, S. E., Trujillo, M. S., Dansie, L. E., Ethell, I. M., & Razak, K. A. (2011). Minocycline treatment reverses ultrasonic vocalization production deficit in a mouse model of Fragile X Syndrome. *Brain research, 1439*, 7–14.

Sansone, S. M., Widaman, K. F., Hall, S. S., Reiss, A. L., Lightbody, A., Kaufmann, W. E., et al. (2012). Psychometric study of the aberrant behavior checklist in Fragile X syndrome and implications for targeted treatment. *Journal of autism and developmental disorders, 42*(7), 1377–1392.

Siller, S. S., & Broadie, K. (2011). Neural circuit architecture defects in a Drosophila model of fragile X syndrome are alleviated by minocycline treatment and genetic removal of matrix metalloproteinase. *Disease models & mechanisms, 4*(5), 673–685.

Smith, K., & Leyden, J. J. (2005). Safety of doxycycline and minocycline: a systematic review. *Clinical therapeutics, 27*(9), 1329–1342.

Sullivan, S. D., Welt, C., & Sherman, S. (2011). FMR1 and the continuum of primary ovarian insufficiency. *Seminars in Reproductive Medicine, 29*, 299–307.

Tassone, F., Hagerman, R. J., Taylor, A. K., Gane, L. W., Godfrey, T. E., & Hagerman, P. J. (2000). Elevated levels of FMR1 mRNA in carrier males: A new mechanism of involvement in the fragile-X syndrome. *American journal of human genetics, 66*(1), 6–15.

Tassone, F., Long, K. P., Tong, T., Lo, J., Gane, L., Berry-Kravis, E., et al. (2012). FMR1 CGG allele size and prevalence ascertained through newborn screening in the United States. *Genome medicine, 4*, 100. doi:10.1186/gm401

Thomas, A. M., Bui, N., Perkins, J. R., Yuva-Paylor, L. A., & Paylor, R. (2012). Group I metabotropic glutamate receptor antagonists alter select behaviors in a mouse model for fragile X syndrome. *Psychopharmacology (Berlin)*, *219*, 47e58.

Utari, A., Chonchaiya, W., Rivera, S. M., Schneider, A., Hagerman, R. J., Faradz, S. M., et al. (2010). Side effects of minocycline treatment in patients with fragile X syndrome and exploration of outcome measures. *American journal on intellectual and developmental disabilities*, *115*(5), 433–443.

Wananukul, S., Voramethkul, W., Kaewopas, Y., Hanvivatvong, O. (2005). Prevalence of positive antinuclear antibodies in healthy children. *Asian pacific journal of allergy immunology*, *23*, 153–157.

Watson, D., Hoeft, F., Garrett, A. S., Hall, S. S., & Reiss, A. L. (2009). Aberrant brain activation during gaze processing in boys with fragile X syndrome. *Archives of general psychiatry*, *65*, 1315–1323.

Winarni, T. I., Schneider, A., Borodyanskara, M., & Hagerman, R. J. (2012a). Early intervention combined with targeted treatment promotes cognitive and behavioral improvements in young children with fragile X syndrome. *Case Reports in Genetics*, *2012*, 280813:1–4. doi: 10.1155/2012/280813

Winari, T. I., Chonchaiya, W., Adams, E., Au, J., Yi Mu, Rivera, S. M., Nguyen, D. V., Hagerman, R. J. (2012b). Sertraline may improve language developmental trajectory in young children with fragile X syndrome: a retrospective chart review. *Autism Research and Treatment*, 2012; Epub 2012 May 31. doi:10.1155/2012/104317.

Wirojanan, J., Jacquemont, S., Diaz, R., Bacalman, S., Anders, T. F., Hagerman, R. J., & Goodlin-Jones, B. L. (2009). The efficacy of melatonin for sleep problems in children with autism, fragile X syndrome, or autism and fragile X syndrome. *Journal of Clinical Sleep Medicine*, *5*(2), 145–150.

CHAPTER 10

Angelman Syndrome

MARY JACENA LEIGH, LINDSEY PARTINGTON,
AND EDWIN WEEBER

INTRODUCTION

"M" is an eight-year-old girl. She is the product of a full-term pregnancy,
and her developmental delays were noted at a young age. She has seizures,
which were difficult to control, but a modified ketogenic diet and antiepi-
leptics have helped. She uses three words—"Mama," "oh ma" for Grandma
and "uh uh" for no. She also uses signs. She has gastroesophageal reflux
and difficulties with sleep. Her parents come to you asking about targeted
treatments for Angelman syndrome (Figure 10.1).

CLINICAL DESCRIPTIONS AND STANDARD TREATMENT

History of Characterization of Syndrome

In 1965, Dr. Angelman described three cases of children with similar
features, including intellectual disabilities, unusual jerking movements,
seizures, and episodes of inappropriate laughter (Angelman, 1965). He
referred to them as "puppet children." The term "happy puppet syndrome"
was used in the past, but use of this term today is discouraged.

Epidemiology

Angelman syndrome (AS) is estimated to affect approximately 1/10,000
to 1/20,000 individuals according to population-based studies (Kyllerman,
1995; Petersen, Brondum-Nielsen, et al., 1995; Buckley, Dinno, et al., 1998).

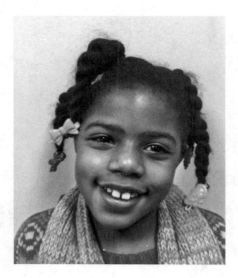

Figure 10.1:
Eight-year-old girl with Angelman Syndrome.

Consensus Criteria

In 1995, consensus criteria for the diagnosis of Angelman syndrome were published. The criteria were updated in 2005. These include:

- Consistent features (present in 100%): Severe developmental delays, movement or balance disorders (typically ataxia or tremulous limb movements), unique behaviors (frequent laughing or smiling, happy demeanor, easily excitable, uplifted hand-flapping or waving movements, hypermotoric behavior), and speech impairment (none to a few words, and receptive and nonverbal communications skills are more developed than verbal skills).
- Frequently seen features (>80%): Microcephaly usually by age two, seizures (onset usually <3 years of age), EEG abnormalities.
- Associated features (20–80%): Flat occiput; occipital groove; tongue protrusions and thrusting, sucking, or swallowing disorders; feeding problems and/or truncal hypotonia in infancy; prognathism; wide mouth; widely spaced teeth; frequent drooling; excessive chewing/mouthing; strabismus; hypopigmented skin, light hair and eye color (in cases caused by a deletion); hyperactive deep-tendon reflexes in the lower extremities; uplifted flexed-arm position during ambulation; wide-based gait; increased heat sensitivity; diminished need for sleep and abnormal sleep cycles; fascination with water, crinkly papers, and plastics; obesity in

older children; scoliosis; constipation; and abnormal food-related behaviors (Williams, Angelman, et al., 1995; Williams, Beaudet, et al., 2006).

Description of Selected Physical Features

Ataxic gait: Individuals with Angelman syndrome have difficulties with motor control. They may have a wide-based gait and hold their arms in a flexed position when walking. Studies comparing children with AS to other children with either learning disabilities, epilepsy, or motor dysfunction, find that children with AS more frequently have stiff lower limbs, distal lower extremity spasticity, an ataxic-like gait, as well as asymmetrical muscle strength (Beckung, Steffenburg, et al., 2004).

Microcephaly: Individuals with AS may have slow or delayed growth in head circumference, which results in relative or absolute microcephaly by two years of age.

Description of Selected Developmental/Behavioral Features

Developmental delays: The developmental milestones are delayed, usually by 12 months of age. Expressive language delays are typically more severe than receptive language delays. A study of 20 children ages 2–14 with AS showed that most of the children studied used fewer than five words (Andersen, Rasmussen, et al., 2001). The typical developmental level found on standardized testing for individuals with AS up to 14 years of age was 18–24 months (Andersen, Rasmussen, et al., 2001; Peters, Goddard-Finegold, et al., 2004). Adaptive behavior has been found to be strongly correlated to cognitive level, showing strength in social skills and weakness in motor skills, but there is still an overall delay (Peters, Goddard-Finegold, et al., 2004). Gross motor milestones are often delayed, with sitting occurring after 12 months of age and walking starting at 3–5 years (Williams, Driscoll, et al., 2010).

Autism spectrum disorders: Chromosome 15q11-q13 abnormalities are commonly associated with autism spectrum disorders (ASD) (Hogart, Wu, et al., 2010). However, studies have suggested that it is the severe cognitive delays that underlie the social and communication deficits seen in individuals with AS who meet algorithm definitions of autism spectrum disorders on the Autism Diagnostic Observation Schedule (ADOS), in contrast to the specific social and communication deficits seen in autism (Trillingsgaard & Østergaard, 2004).

Description of Selected Associated Medical Conditions

Seizures: Epilepsy is a frequent clinical feature of AS, with more than 80% of AS-affected individuals experiencing epileptic seizures with abnormal EEG activity. Individuals with AS may have any type of seizure. Seizure severity is worse around four years of age. Severity decreases with age, but usually continues to adulthood (Williams, Beaudet, et al., 2006).

EEG abnormality: Abnormalities in the EEG may occur without association with clinical seizures. The abnormalities usually occur in the first two years of life. In a study of over 100 individuals with AS, abnormalities noted include intermittent delta waves, interictal epileptiform discharges, intermittent rhythmic theta waves, and posterior rhythm slowing. Centro-occipital and centro-temporal delta waves decreased with age (p = 0.01, p = 0.03). Although there were no specific correlations found between genotypes and EEG patterns, the authors were able to put together a classification tree that suggested relationships that allowed prediction of genotypes based on EEG, including deletions class-1 (5.9 Mb) in patients with intermittent theta waves in <50% of EEG and interictal epileptiform abnormalities and uniparental disomy (UPD). UBE3A mutation or imprinting defects were typically seen in AS patients with intermittent theta in <50% of EEGs without interictal epileptiform abnormalities (Vendrame, Loddenkemper, et al., 2012).

Sleep: Individuals with AS have a decreased need for sleep, typically seen between the ages of 2–6 years of age, which improves with age. Reports have also shown increased sleep-onset latency, frequent awakenings, decreased rapid eye movement (REM) sleep, and periodic leg movements (Pelc, Cheron, et al., 2008).

Time Course of Development in AS

The developmental delays associated with AS typically first appear around six months of age, but some of the unique characteristics of AS may not be evident until one year of age (Williams, Driscoll, et al., 2010). Puberty typically occurs at the normal time and fertility is preserved. Most individuals live at home or in a home-like setting with assistance. The lifespan of individuals with AS may be decreased by 10–15 years (Williams, Driscoll, et al., 2010).

Differential Diagnosis

In 2001, Williams and colleagues reported on conditions that may mimic AS. These include chromosomal disorders, single gene disorders, and symptom complexes. Chromosomal disorders may include 22q13.3 terminal deletions, as individuals with these deletions have severe speech delays and intellectual disability, but seizures in the minority. Another is Prader Willi syndrome, as it represents the maternal deletion of the same 15q11-13 region, but it has quite different clinical characteristics, including hypotonia in infancy, hyperphagia, and obesity. Mowat Wilson syndrome also has some similarities to AS, such as severe intellectual disability and seizure disorder, but is also associated with congenital heart disease and genitourinary disease. It has distinctive physical features and may be associated with Hirschsprung's disease (Mowat, Croaker, et al., 1998).

Single gene disorders exhibiting phenotypic overlap with AS include Rett syndrome, which is associated with hypotonia, seizures, microcephaly, and abnormal gait. However, individuals with AS have more advanced cognitive skills. Individuals with alpha-thalassemia retardation syndrome, X-linked, have severe intellectual disability and sometimes no laboratory evidence for alpha-thalessemia. Methylene tetrahydrofolate reductase deficiency may present with seizures, ataxia, and a happy affect (Arn, Williams, et al., 1998). Gurrieri syndrome may also have early onset seizures, absent speech, and intellectual disability, but it is also associated with bone dysplasia (Battaglia & Gurrieri, 1999). Pitt Hopkins syndrome, which involves the transcription factor 4 (TCF4) mutations, is associated with severe intellectual disability and breathing abnormalities (Marangi, Ricciardi, et al., 2011). Symptom complexes that involve brain and nervous system functions, such as movement, learning, speech, seizure, and thinking, may be misdiagnosed as AS. These can include cerebral palsy, Lennox-Gastaut syndrome, static or mitochondrial encephalopathy, and autism spectrum disorders (Williams, Lossie, et al., 2001).

Treatment of Symptoms

Medical

Treatment of reflux: For gastroesophageal reflux, treatments include medications such as proton pump inhibitors and H2 blockers. For serious cases of reflux, surgery may be required.

Treatment of seizures: Antiepileptic drugs (AEDs) are commonly prescribed to AS patients to help control seizure activity. The most commonly prescribed AEDs are valproic acid, clonazepam, phenobarbital, topiramate, and lamotrigine. Valproic acid in combination with clonazepam or another benzodiazepine has consistently been reported as the most effective antiepileptic regimen for AS patients, with minimal adverse reactions (Laan, van Haeringen, et al., 1999; Ostergaard & Balslev, 2001; Thibert, Conant, et al., 2009). A recent review of AEDs in the largest AS population size to date reported that newer AEDs, specifically topiramate, lamotrigine, and levetiracetam, were comparable to valproic acid and clonazepam in terms of efficacy and tolerability (Thibert, Conant, et al., 2009). Lastly, studies consistently show that treatment with carbamazepine may cause seizure exacerbation and should be avoided in the AS population (Laan, van Haeringen, et al., 1999; Ostergaard & Balslev, 2001; Thibert, Conant, et al., 2009). A low glycemic index diet has been reported to reduce seizure frequency by 90% in five individuals who were on the low glycemic index diet for one year (Thibert, Pfeifer, et al., 2012). Corticosteroids were reported to be helpful in four patients to decrease the frequency of seizures as well as result in EEG changes (Forrest, Young, et al., 2009). The ketogenic diet was reported to be helpful in a case report (Evangeliou, Doulioglou, et al., 2010).

Therapy

Speech therapy is important to develop communication, including nonverbal communication. Physical therapy is often recommended due to the gross motor difficulties encountered by individuals with AS. Occupational therapy is also helpful for fine motor deficits. Behavioral modification therapy can be effective to treat self-injurious or disruptive behaviors (Williams, Driscoll, et al., 2010).

Sleep: Melatonin supplementation to aid sleep difficulties associated with AS has been evaluated in a double-blind trial in eight children with AS. Treatment with 2.5 to 5 mg of melatonin at night led to improvement in sleep onset, decreased sleep latency, increased total sleep time, and also reduced night awakenings (Braam, Didden, et al., 2008). Behavioral treatment, including sleep environment, sleep-wake schedule, and parent–child interactions, was shown to be helpful in a recent study in which parents showed high satisfaction (Allen, Kuhn, et al., 2013). However, sometimes more potent sleep agents are needed, such as clonidine.

MOLECULAR, EPIGENETIC, AND NEUROBIOLOGICAL ASPECTS

Molecular

Chromosome 15q11.2-q13

Chromosome 15q11.2-13 spans 4Mb and contains a unique cluster of imprinted genes that when altered can produce at least three distinct disorders. Disruption of paternal 15q11.2-13 results in Prader-Willi syndrome; deficiencies in maternal 15q11.2-13 results in Angelman syndrome; and specific maternal duplication is believed to lead to autism (Grafodatskaya, Chung et al., Lalande & Calciano, 2007). The *UBE3A* allele resides in the 15q11.2-13 region and spans approximately 120 kb of genomic DNA consisting of 16 exons. The last two nucleotides of exon 7 are included as the AT of the ATG start codon necessary for all three isoforms of protein. The *UBE3A* coding region is approximately 60 kb, and the gene encodes all three known protein isoforms (UBE3A I, II, and III) (Sartori, Anesi, et al., 2008). There are four known genetic mechanisms that result in AS (Classes 1–4, described below), and a subset of patients with a clinical diagnosis have no identifiable cytogenetic or molecular abnormality of the AS locus (Class 5) (Clayton-Smith & Laan, 2003; Lalande & Calciano, 2007).

UBE3A *Deletion*

The highest frequency of known genetic causes of AS is a maternally derived interstitial deletion of 15q11-13, occurring in approximately 70–75% of diagnosed patients. The majority are *de novo* deletions of genetic material, including the *UBE3A* gene on the maternal chromosome 15q11-13. These cases are designated as Class I (Kaplan, Wharton, et al., 1987; Magenis, Toth-Fejel, et al., 1990). Type I deletions are the larger deletions that total approximately 4–6 Mb, spanning breakpoint 1 (BP1) or BP2 to distal BP3 (Valente, Varela, et al., 2013). Type II deletions are smaller, consisting of approximately 500kb that span BP2 and BP3. Closer examination of Type I deletions reveal that even larger deletions are possible. These Type I deletions can occur between BP1 or BP2 to BP4, BP4A, or BP5 and can be a 9Mb deletion or greater; however, these larger-deletion patients represent fewer than 5% of the those with a Type I deletion.

Uniparental Disomy

Imprinted alleles in the 15q11.2-13 region show differential methylation patterns based on paternal or maternal legacy. Uniparental disomy (UPD) (designated as Class II) represents ~5% of AS patients and occurs when a child receives both copies of an entire or partial chromosome from one parent. Mechanisms for UPD primarily occur from non-disjunction events due to the disruption of segregation in either meiosis I or meiosis II (Buiting, 2010). Specifically in the case of AS, trisomic zygote rescue, gamete complementation, compensatory UPD, or mitotic errors can each result in duplication of the paternal chromosome 15 and subsequent silencing of both *UBE3A* alleles (Robinson, Wagstaff, et al., 1993).

Imprinting Center Defects

Patients who do not have deletions (Class I) or UPD (Class II), but exhibit abnormal gene methylation, comprise 3–5% of diagnosed AS patients and are shown to have imprinting defects (Class III) (Buiting, 2010). Within the 15q11.2-13 is a region identified as the imprinting center (IC). The IC controls the methylation state of imprinted genes. The Angelman/Prader Willi IC governs the switch from non-methylation to methylation of the genes within the 15q11.2-13 region, or vice versa, during gametogenesis and retention of parental lineage (Boyes, Wallace, et al., 2006; Dagli, Buiting, et al., 2012). In half of the patients with Class III alterations, a genetic mutation in the IC can be identified, usually due to a deletion of varying size (5–200kb). Interestingly, in the remaining 50% of those patients, the genetic cause for the disruption is unknown and is not associated with familial AS inheritance.

UBE3A Mutation

The patients who fall into Class IV are those with mutations specific to the *UBE3A* allele and they represent 7–10% of diagnosed AS patients. Over 40 specific mutations throughout the entire coding region have been identified, with notable groups of mutations associated with exons 9 and 16. Importantly, exon 16 contains the highly conserved HECT (*H*omologous to the *E*6-AP [UBE3A] *C*arboxyl *T*erminus) domain that imparts the catalytically functional domain of the UBE3A enzyme (Boyes, Wallace, et al., 2006). Frameshift and nonsense mutations account for most of the identified genetic alterations, but splice-site mutations and missense mutations can occur as well. The majority of mutations are *de novo*, resulting in ~80% of sporadic cases and ~20% familial (Clayton-Smith & Laan, 2003; Dagli, Buiting, et al., 2012).

Clinically Diagnosed

The remaining Class V patients represent those without an identifiable genetic abnormality, but who exhibit multiple phenotypic characteristics of AS. The standard is to diagnose through the combination of clinical features and molecular genetic testing. However, in the absence of conclusive molecular data, the multiple biological and behavioral symptoms of AS coupled with the wide variation in their severity often lead to misdiagnoses.

Phenotypical Differences Among the Various Classes of AS

Genotype–phenotype correlations have been made between the classes of AS, but they have been complicated due to overlapping clinical features for all the different mechanisms. Individuals with the large chromosomal deletions (Class I or Class II) tend to have a more severe phenotype, which seems likely to be due to haploinsufficiency of genes around *UBE3A*. They are more likely to have microcephaly, seizures, and greater problems with language than those with AS due to other causes. There has also been correlation between hypopigmentation of the skin, hair, and iris as well as lower weight in those with large deletions. Individuals with AS due to IC defects and uniparental disomy have relatively more advanced language and developmental skills (Dagli, Buiting, et al., 2012). Studies have noted that individuals with UPD have better growth and are less likely to have microcephaly, ataxia, and seizures (Lossie, Whitney, et al., 2001; Saitoh, Wada, et al., 2005).

Diagnosis of Condition

To diagnose AS, methylation studies of chromosome 15q11-q13 are the most sensitive single approach. They will detect deletions, uniparental disomy, or IC defects, and further testing can clarify the specific mechanism. There are two different types of methylation studies—methylation specific polymerase chain reaction (MS-PCR) and methylation sensitive multiplex ligation-dependent probe amplification (MS-MLPA). MS-PCR will confirm a diagnosis, but it will not distinguish between deletions, uniparental disomy, or IC defects. Usually, a subsequent microsatellite, fluorescence in situ hybridization (FISH) analysis, or microarray study will be necessary to confirm the cause of AS. For MS-MLPA, a positive result confirms the diagnosis and a deletion. If a deletion is not present, a microsatellite or microarray study can be done to confirm AS due to UPD or IC defect.

If the methylation studies are negative, testing for mutations of the *UBE3A* gene is generally the next step (Ramsden, Clayton-Smith, et al., 2010). If testing is negative, consensus criteria for the clinical diagnosis of AS have been developed for a clinical diagnosis, as mentioned above. After the diagnosis is confirmed, parental studies are recommended to identify balanced rearrangements, and genetic counseling should be provided to the families.

TARGETED TREATMENT INFORMATION, ANIMAL AND HUMAN STUDIES

Topoisomerase Inhibitors

In all instances of AS with a molecular diagnosis, the silenced paternal allele is intact. This makes the reactivation of the paternal allele to a functioning UBE3A protein producer an attractive therapeutic target. Recently, researchers have identified compounds that belong to a broad class of drugs known as topoisomerase inhibitors that increase paternal expression of *Ube3a*. Topoisomerase inhibitors are widely used in cancer therapy as chemotherapeutics (Moukharskaya & Verschraegen, 2012) and cause replicating cells to undergo apoptosis by inducing double strand breaks that stall the replication fork.

Animal Studies

The mouse and human *Ube3a* are orthologous, as the general organizations of the regions are similar and undergo maternal imprinting, making the mouse an attractive model system in which to perform research (Jiang, Armstrong, et al., 1998). It should be noted that there are two distinct mouse models of AS using different strategies to disrupt *Ube3a*. One of these models utilized an Epstein-Barr virus *latent membrane protein* 2A (*Lmp2a*) transgenic insertion to remove the entire equivalent AS critical region (Albrecht, Sutcliffe, et al., 1997; Gabriel, Merchant, et al., 1999). The other created a maternal gene knockout in *Ube3a* via a null mutation in intron 2 (Jiang, Armstrong, et al., 1998). While both of these mouse models effectively disrupt maternal *Ube3a* expression, the null mutation model (Ube3a m-/p+) has become the prominently used model for basic research and testing of potential therapeutics. The Ube3a m-/p+ mouse exhibits cognitive defects, motor coordination problems, and increased seizure propensity, as well as disruption of hippocampal, cerebellar, and cortical synaptic function. It was shown that direct infusion of topotecan, an FDA-approved member of the topoisomerase inhibitor family, into the central nervous system (CNS) resulted in paternal expression of functionally active *Ube3a* (Huang, Allen et al.). The unsilencing effect was observed in the hippocampus, neocortex, striatum, cerebellum, and spinal cord. In the spinal cord, paternal *Ube3a* expression remained for up to three months following treatment. The mechanism underlying topotecan's actions appears to be through the disruption of the paternal *Ube3a* antisense. This disruption would allow the paternal transcript to be produced and subsequent native UBE3A protein translation. This could represent a viable therapeutic strategy if protein concentration and gene regulation was equivalent to that measured with the maternal allele. It is not yet established whether topotecan treatment is effective in recovering the above described phenotypes in the AS mouse model.

Human Studies

Although an important demonstration of the proof of concept for reactivation of the paternal *Ube3a* allele, a potential challenge to the further development of topotecan as a pediatric therapy for AS lies in historical accounts of its numerous deleterious side effects. The most severe side effects are hematological, with nearly all patients taking the medication for cancer treatment developing thrombocytopenia with associated increased bleeding (Sheng, Miao, et al., 2011). To date, there are no human clinical trials examining the efficacy of topotecan or other topoisomerase inhibitors in Angelman syndrome.

Minocycline

Minocycline is a semi-synthetic tetracycline derivative that has broad-spectrum antibiotic properties and can easily cross the blood–brain barrier (BBB). Minocycline is a well-characterized molecule that is FDA approved, and it has been used in clinical practice and in experimental models for more than 30 years. The most common side effects of extended minocycline treatment include teeth discoloration, gastrointestinal irritability, and increased susceptibility to candidiasis.

Animal Studies

In unpublished studies, three-week treatment of adult AS mice with minocycline resulted in marked improvement in motor coordination, cognition, and hippocampal synaptic function. Specifically, a normalization of accelerating rotorod performance following eight training sessions and a recovery in associative fear-conditioned learning and memory were observed. It is unclear which specific molecular mechanism is underlying these results; however, minocycline has previously been reported to result in biochemical effects in the CNS, including, but not limited to, inhibition of caspase-1 and caspase-3, inducible nitric oxide synthetase (iNOS), P38 mitogen-activated protein kinase (MAPK), matrix metalloproteinases (MMPs), and reduced microglial-dependent inflammation (Zhu, Stavrovskaya, et al., 2002; Wei, Zhao, et al., 2005; Vincent & Mohr, 2007). Notably, the AS mouse model has significantly decreased spine density in the hippocampus, cerebellum, and cortex (Dindot, Antalffy, et al., 2008). It is well established that alterations in spine density, maturation, or shape can disrupt synaptic function, and this may contribute to the cognitive and behavioral phenotypes observed in the AS mouse model. It has already been demonstrated that minocycline can rescue defects in dendritic spine maturation in an animal model for fragile X syndrome (Bilousova, Dansie, et al., 2009; Hagerman, Lauterborn, et al., 2012; see Chapter 9) and may be achieving amelioration of the major phenotypes in the AS animal model by a similar mechanism. Reduced post-synaptic calcium may play into this mechanism through previously reported reduced calcium-calmodulin protein kinase II (CaMKII) activity (Figure 10.2a). CaMKII can modify synaptic function in a number of ways. First, CaMKII is responsive to calcium influx through normal synaptic activity and can control 2-amino-3-(3-hydroxy-5-methyl-isoxazol-4-yl) propanoic acid (AMPA) receptor insertion. CaMKII can also target N-methyl-D-aspartate (NMDA) receptors and modify calcium conductance through subunit phosphorylation. Furthermore, calcium-calmodulin activity is linked to spine formation and spine morphology through the MMP-9–intercellular adhesion molecule 5 (ICAM5)–cofilin pathway. It is unclear if this pathway is involved in AS neuronal spine defects, or how minocycline may be working in the AS mouse. However, one model suggests that Ube3a deficiency results in the upregulation of the inactive form of MMP-9, and minocycline reduces the levels of this MMP-9 species, thus increasing the signal to initiate synaptic remodeling (Figure 10.2b).

Human Studies

There is interest in using minocycline alone or in combination with other drugs to treat stroke and ischemia, Alzheimer's disease, schizophrenia (Chapter 3), bipolar disorder, autism (Chapter 2), and fragile X syndrome

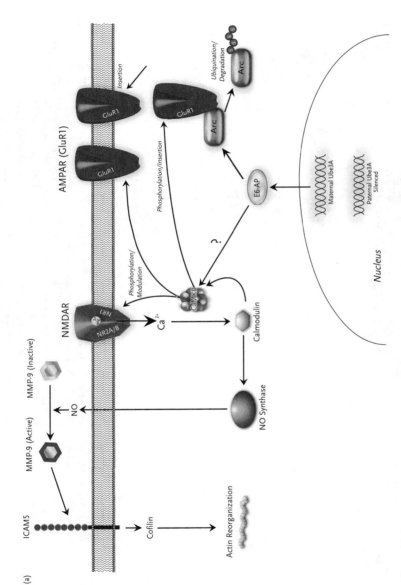

Figure 10.2a:
Under normal conditions, synapses are maintained through spontaneous activity. Calcium influx through N-methyl-D-aspartate (NMDA) receptors forms an active complex with calmodulin. Increased synaptic activity results in increased calcium-calmodulin, which in turn stimulates a rapid release of post-synaptic nitric oxide (NO) from the intracellular to the extracellular environment where activation of matrix metalloproteinase-9 (MMP-9) occurs. One target of MMP-9 is the intercellular adhesion molecule 5 (ICAM5). This results in changes in actin polymerization, in part through the activation of cofilin. This process underlies synapse morphological changes and indirectly, the ability to increase spine density through increased global activity.

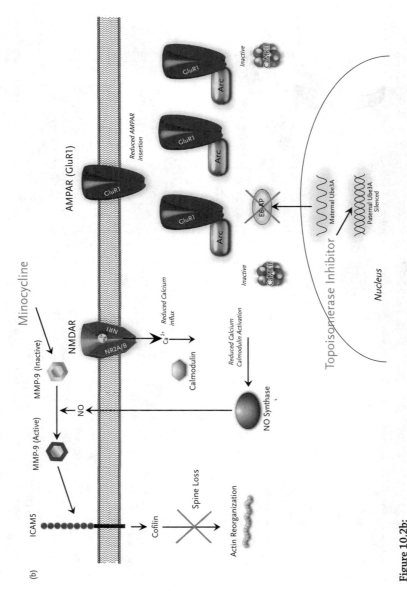

Figure 10.2b:

In Angelman syndrome (AS), there is a significant lack of synaptic available calmodulin protein kinase II (CaMKII) and reduced CaMKII activity. Arc, a target of UBE3A, is increased in AS, resulting in the internalization of 2-amino-3-(3-hydroxy-5-methyl-isoxazol-4-yl)propanoic acid AMPA receptors. Reduced AMPA receptor-dependent synaptic depolarization results in reduced NMDA receptor conductance, calcium-calmodulin complex and NO release in response to synaptic activity.

*Topotecan acts on double-stranded DNA and is shown to alleviate antisense silencing of the paternal *Ube3a* allele. Increased Ube3a would reduce ARC levels and restore the normal complement of membrane-associated AMPA receptors.

**Minocycline is known to reduce MMP-9 levels and activity.

(Chapter 9), with ongoing human trials (see clinicaltrials.gov). Based upon the mouse studies described, a single-arm, non-placebo-control human trial began in 2012 to test the effects of minocycline on the symptoms of AS in a population of children 4 to 14 years of age (Clinical Trial # NCT01531582). The clinical trial ended in early 2013, and published results are unavailable. However, post-trial reports reveal that minocycline treatment showed positive effects for multiple clinical outcomes, including increased communication (both verbal and nonverbal), better attention, decreased aberrant behavior, and a significant normalization of the abnormal EEG.

Promethylation Dietary Supplements

Recently, promethylation dietary supplements, such as folic acid and betaine, have been investigated as a potential targeted treatment for AS. The rationale for treatment with promethylation dietary supplements was that increased methyl donors in the diet may increase DNA methylation and activate the paternally inherited, unmethylated *UBE3A* allele (Peters, Bird, et al., 2010).

Animal Studies

Animal studies have shown that feeding a methyl-donor-supplemented diet to pregnant agouti mice results in coat color alterations of mouse pups. Changes in agouti coat color alleles are associated with changes in DNA methylation as a result of maternal diet (Wolff, Kodell, et al., 1998; Cooney, Dave, et al., 2002).

Human Studies

In humans, intake of folic acid has been used in postmenopausal women and in individuals with hyperhomocystinemia to treat changes in DNA methylation of blood lymphocytes and inappropriate biallelic gene expression, respectively (Jacob, Gretz, et al., 1998; Ingrosso, Cimmino, et al., 2003). Thus, it was believed that high-dose intake of promethylation supplements in the diet may increase DNA methylation and rescue the AS phenotype caused by lack of the maternal *UBE3A* allele (Peters, Bird, et al., 2010).

Peters and colleagues conducted a 12-month, double-blind, placebo-controlled trial with subjects receiving either active treatment with folic acid and betaine or placebo. The folic acid dose was 15 mg once daily. The betaine dose was weight-based, with those under 30 kg receiving 2 g, three times daily, and those at or above 30 kg receiving 3 g, four times daily. All subjects in the active and placebo groups received a pediatric multivitamin, taken once daily, containing 400 µg folic acid. Subjects took either a half tablet or full tablet based on weight. Enrolled subjects were between the ages of 5 months to 14 years, and all had a confirmed AS diagnosis. Subjects were evaluated at baseline and after one year of treatment with complete medical history, physical and neurological examinations, formal developmental assessments, laboratory investigations, EEG studies, and parental reports. Outcome measures were changes in biochemical measurements, seizure onset, changes in formal developmental assessment scores, and changes in parental reports. There were no significant differences between treatment and placebo group in any of the outcome variables; although trends suggested improvement in some developmental areas for younger subjects (Peters, Bird, et al., 2010).

Following this trend, a second trial was completed, with a younger AS population. Study design changes included changing the promethylation dietary regimen to incorporate L-5-methyltetrahydrofolate instead of folic acid to address concerns of accumulation of unmetabolized folic acid as well as adding creatine and vitamin B_{12} to increase the availability of S-adenosylmethionine for DNA methylation. Subjects were limited to AS patients who were younger than age 6. The study was a one-year non-randomized open-label clinical trial of L-5-methyltetrahydrofolate (0.5 mg/kg/day, maximum 8 mg/day), creatine (200 mg/kg/day, maximum 5 g/day), betaine (100–200 mg/kg/day), and vitamin B_{12} (1 mg/day). Subjects were evaluated at baseline and after one year of treatment with complete medical history, physical and neurological examinations, formal developmental assessments, laboratory investigations, and EEG studies. Outcome variables were changes in formal developmental assessment scores and changes in blood biochemical parameters, all relative to baseline scores and measurements. Statistical analysis found no significant differences between pre-treatment and post-treatment scores on cognitive and language abilities, as well as no significant differences between pre-treatment and post-treatment measurements of global DNA methylation. With lack of efficacy seen in both trials, use of promethylation dietary supplements is not endorsed as an effective treatment for AS (Bird, Tan, et al., 2011).

Levodopa

Another targeted treatment being investigated for AS is Levodopa (L-dopa). Levodopa is indicated for the clinical treatment of Parkinson's disease as a dopamine agonist.

Animal Studies

Parkinson's disease (PD) animal studies have shown lowered dopamine levels in the striatum, resulting in an abnormal increase of phosphorylation of αCaMKII, the combination of both abnormalities leading to motor function deficits. Administration of Levodopa reversed the effects of excess phosphorylation of αCaMKII, subsequently leading to improved motor function (Picconi, Gardoni, et al., 2004; Brown, Deutch, et al., 2005). Similar abnormalities have been found in AS animal studies (Weeber, Jiang, et al., 2003; van Woerden, Harris, et al., 2007; Mulherkar & Jana, 2010; Riday, Dankoski, et al., 2012).

AS mice lacking the maternal ube3a ($ube3a^{m-/p+}$ mice) have reduced dopamine cell numbers in the substantia nigra, impaired dopaminergic functioning in the striatum, and increased levels of phospho αCaMKII as compared to wild-type mice. These abnormalities manifest behaviorally as significantly worse performance in nigrostriatal and basal ganglia motor ability paradigms (Mulherkar & Jana, 2010). $Ube3a^{m-/p+}$ mice have shown pathway-specific dopaminergic deficits with increased dopamine mesolimbic release and decreased nigrostriatal dopamine release compared to wild-type mice. These pathways exhibited dopaminergic dysregulation during drug-induced or electrical stimulation that resembled dopaminergic dysregulation seen in mouse models of human mutations in patients with autosomal recessive familial PD (Riday, Dankoski, et al., 2012). Furthermore, $ube3a^{m-/p+}$ mice have increased levels of phospho αCaMKII levels in the hippocampus, which may result in behavioral deficits in AS (Weeber, Jiang, et al., 2003; van Woerden, Harris, et al., 2007). These behavioral deficits were reversed in $ube3a^{m-/p+}$ mice when a mutation blocking the phosphorylation of αCaMKII was introduced (van Woerden, Harris, et al., 2007). While there have been no published studies examining the use of Levodopa in AS animal models directly, the similarities between AS and PD mouse models suggest that it may be an effective treatment.

Human Studies

To date, there has been one published case report on the use of Levodopa as treatment for two adult AS patients (Harbord, 2001). Two AS patients, a 23-year-old male and a 43-year-old female, both presented signs of early-onset Parkinsonism with resting tremor, cogwheel rigidity, bradykinesia, and lower limb spasticity, in addition to typical AS motor deficits. Both patients had dramatic improvement of symptoms after starting Levodopa/Carbidopa (100 mg/10 mg), suggesting that the medication may be an effective treatment option. Currently, a clinical trial of Levodopa/ Carbidopa is being conducted to examining tolerability and efficacy of Levodopa/Carbidopa in children with AS (Tan, W-H, http://clinicaltrials. gov/ct2/show/NCT01281475). The study is presently ongoing, and results have not yet been published.

Future Research

Recent research investigating the role of *UBE3A* in nervous system development has found *UBE3A* to be an activity-regulated gene that controls the function of the synaptic protein Arc. Disruption of *UBE3A* results in the dysregulation of neuronal Arc, and, subsequently, impairs AMPA receptors and synaptic functioning. Arc is translationally inhibited by the fragile X mental retardation 1 protein (FMRP), indicating a potential commonality between AS and FXS. It is not known at this time if fragile X syndrome (FXS) therapeutic strategies would be of benefit to AS treatment, although the use of minocycline appears to be helpful for both disorders (Chapter 9) (Leigh, Nguyen, et al., 2013); and further research is needed (Greer, Hanayama, et al., 2010; Philpot, Thompson, et al., 2011).

In summary, Angelman syndrome is a genetic disorder characterized by features including developmental delays especially in expressive language, ataxia, and a happy demeanor. Traditional treatments targeted specific behaviors or physical symptoms such as seizures. Discovery of the cause of AS—disruption of the maternal *UBE3A* gene through deletions, mutations, and uniparental disomy—have led to the development and testing of targeted treatments, including topoisomerase inhibitors, minocycline, promethylation agents, and Levodopa both in animal models and in individuals with AS. The future is promising for individuals with AS.

DISCLOSURES

Conflicts of interest: The authors have no conflict of interest to disclose.

REFERENCES
Albrecht, U., Sutcliffe, J. S., et al. (1997). Imprinted expression of the murine Angelman syndrome gene, *Ube3a*, in hippocampal and Purkinje neurons. *Nature Genetics*, 17(1), 75–78.
Allen, K. D., Kuhn, B. R., et al. (2013). Evaluation of a behavioral treatment package to reduce sleep problems in children with Angelman syndrome. *Research in Developmental Disabilities*, 34(1), 676–686.

Andersen, W. H., Rasmussen, R. K., et al. (2001). Levels of cognitive and linguistic development in Angelman syndrome: a study of 20 children. *Logopedics Phoniatric Vocology*, *26*(1), 2–9.

Angelman, H. (1965). "Puppet" children, a report on three cases. *Developmental Medicine & Child Neurology*, *7*, 681–688.

Arn, P. H., Williams, C. A., et al. (1998). Methylenetetrahydrofolate reductase deficiency in a patient with phenotypic findings of Angelman syndrome. *American Journal of Medical Genetics*, *77*(3), 198–200.

Battaglia, A., & Gurrieri, F. (1999). Case of apparent Gurrieri syndrome showing molecular findings of Angelman syndrome. *American Journal of Medical Genetics*, *82*(1), 100.

Beckung, E., Steffenburg, S., et al. (2004). Motor impairments, neurological signs, and developmental level in individuals with Angelman syndrome. *Developmental Medicine & Child Neurology*, *46*(4), 239–243.

Bilousova, T. V., Dansie, L., et al. (2009). Minocycline promotes dendritic spine maturation and improves behavioural performance in the fragile X mouse model. *Journal of Medical Genetics*, *46*(2), 94–102.

Bird, L. M., Tan, W. H., et al. (2011). A therapeutic trial of pro-methylation dietary supplements in Angelman syndrome. *American Journal of Medical Genetics A*, *155A*(12), 2956–2963.

Boyes, L., Wallace, A. J., et al. (2006). Detection of a deletion of exons 8–16 of the UBE3A gene in familial Angelman syndrome using a semi-quantitative dosage PCR based assay. *European Journal of Medical Genetics*, *49*(6), 472–480.

Braam, W., Didden, R., et al. (2008). Melatonin for chronic insomnia in Angelman syndrome: a randomized placebo-controlled trial. *Journal of Child Neurology*, *23*(6), 649–654.

Brown, A. M., Deutch, A. Y., et al. (2005). Dopamine depletion alters phosphorylation of striatal proteins in a model of Parkinsonism. *European Journal of Neuroscience*, *22*(1), 247–256.

Buckley, R. H., Dinno, N., et al. (1998). Angelman syndrome: are the estimates too low? *American Journal of Medical Genetics*, *80*(4), 385–390.

Buiting, K. (2010). Prader-Willi syndrome and Angelman syndrome. *American Journal of Medical Genetics C Semin Med Genet*, *154C*(3), 365–376.

Clayton-Smith, J., & Laan, L. (2003). Angelman syndrome: a review of the clinical and genetic aspects. *Journal of Medical Genetics*, *40*(2), 87–95.

Cooney, C. A., Dave, A. A., et al. (2002). Maternal methyl supplements in mice affect epigenetic variation and DNA methylation of offspring. *Journal of Nutrition*, *132*(8 Suppl), 2393S–2400S.

Dagli, A., Buiting, K., et al. (2012). Molecular and clinical aspects of Angelman syndrome. *Molecular Syndromology*, *2*(3–5), 100–112.

Dindot, S. V., Antalffy, B. A., et al. (2008). The Angelman syndrome ubiquitin ligase localizes to the synapse and nucleus, and maternal deficiency results in abnormal dendritic spine morphology. *Human Molecular Genetics*, *17*(1), 111–118.

Evangeliou, A., Doulioglou, V., et al. (2010). Ketogenic diet in a patient with Angelman syndrome. *Pediatrics International*, *52*(5), 831–834.

Forrest, K. M., Young, H., et al. (2009). Benefit of corticosteroid therapy in Angelman syndrome. *Journal of Child Neurology*, *24*(8), 952–958.

Gabriel, J. M., Merchant, M., et al. (1999). A transgene insertion creating a heritable chromosome deletion mouse model of Prader-Willi and Angelman syndromes. *Proceedings of the National Academy of Sciences of the USA*, *96*(16), 9258–9263.

Grafodatskaya, D., Chung, B., et al. Autism spectrum disorders and epigenetics. *Journal of the American Academy of Child & Adolescent Psychiatry*, *49*(8), 794–809.

Greer, P. L., Hanayama, R., et al. (2010). The Angelman syndrome protein Ube3A regulates synapse development by ubiquitinating Arc. *Cell*, *140*(5), 704–716.

Hagerman, R., Lauterborn, J., et al. (2012). Fragile X syndrome and targeted treatment trials. *Results and Problems in Cell Differentiation*, *54*, 297–335.

Harbord, M. (2001). Levodopa-responsive Parkinsonism in adults with Angelman syndrome. *Journal of Clinical Neuroscience*, *8*(5), 421–422.

Hogart, A., Wu, D., et al. (2010). The comorbidity of autism with the genomic disorders of chromosome 15q11.2-q13. *Neurobiology of Disease*, *38*(2), 181–191.

Huang, H. S., Allen, J. A., et al. Topoisomerase inhibitors unsilence the dormant allele of *Ube3a* in neurons. *Nature*, *481*(7380), 185–189.

Ingrosso, D., Cimmino, A., et al. (2003). Folate treatment and unbalanced methylation and changes of allelic expression induced by hyperhomocysteinaemia in patients with uraemia. *Lancet*, *361*(9370), 1693–1699.

Jacob, R. A., Gretz, D. M., et al. (1998). Moderate folate depletion increases plasma homocysteine and decreases lymphocyte DNA methylation in postmenopausal women. *Journal of Nutrition*, *128*(7), 1204–1212.

Jiang, Y. H., Armstrong, D., et al. (1998). Mutation of the Angelman ubiquitin ligase in mice causes increased cytoplasmic p53 and deficits of contextual learning and long-term potentiation. *Neuron*, *21*(4), 799–811.

Kaplan, L. C., Wharton, R., et al. (1987). Clinical heterogeneity associated with deletions in the long arm of chromosome 15: report of 3 new cases and their possible genetic significance. *American Journal of Medical Genetics*, *28*(1), 45–53.

Kyllerman, M. (1995). On the prevalence of Angelman syndrome. *American Journal of Medical Genetics*, *59*(3), 405; author reply 403–404.

Laan, L. A., van Haeringen, A., et al. (1999). Angelman syndrome: a review of clinical and genetic aspects. *Clinical Neurology & Neurosurgery*, *101*(3), 161–170.

Lalande, M., & Calciano, M. A. (2007). Molecular epigenetics of Angelman syndrome. *Cellular & Molecular Life Sciences*, *64*(7-8), 947–960.

Leigh, M. J., Nguyen, D. V., et al. (2013). A randomized double-blind, placebo-controlled trial of minocycline in children and adolescents with fragile X syndrome. *Journal of Developmental & Behavioral Pediatrics*, *34*(3), 147–155.

Lossie, A. C., Whitney, M. M., et al. (2001). Distinct phenotypes distinguish the molecular classes of Angelman syndrome. *Journal of Medical Genetics*, *38*(12), 834–845.

Magenis, R. E., Toth-Fejel, S., et al. (1990). Comparison of the 15q deletions in Prader-Willi and Angelman syndromes: specific regions, extent of deletions, parental origin, and clinical consequences. *American Journal of Medical Genetics*, *35*(3), 333–349.

Marangi, G., Ricciardi, S., et al. (2011). The Pitt-Hopkins syndrome: report of 16 new patients and clinical diagnostic criteria. *American Journal of Medical Genetics A*, *155A*(7), 1536–1545.

Moukharskaya, J., & Verschraegen, C. (2012). Topoisomerase 1 inhibitors and cancer therapy. *Hematology/Oncology Clinics of North America*, *26*(3), 507–525, vii.

Mowat, D. R., Croaker, G. D., et al. (1998). Hirschsprung disease, microcephaly, mental retardation, and characteristic facial features: delineation of a new syndrome and identification of a locus at chromosome 2q22-q23. *Journal of Medical Genetics*, *35*(8), 617–623.

Mulherkar, S. A., & Jana, N. R. (2010). Loss of dopaminergic neurons and resulting behavioural deficits in mouse model of Angelman syndrome. *Neurobiology of Disease, 40*(3), 586–592.

Ostergaard, J. R., & Balslev, T. (2001). Efficacy of different antiepileptic drugs in children with Angelman syndrome associated with 15q11-13 deletion: the Danish experience. *Developmental Medicine & Child Neurology, 43*(10), 718–719.

Pelc, K., Cheron, G., et al. (2008). Are there distinctive sleep problems in Angelman syndrome? *Sleep Medicine, 9*(4), 434–441.

Peters, S. U., Bird, L. M., et al. (2010). Double-blind therapeutic trial in Angelman syndrome using betaine and folic acid. *American Journal of Medical Genetics A, 152A*(8), 1994–2001.

Peters, S. U., Goddard-Finegold, J., et al. (2004). Cognitive and adaptive behavior profiles of children with Angelman syndrome. *American Journal of Medical Genetics A, 128A*(2), 110–113.

Petersen, M. B., Brondum-Nielsen, K., et al. (1995). Clinical, cytogenetic, and molecular diagnosis of Angelman syndrome: estimated prevalence rate in a Danish county. *American Journal of Medical Genetics, 60*(3), 261–262.

Philpot, B. D., Thompson, C. E., et al. (2011). Angelman syndrome: advancing the research frontier of neurodevelopmental disorders. *Journal of Neurodevelopmental Disorders, 3*(1), 50–56.

Picconi, B., Gardoni, F., et al. (2004). Abnormal Ca2+-calmodulin-dependent protein kinase II function mediates synaptic and motor deficits in experimental Parkinsonism. *Journal of Neuroscience, 24*(23), 5283–5291.

Ramsden, S. C., Clayton-Smith, J., et al. (2010). Practice guidelines for the molecular analysis of Prader-Willi and Angelman syndromes. *BMC Medical Genetics, 11*, 70.

Riday, T. T., Dankoski, E. C., et al. (2012). Pathway-specific dopaminergic deficits in a mouse model of Angelman syndrome. *Journal of Clinical Investigation, 122*(12), 4544–4554.

Robinson, W. P., Wagstaff, J., et al. (1993). Uniparental disomy explains the occurrence of the Angelman or Prader-Willi syndrome in patients with an additional small inv dup(15) chromosome. *Journal of Medical Genetics, 30*(9), 756–760.

Saitoh, S., Wada, T., et al. (2005). Uniparental disomy and imprinting defects in Japanese patients with Angelman syndrome. *Brain & Development, 27*(5), 389–391.

Sartori, S., Anesi, L., et al. (2008). Angelman syndrome due to a novel splicing mutation of the *UBE3A* gene. *Journal of Child Neurology, 23*(8), 912–915.

Sheng, C., Miao, Z., et al. (2011). New strategies in the discovery of novel non-camptothecin topoisomerase I inhibitors. *Current Medicinal Chemistry, 18*(28), 4389–4409.

Thibert, R. L., Conant, K. D., et al. (2009). Epilepsy in Angelman syndrome: a questionnaire-based assessment of the natural history and current treatment options. *Epilepsia, 50*(11), 2369–2376.

Thibert, R. L., Pfeifer, H. H., et al. (2012). Low glycemic index treatment for seizures in Angelman syndrome. *Epilepsia, 53*(9), 1498–1502.

Trillingsgaard, A., & Østergaard, JR (2004). Autism in Angelman syndrome: an exploration of comorbidity. *Autism, 8*(2), 163–174.

Valente, K. D., Varela, M. C., et al. (2013). Angelman syndrome caused by deletion: A genotype-phenotype correlation determined by breakpoint. *Epilepsy Research, 105*(1–2), 234–239.

van Woerden, G. M., Harris, K. D., et al. (2007). Rescue of neurological deficits in a mouse model for Angelman syndrome by reduction of alphaCaMKII inhibitory phosphorylation. *Nature Neuroscience, 10*(3), 280–282.

Vendrame, M., Loddenkemper, T., et al. (2012). Analysis of EEG patterns and genotypes in patients with Angelman syndrome. *Epilepsy & Behavior, 23*(3), 261–265.

Vincent, J. A., & Mohr, S. (2007). Inhibition of caspase-1/interleukin-1beta signaling prevents degeneration of retinal capillaries in diabetes and galactosemia. *Diabetes, 56*(1), 224–230.

Weeber, E. J., Jiang, Y. H., et al. (2003). Derangements of hippocampal calcium/calmodulin-dependent protein kinase II in a mouse model for Angelman mental retardation syndrome. *Journal of Neuroscience, 23*(7), 2634–2644.

Wei, X., Zhao, L., et al. (2005). Minocycline prevents gentamicin-induced ototoxicity by inhibiting p38 MAP kinase phosphorylation and caspase 3 activation. *Neuroscience, 131*(2), 513–521.

Williams, C. A., Angelman, H., et al. (1995). Angelman syndrome: consensus for diagnostic criteria. Angelman Syndrome Foundation. *American Journal of Medical Genetics, 56*(2), 237–238.

Williams, C. A., Beaudet, A. L., et al. (2006). Angelman syndrome 2005: updated consensus for diagnostic criteria. *American Journal of Medical Genetics A, 140*(5), 413–418.

Williams, C. A., Driscoll, D. J., et al. (2010). Clinical and genetic aspects of Angelman syndrome. *Genetics in Medicine, 12*(7), 385–395.

Williams, C. A., Lossie, A., et al. (2001). Angelman syndrome: mimicking conditions and phenotypes. *American Journal of Medical Genetics, 101*(1), 59–64.

Wolff, G. L., Kodell, R. L., et al. (1998). Maternal epigenetics and methyl supplements affect agouti gene expression in Avy/a mice. *Federation of American Societies for Experimental Biology Journal, 12*(11), 949–957.

Zhu, S., Stavrovskaya, I. G., et al. (2002). Minocycline inhibits cytochrome C release and delays progression of amyotrophic lateral sclerosis in mice. *Nature, 417*(6884), 74–78.

CHAPTER 11

Pharmacotherapy for Cognitive Enhancement in Down Syndrome

AARTI RUPARELIA, DAVID PATTERSON,
AND WILLIAM C. MOBLEY

INTRODUCTION

Down syndrome (DS) is a multifaceted genetic condition caused by trisomy of human chromosome 21 (HSA21). The incidence of DS is approximately one in 700 live births worldwide, and it accounts for 15% of the population with intellectual disability (Bittles et al., 2007). Trisomy 21 is caused by nondisjunction of chromosome 21, resulting in chromosomal imbalance. DS leads to the overexpression of many (approximately 350–500) genes; a number of which are known to play a role in regulating neuronal cell number, gene transcription, mRNA translation, and protein function. Consequently, triplication of these genes in DS creates a multitude of possibilities for changes in the structure and function of several organ systems. The increased expression of HSA21 genes is not ubiquitous, with discrepancies in expression levels in different tissues, which give rise to phenotypical variations that characterize DS (Hattori et al., 2000).

Cognitive impairment is a hallmark phenotype that occurs invariably in DS; however, a prototypical cognitive profile in DS is difficult to identify due to variance in the prevalence, severity, and expressivity of cognitive function among individuals with DS. Individuals with DS show reduced brain volume and brachycephaly, with the hippocampus, frontal cortex, and cerebellum displaying disproportionate impairments (Wisniewski, 1990). In DS, prenatal brains display delayed and disorganized cortical development, with reduced dendritic arborization and fewer synapses (Marin-Padilla, 1976). Neuronal, dendritic, and synaptic impairments are further exaggerated during childhood and adulthood (Takashima et al., 1989). Additionally, individuals with DS are highly susceptible to early-onset Alzheimer's disease (AD); by the age of 65 years, over 75% have a clinical diagnosis of dementia (Masters et al., 1985). The age-linked neuropathology of DS is essentially identical to that of AD, featuring deposits of misfolded proteins, with extracellular amyloid-β (Aβ) plaques and intracellular hyperphosphorylated Tau in neurofibrillary tangles (NFTs) (Mann & Esiri, 1989). AD-related hallmark features also include diffuse brain atrophy and endocytic perturbations. The latter is evident even in very young people with DS (Cataldo et al., 2003).

Studies of mouse models of DS have been instrumental in extending our understanding about the clinical manifestation of DS. The Ts65Dn mouse model is the most widely studied DS mouse model and is trisomic for approximately 122 genes that correspond to the distal end of HSA21 (Davisson et al., 1993). Ts65Dn mice recapitulate several DS phenotypes, including perturbed brain anatomy and neurodevelopment, impaired dendritic arborization and synaptic plasticity, and neurodegeneration.

Significant advances in scientific research, medical technology, and social intervention have led to a marked increase in life expectancy of people with DS in developed countries (Bittles et al., 2007). However, the increase in longevity is linked with a greater prevalence of the disorder and increasing challenges with respect to addressing cognitive decline in an aging DS population. The development of targets for pharmacotherapies to enhance cognitive functioning in DS is essential. Similarities in neuropathology between AD and DS have led to clinical trials in DS using therapeutic interventions targeted for improving cognitive decline in AD. Unfortunately, these trials have been disappointing. Findings from studies with Ts65Dn mice have suggested promising targets for pharmacotherapeutic intervention. This chapter reviews recent progress in target discovery and pharmacotherapeutic interventions to enhance cognition in DS.

Strategies for Defining Therapeutic Targets in Down Syndrome

Less than 10 years ago, the suggestion that one could rationally attempt to discover a treatment for cognitive deficits in DS would have been met with a great deal of skepticism. A critique would have stated that the disorder, due to the presence of an additional entire chromosome, was "too complex to understand," "too difficult to study," and, in any case, by the time a child was born, it was "too late to treat." However, seemingly rational at the time, all of those assertions have proven to be inaccurate, largely because of the important new tools and concepts that have benefitted research in DS. The complete sequencing of the human genome as well as continuing studies to define the genes and regulatory sequences on HSA21 have given important new insights into gene number and complexity, as well as provided tools to manipulate genes and genetic segments. With this has come an increasing number and quality of mouse models in which to test hypotheses. An increasingly large number of segmentally trisomic mice now exist that carry mouse homologues of HSA21, thus allowing studies to test the role of segments and individual genes in creating well-defined phenotypes. In addition, advances in the technological resources for the neurosciences have proliferated, with tools now available to interrogate structure and function as never before. Finally, early successes in deciphering phenotypes, genes, and mechanisms have encouraged the view that investigators can now enter this field of study with realistic expectations that their work will be productive. Taken together, the view increasingly held is that DS can be studied, mechanisms and underlying genes deciphered, and treatment targets defined and tested.

The question remains as to how best to conduct a research program in cognition in DS. At least three general strategies have been used. In principle, they are used interchangeably and in combination. In the first strategy, one relies heavily on the findings from human studies, including neuropathological observations, to create a testing paradigm that attempts to replicate the changes and then to reverse the changes and elucidate underlying mechanisms. The test assays may be studies *in vivo*, using animal tissues, or *in vitro*, using human or animal cells. As one possible example, evidence for increased free radical production in the human and DS brain might suggest studies to treat human cells with free radical scavengers in an attempt to rescue apparent changes (Lott et al., 2011). Studies to define the underlying mechanism might follow with an evaluation of the oxidative changes in various molecular species and their responses to treatment.

A second strategy focuses on linking phenotypes present in humans or in mouse models to underlying mechanisms—both molecular and cellular. One example of this approach was the demonstration that increased inhibitory neurotransmission appears to play a defining role in the reduced synaptic plasticity and cognitive deficits present in mouse models of DS. The follow-on here has been to decipher which elements of the GABAergic system are perturbed, an effort that is largely responsible for an ongoing clinical trial in DS (Roche, 2011).

Finally, based on the fact that all changes in cognitive function must arise directly or indirectly from an increase in the dose of a gene(s) or regulatory sequence(s) on HSA21, studies to link relevant phenotypes to specific genes have proven quite useful. The most clear-cut example of this is the identification of APP gene dose as necessary for the changes of AD in both mouse models (Salehi et al., 2006, Salehi et al., 2009) and, with increasing clarity, in humans (Prasher et al., 1998). It is worth noting a strategy that we see as very useful in defining the relevant gene(s). Initially envisioned in the context of DS, this approach argues that a search begins with the definition of highly quantitative robust phenotypes, followed by attempts to link one or more to a specific genetic segment. If possible, one then proceeds to define candidate genes and to make mice in which increased dose for just the candidate is reduced to disomic levels. Phenotypes that are no longer present give evidence that the candidate was necessary. Follow-on experiments ask if the same gene, introduced in one extra copy on the euploid background, recreates the phenotype; if so, increased dose for this gene is also sufficient to create the phenotype. Working in this way, it is possible to identify genes of interest with confidence and to understand to what extent they add to or dominate the production of changes of interest. Studies to date encourage the view that individual genes will be shown to play important roles and can serve as therapeutic targets. In practice, this may prove adequate for enhancing function. But it is also likely that most phenotypes result from the contribution of more than one gene and that fully correcting them may well require targeting several genes. In summary, as work proceeds, the continued use of these strategies, and especially the mapping of phenotype–genotype correlations using mouse models, can be predicted to lead to an increasing harvest of treatments for enhancing cognition in children and adults with DS.

THERAPEUTIC STRATEGY I: EXPLORING AND TREATING NEUROPATHOLOGICAL HALLMARKS IN DOWN SYNDROME

Basal Forebrain Cholinergic Neuron Degeneration

Basal forebrain cholinergic neurons (BFCNs) provide the major cholinergic innervation to the hippocampus and cortex and therefore play a major role in attention and cognition processing. Characteristic cholinergic hallmarks of individuals with AD and DS are the progressive loss of BFCNs, neocortical deficits in choline acetyltransferase, and reduced choline uptake and acetylcholine (ACh) release. This "cholinergic hypothesis" has been the main thrust of pharmacological intervention in AD. Selective cholinesterase inhibitors (ChEIs), such as galantamine and donepezil, have been developed as promnesic agents, with the aim of enhancing the central cholinergic system. These inhibitors increase the availability of ACh to post-synaptic receptors by limiting its breakdown in the synapse. Indeed, several studies have shown that administration of ChEIs have improved cognition and function in individuals with AD. However, evidence of the efficacy of ChEIs in treating cognitive dysfunction in DS is surprisingly limited.

Galantamine

Galantamine is an alkaloid found in plant extracts that also acts at the nicotinic cholinergic receptors, thereby augmenting the effect of increased ACh in improving cholinergic transmission. Galantamine is well tolerated and enhances cognitive, functional, and behavioral symptoms of patients with mild to moderate AD (Tariot et al., 2000). The efficacy and tolerability of galantamine treatment in DS has not yet been examined.

Recently, galantamine was administered to the Ts65Dn mouse model (de Souza et al., 2011). Mice heavily depend on their olfactory senses to inform learning and memory. Interestingly, people with AD and DS show a significant impairment in olfactory function compared to the general population (Murphy, 1999). Ts65Dn mice exhibit significant deficits in an olfactory associative learning paradigm, which was rescued with galantamine treatment for 10 days (de Souza et al., 2011). These findings encourage the view that administration of galantamine may enhance cholinergic neurotransmission in DS. However, further studies to understand the mechanism of action would be necessary before translating into a clinical trial. Correspondingly, evidence of efficacy in clinical trials is needed before making recommendations regarding use of galantamine in people with DS.

Donepezil

Donepezil is well tolerated and has been approved for the treatment of mild to severe AD in the general population to improve cognition and language, and enhance function and daily activities (Winblad et al., 2006). Treatment benefits in cognition and global function were observed in individuals with DS who had AD (Prasher et al., 2003). Treatment with donepezil also led to an improvement in expressive language in clinical trials in adults and children with DS (Heller et al., 2004, Heller et al., 2003).

A large, multicenter clinical trial was conducted to assess the safety and functional efficacy of donepezil on cognition in young adults (18–25 years old) with DS who had no signs of AD (Kishnani et al., 2009).

Despite being well tolerated and safe, the cognitive-enhancing efficacy of donepezil intervention was limited. A Phase II trial (Clinical Trials Registry NCT00754052) reported that early donepezil treatment in children and adolescents with DS is well tolerated; however, it did not demonstrate any benefits in improving cognition or function (Kishnani et al., 2010). Even though donepezil may be effective for treating language impairments, at this time no recommendation can be made for its therapeutic intervention to treat cognitive dysfunction in children and adolescents with DS.

Locus Coeruleus Degeneration

Contextual discrimination requires input from the sensory and the modulatory afferent systems. Sensory information originates from the entorhinal cortex, whereas modulatory inputs extensively innervate the hippocampus from various neuronal populations, including BFCN, norepinephrine (NE)-containing neurons of the locus coeruleus (LC), and serotonergic neurons of the raphe nuclei. The LC is the sole source of norepinephrinergic inputs that engage β–adrenergic receptors in the hippocampus, which is essential for successful contextual discrimination. In AD, NE concentrations are drastically reduced, and LC neurons undergo extensive degeneration (Grudzien et al., 2007).

L-DOPS and Xamoterol

L-DOPS (L-Threo-3,4-dihydroxyphenylserine) is an NE prodrug used in clinical trials for the treatment of neurogenic orthostatic hypotension associated with movement disorders and autonomic neuropathies (Kaufmann, 2008). In Ts65Dn mice, degeneration of LC neurons is prevalent at six months of age, accompanied by changes in LC terminals innervating the hippocampus, which precede the morphological alterations in the soma (Salehi et al., 2009). Reduced NE concentrations are prevalent by 18 months of age. Interestingly, there is an increase in postsynaptic β_1-adrenergic receptors in response to decreasing NE transmission, suggesting that postsynaptic mechanism remained functional amidst LC dysfunction and degeneration. Treatment with L-DOPS completely restored contextual memory and nesting behavior in Ts65Dn mice. NE concentrations were also normalized following L-DOPS treatment. The use of L-DOPS in clinical trials is well tolerated and effective, with mild side effects (Mathias et al., 2001), and suggests that stimulating NE neurotransmission may enhance cognition in DS. Xamoterol, a β_1-adrenergic receptor partial agonist, also targets NE deficiency and improved performance in the contextual fear-conditioning task in Ts65Dn mice (Salehi et al., 2009). In another study, Xamoterol also restored memory deficits in the spontaneous alteration and novel object recognition (NOR) tasks. Administering betaxolol, a selective β_1-adrenergic antagonist, reversed the behavioral improvements, highlighting the critical involvement of the β_1-adrenergic receptors (Faizi et al., 2011).

Formoterol

β_1-adrenergic receptors are likely to induce peripheral cardiovascular side effects; however, many people with DS innately experience cardiovascular abnormalities, so the use of β_2-adrenergic receptors may prove to be safer. Additionally, unlike β1AR receptors, β2AR signaling plays a critical role in the prevention of impaired hippocampal long-term potentiation (LTP) in the presence of Aβ oligomers (Li et al., 2013). Formoterol is a long-acting selective β_2-adrenergic receptor. Acute treatment with formoterol in six-month-old Ts65Dn mice improved contextual learning in a fear-conditioning test and reduced hyperactivity in an open-field activity test (Dang et al., 2013). Formoterol treatment also increased synaptophysin (SYN) immunoreactivity, suggesting an improvement in synaptic density, and increased dendritic complexity and synaptic strength. An improvement in microglia load was also observed, suggesting that an increase in NE levels could restore microglial functions.

Together, these findings highlight the importance of NE neurotransmission and highlight β_2-adrenergic receptor signaling as an attractive strategy in mediating hippocampal-dependent contextual memory in people with DS. However, it will be important to test such agents in clinical trials of people with DS before they can be recommended.

THERAPEUTIC STRATEGY II: EXPLORING AND TREATING PERTURBED PHYSIOLOGICAL MECHANISMS IN DOWN SYNDROME

GABAergic Neurotransmission

Ts65Dn mice exhibit a 30% decrease in the number of asymmetrical synapses in the temporal cortex, suggesting a selective decrease in the number of excitatory synapses and synaptic connectivity (Belichenko et al.,

2004). In more recent studies in hippocampus, there was no decrease in the number of asymmetrical and symmetrical synapses, but an increase in the size of symmetrical synapses at a critical time point in the development of neuronal circuitry (Mitra et al., 2012). These data and other physiological studies are evidence of excessive γ-aminobutryic acid (GABA)-mediated inhibition impairing LTP induction in the hippocampus (Belichenko et al., 2004, Hanson et al., 2007, Kleschevnikov et al., 2004). The GABA$_A$ receptor chloride channel is the primary inhibitory neurotransmitter receptor. Several pharmacological interventions have aimed to modulate the excitatory–inhibitory imbalance by decreasing excessive inhibition of GABAergic neurotransmission.

Picrotoxin

The efficacy of picrotoxin (PTX), a non-competitive GABA$_A$ antagonist, was assessed to rescue declarative memory in Ts65Dn mice (Fernandez et al., 2007). As GABA$_A$ antagonists are prototypically anxiogenic and convulsant, a four-week crossover study was conducted in which 3–4-month-old Ts65Dn mice and controls were assigned to groups receiving daily intraperitoneal injections of PTX at non-epileptic doses, or saline. At the two-week midpoint, mice that had been chronically administered PTX were switched onto a saline regimen, whereas mice that initially received saline either continued to receive daily saline or began daily injections of PTX. Ts65Dn mice injected with saline in either the first half or throughout the entire experimental period did not show novelty discrimination above chance levels in a NOR task. However, Ts65Dn mice treated with PTX showed a marked improvement in the NOR task. Unexpectedly, Ts65Dn mice that had received chronic PTX administration during the first half of the experimental period maintained their improved performance for up to two weeks later.

Pentylenetetrazol

The efficacy of pentylenetetrazole (PTZ), another non-competitive GABA$_A$ antagonist, was also evaluated in Ts65Dn mice (Fernandez et al., 2007). Chronic oral PTZ treatment in Ts65Dn reversed the deficits seen in the NOR task and a spontaneous alteration task, suggesting a restoration of declarative memory. Consistent with the post-drug recovery in cognition observed with PTX, Ts65Dn mice treated with PTZ showed a sustained improvement in cognitive performance in the NOR task for up to two months after termination of the drug regimen. Accompanying these behavioral findings, increased LTP in the dentate gyrus (DG) persisted for up to three months. In another study, chronic administration of PTZ in four-month-old Ts65Dn mice normalized spatial learning and memory deficits in the Morris Water Maze (MWM), without affecting sensorimotor or locomotor activity (Rueda et al., 2008a).

These studies suggest that chronic administration of non-competitive GABA$_A$ antagonists ameliorate declarative memory deficits in Ts65Dn mice and that the effects persist beyond the window of drug treatment. Unfortunately, many have pointed to the concern that these drugs have convulsant, pro-convulsant, and anxiogenic effects, which may preclude their use as cognitive enhancers in people with DS, particularly as people with DS are more susceptible to convulsions (Menendez, 2005).

α5 Inverse Agonist

An alternative to GABA$_A$ antagonists are GABA$_A$ inverse agonists (also known as negative allosteric modulators), which act at the benzodiazepine recognition site of GABA$_A$ receptors to decrease the efficacy of GABAergic neurotransmission. The α5 subunit of the benzodiazepine receptor is highly expressed in the hippocampus, and reduced expression of the α5 subunit facilitated cognitive performance in hippocampal-dependent tasks (Collinson et al., 2006).

RO4938581 (F. Hoffman–La Roche), a benzodiazepine site ligand with inverse agonism selective to the α5 subunit, specifically decreases GABAergic neurotransmission and enhances cognition and LTP without adverse pro-convulsive or anxiogenic effects in rats and monkeys (Ballard et al., 2009). Chronic treatment with RO4938581 in Ts65Dn mice improved cognition in a modified version of the MWM and rescued deficient hippocampal LTP (Martinez-Cue et al., 2013). RO4938581 treatment also restored cell proliferation levels and normalized neurogenesis of matured neurons. The density of GABAergic synaptic markers in the inner molecular layer of the DG was also normalized, suggesting a reduction in GABA-mediated over-inhibition. RO4938581 treatment in Ts65Dn also improved attention and hyperactivity without inducing anxiety or convulsions. These findings suggest that RO4938581 can reverse cognitive, electrophysiological, and morphological deficits in Ts65Dn mice without inducing overt side effects.

Another α5-selective inverse agonist, α5IA, was also assessed in Ts65Dn mice (Braudeau et al., 2011a). Acute and chronic treatment with α5IA did not induce convulsant, pro-convulsant, or anxiogenic effects, and did not cause histological alterations or toxicity. Daily intraperitoneal injections of α5IA, immediately before a trial, rescued MWM spatial-reference learning deficits and alleviated inadequate navigation strategies in Ts65Dn mice. Impaired object-recognition memory was also rescued.

Long-term memory requires the activation of immediate early genes (IEGs), and memory of new information requires a specific pattern of IEG expression. The induction levels of four IEGs that are typically expressed after behavioral stimulation (*Arc, Homer1, c-Fos,* and *EGR2*) were reduced in Ts65Dn mice compared to controls, suggesting impaired induction (Braudeau et al., 2011a, Braudeau et al., 2011b). Chronic α5IA treatment for 12 days globally increased the expression of these IEGs, particularly of *Arc* and *c-Fos*. Additionally, α5IA treatment normalized the expression levels of *Sod1*, a trisomic gene in DS. Overexpression of *Sod1* in transgenic mice upregulates GABAergic neurotransmission by impairing LTP and hippocampal neurogenesis, and also enhances sensitivity to degeneration and apoptosis. The restoration of IEG expression levels and normalization of *Sod1* levels may contribute to the effect of α5IA treatment in Ts65Dn mice.

On the basis of these developments, with the ultimate aim of enhancing cognition by reducing GABAergic neurotransmission, Roche announced the commencement of a Phase I clinical trial to assess safety of a drug selective for the α5 subunit of $GABA_A$ receptors (Roche, 2011). It is still in its early stages, and it will be exciting to follow the results of this trial. In this regard, it is noteworthy that the first clinical trial of α5IA as a cognitive enhancer was found safe and tolerable to reduce the amnesic effect of alcohol in the non-DS population (Nutt et al., 2007).

Glutamatergic Neurotransmission

Learning and memory deficits in hippocampal-dependent tasks may also be attributable to abnormal N-methyl-D-aspartate (NMDA) receptor signaling. Physiological glutamate-mediated activation of the NMDA receptor is necessary for normal cognitive functioning; however, pathological activation may contribute to the neuronal death in AD and DS. The view that excessive NMDA activation may contribute to neurodegeneration was an important stimulus for efforts to modulate this channel therapeutically in people with AD.

Memantine is a low-affinity uncompetitive antagonist of glutamate NMDA receptors. Memantine is approved for decreasing clinical deterioration in moderate to severe AD, is well tolerated, and does not appear to interfere with the acquisition or processing of cognitive information (Reisberg et al., 2003).

Acute memantine treatment in 4–6-month-old Ts65Dn mice rescued contextual memory in a fear conditioning test (Costa et al., 2008). These data are evidence that memantine effects are mediated, at least in part, by a mechanism(s) distinct from that which protects against neurodegeneration. Ts65Dn mice show increased APP expression in the hippocampus and cortex, reduced granule cell density in the DG, and reduced VGLUT1 levels, a marker of glutamatergic synapses (Rueda et al., 2010). Oral treatment with memantine for nine weeks in nine-month-old Ts65Dn mice slightly reduced APP levels, normalized VGLUT1 levels in the hippocampus, and improved spatial learning in the MWM. However, there was no effect on decreased density of hippocampal granule cells. Ts65Dn brain slices exhibited exaggerated NMDA-mediated LTD in the CA1 region, which is crucial for regular synaptic plasticity and memory formation. Acute pharmacological application of memantine restored LTD levels (Scott-McKean & Costa, 2011), thereby further supporting the view that changes in NMDA signaling may be implicated in reduced synaptic plasticity. Chronic memantine treatment in 10-month-old Ts65Dn mice improved spatial reference memory in the MWM and rescued object discrimination ability in the NOR task; however, still impaired was long-term memory in the NOR paradigm and activity in the spontaneous alteration task (Lockrow et al., 2011).

Memory function may be mediated by brain-derived neurotrophic factor (BDNF); in some studies, decreased BDNF levels have been documented in AD and DS brains (Connor et al., 1997). Chronic memantine administration increased BDNF protein levels and *Bdnf* mRNA levels by 30% in the Ts65Dn hippocampus. Histopathological analyses revealed no morphological changes, which was indicative of protection from neurodegeneration or alleviation of microglial activation (Lockrow et al., 2011). Whether or not memantine effects on BDNF gene expression contribute to cognitive benefits has not yet been addressed.

Based on studies in Ts65Dn mice, and the parallels between the neuropathological hallmarks for DS and AD, a clinical trial assessed the safety and efficacy of 52-week memantine treatment for dementia in adults older than 40 years with DS (Hanney et al., 2012). Unfortunately, memantine conferred no significant benefit on cognition, behavior, or function, irrespective of a formal diagnosis of dementia. More recently, a pilot study assessed the neuroprotective role of early treatment with memantine in young adults with DS between 18–32 years of age (Boada et al., 2012). No therapeutic treatment effects were observed. Thus, despite memantine's efficacy in those with moderate to severe AD, and mouse studies exhibiting promising benefits, these trials indicate that memantine is not an effective treatment for progressive cognitive decline or dementia in people with DS. The discrepancy between clinical efficacy in DS and AD is interesting and unexplained. At the very least it suggests the existence of differences in the activity of cognitive circuits impacted by AD-related pathogenesis in the two conditions.

Neurogenesis

Neurogenesis comprises the proliferation and differentiation of neurons. Present in the developing brain, neurogenesis continues to occur throughout adulthood within the subgranular layer (SGL) of the lateral ventricles of the DG and the subventricular zone (SVZ) of the DG. Neurogenesis can be adversely affected by stress and depression; chronic use of antidepressants, such as fluoxetine, a selective serotonin reuptake inhibitor (SSRI), has been shown to counter the behavioral aspects of depression (Santarelli et al., 2003). Moreover, a defective serotonergic system is observed in DS, characterized by reduced serotonin (5-HT) receptor levels, which are crucial for regulating neurogenesis (Banasr et al., 2004).

Fluoxetine

Fluoxetine is readily available, widely used, and has no adverse effects on somatic development (Bairy et al., 2007). To alleviate hippocampal neurogenesis impairments observed in DS, Ts65Dn mice were treated with fluoxetine for 24 days (Clark et al., 2006). In Ts65Dn mice, 70% of the newborn cells in the SGL had altered morphology, suggesting impaired neurogenesis, and the number of newly born neurons migrating to the granule cell layer (GCL) was reduced. Chronic treatment with fluoxetine in Ts65Dn mice restored hippocampal neurogenesis by inducing a 60% increase of newborn cells in the SGL and in the GCL, accompanied by normalized nuclear morphology.

Neurogenesis in the DG occurs mainly early in the postnatal period, thus the potential of early pharmacotherapy with fluoxetine to improve neurogenesis defects in DS was explored (Bianchi et al., 2010b). Ts65Dn mice received daily fluoxetine injections from postnatal day (P) 3 to P15. Chronic treatment with fluoxetine increased the number of mature cells in the SGL and SVZ of the lateral ventricle, and increased cell proliferation by 110%. Significantly, at P45, a month after cessation of treatment, mice showed an increase in the number of surviving cells that had migrated to the GCL. Moreover, fluoxetine treatment increased the absolute number of new neurons and new astrocytes in the DG, and granule cell number and density. It also increased the expression of 5-HT1A receptors in the hippocampus and hippocampal neurospheres, and increased BDNF levels to normal. Furthermore, behavioral deficits in a contextual fear-conditioning task were rescued.

Interestingly, adult-onset fluoxetine treatment in 5–7-month-old Ts65Dn mice did not reverse spatial learning and memory deficits in the MWM (Heinen et al., 2012). Additionally, increased mortality and handling-induced seizures were observed. However, these negative results may be explained by a higher drug dosage and the late onset of treatment. This suggests that a clinically relevant drug dose of fluoxetine may restore neurogenesis when administered during a crucial window for hippocampal development and corticogenesis. A caveat is that fluoxetine addresses a number of targets; its actions cannot be viewed as due only to its SSRI effects. More specifically, enhancing 5-HT signaling would help define the extent to which this system is responsible for defective neurogenesis.

Connectivity

Dendritic abnormalities are seen in DS and may contribute to deficits in synaptic plasticity deficits and impaired learning and memory. Fluoxetine has previously been shown to improve dendritic spine maturation and stimulate synaptic plasticity (Wang et al., 2008). The efficacy of early fluoxetine pharmacotherapy (P3 to P15) was assessed for rescuing dendritic pathology and connectivity (Guidi et al., 2013). Hypotrophic dendritic arbors, reduced DG spine density and decreased innervation were observed in granule cells in Ts65Dn mice. Specifically, newborn granule cells showed long branches of low order and fewer branches of intermediate and higher order dendritic trees. Fluoxetine treatment restored the aberrant dendritic tree and its architecture, and increased the spine density and innervation in Ts65Dn mice.

Hippocampus-dependent memory functions require intact connectivity from the entorhinal cortex via its axons travelling in the perforant path.

Perforant path axons innervate the middle and outer third of the molecular layer of the DG and use glutamate as a neurotransmitter (Banasr et al., 2004). It is plausible that reduced connectivity is one consequence of severe dendritic hypotrophy. Indeed, Dang and colleagues show reduced granule cell dendrite complexity in Ts65Dn mice (Dang et al., 2013). Additionally, in these mice the hippocampus shows reduced levels of SYN, a synaptic vesicle glycoprotein that is a marker of presynaptic terminals (Guidi et al., 2013). Ts65Dn mice also show reduced co-localization of SYN and vesicular glutamate transporter 1 (VGLUT1) in the inner, middle, and outer third of the molecular layer, suggesting attenuation of excitatory afferents and connectivity. Treatment with fluoxetine in these mice increased SYN levels and the co-localization of SYN and VGLUT1 in all zones of the molecular layer. 5-HT is also essential for the dendritic development of granule cells, especially during the immediate postnatal weeks. Treatment with fluoxetine not only restored 5-HT1A levels in P2-P15 Ts65Dn mice, but also 5-HT levels at P45, thereby further implicating the importance of the serotonergic system in dendritic formation and maturation of granule cells.

Long-term declarative memory requires processing of neocortical signals from the entorhinal cortex that are relayed through a trisynaptic circuit; granule cells of the DG to the pyramidal neurons in the CA3 region and through to pyramidal neurons in the CA1 region. The CA3 is proposed to be pivotal for pattern completion and separation during memory storage. DG neurons send their axons, the mossy fibers, to the CA3 and form a layer called the *stratum lucidum*. The mossy fibers form synapses on the thorny excrescences that cover the proximal apical dendritic shaft of CA3 pyramidal neurons. Additionally, these axons form thin philopodial extensions and small en passant boutons onto inhibitory interneurons located within the stratum lucidum. In Ts65Dn mice, the reduced density of granule cells may lead to a reduction of excitatory signals transferred to the CA3 region, and contribute to the deficits in memory performance. Indeed, the thickness of the mossy fiber bundle and the density of spines forming the thorny excrescences in the stratum lucidum were reduced in Ts65Dn mice. Additionally, reduced SYN and VGLUT levels suggested fewer synaptic terminals and glutamatergic terminals in the stratum lucidum (Stagni et al., 2013). Fluoxetine treatment rescued all these phenotypes. Moreover, electrophysiological assessments that evaluated the functional effectiveness of these new connections showed that fluoxetine treatment normalized the reduced basal excitatory and inhibitory input to CA3 pyramidal neurons.

The data suggest that the serotonergic system and BDNF levels may be mechanisms through which fluoxetine exerts its benefits on cell proliferation, survival, and cognition. Thus, the possibility that enhancing

5-HT signaling may prove effective in DS is worthy of additional research investments.

Lithium

The SVZ produces principal neurons and interneurons that populate the cortical mantle during fetal development; it retains neurogenic potential across the lifespan. Lithium is a mood stabilizer commonly used to treat disorders of affect, and has been shown to increase adult neurogenesis in mice (Malberg et al., 2000). Lithium was administered for one month to assess possible benefits on impaired neurogenesis in 12-month-old Ts65Dn mice (Bianchi et al., 2010a). Ts65Dn mice showed a 40% reduction in the number of proliferating cells in the SVZ. Treatment with lithium increased the number of proliferating cells in Ts65Dn mice by 66%, and increased the pool of proliferating cells in the SVZ.

In a recent study, lithium treatment rescued adult neurogenesis by fully restoring the number of maturing newborn cells in 5–6-month-old Ts65Dn mice (Contestabile et al., 2013). The failure to elicit LTP in Ts65Dn hippocampal slices after high-frequency stimulation of the medial perforant path was reestablished following four weeks of lithium treatment, raising the possibility that lithium-rescued newborn neurons were physiologically functional. A full recovery of long-term explicit memory was also observed in the contextual fear-conditioning, object location, and NOR tasks, all of which rely on hippocampal adult neurogenesis. The Wnt/β-catenin signaling pathway is integral for regulating DG adult neurogenesis, and lithium stimulation activated this canonical pathway to induce hippocampal neural precursor cell proliferation and restore adult neurogenesis.

These studies further encourage the view that currently existing pharmaceuticals, such as antidepressants and other mood stabilizers, as well as newly developed pharmaceuticals can be administered to correct the neurogenesis, connectivity, and cognitive impairments in DS. As with other potential therapeutic interventions, additional studies will be needed to guide future clinical trials and ensure that the treatment is safe and effective in DS.

Neurodevelopment

Infants with DS demonstrate delays in achieving developmental motor and sensory milestones. Corresponding to these deficits are reduced brain volume, delayed myelination of neurons, and glial alterations. Neuroprotective peptides have been suggested to enhance neurodevelopment. Vasoactive intestinal peptide (VIP) is a neuropeptide critical for regulating embryonic growth and development. VIP stimulation of astrocytes results in the release of neuroprotective peptides derived from naturally occurring glial proteins, including activity-dependent neuroprotective protein (ADNP) and activity-dependent neurotrophic factor (ADNF).

Increased VIP levels have been reported in the blood of infants with DS. One view is that this change may underlie the growth and developmental delays (Nelson et al., 2006). In nine-month-old Ts65Dn mice, an increase in VIP binding sites, mRNA, and immunoreactivity was observed in several brain regions (Hill et al., 2003). This phenotype is also seen in Ts65Dn mice as young as eight days old. Additionally, astrocytes from neonatal trisomy mouse brains failed to respond to VIP stimulation to produce neuroprotective peptides that promote neuronal survival (Sahir et al., 2006). Treating human DS cortical neurons with the active fragments of ADNP and ADNF, NAPVSIPQ (NAP) and SALLRSIPA (SAL) respectively, resulted in a two-fold increase in neuronal survival, reduced degenerative morphological changes, and enhanced protection from oxidative damage (Busciglio et al., 2007).

Prenatal administration of NAP + SAL to pregnant Ts65Dn mothers between gestational days 8–12 abolished the delay in achieving most of the motor and sensory milestones in Ts65Dn mice, and even accelerated the achievement of developmental milestones in control mice (Toso et al., 2008). Additionally, NAP + SAL treatment restored the downregulated ADNF expression and glial deficits in the neonatal period. Significantly, spatial learning deficits in the MWM were prevented in 8–10-month-old Ts65Dn mice that had been administered prenatal NAP + SAL treatment (Incerti et al., 2012). The authors suggest that NAP + SAL could serve as a prenatal pharmacological intervention. However, additional studies to define the impact of prenatal treatment on DS brain structure and function will be important.

Oxidative Stress

Oxidative stress is an imbalance in the metabolism of free radicals such as reactive oxygen species (ROS). This causes overproduction of hydrogen peroxide, leading to damage in cell and mitochondrial membranes, lipids, proteins, and mitochondrial DNA. Oxidative stress can occur during prenatal and postnatal development, and can modify neurogenesis and induce apoptosis. AD-affected brain regions show increased levels of lipid peroxidation, and NFTs and Aβ plaques co-localize with markers of oxidative stress (Sayre et al., 1997). Increased levels of ROS, DNA damage, and lipid peroxidation have also been documented in the DS brain (Busciglio & Yankner, 1995, Jovanovic et al., 1998). In DS, a role for the overexpression of the HSA21 gene, *SOD1*, which encodes the superoxide dismutase enzyme that is responsible for changing oxygen free radicals into hydrogen peroxide, may help explain these findings. Neuronal survival has been reported to be restored using antioxidants, suggesting that antioxidant therapy may improve learning and memory abnormalities in DS.

SGS-111

SGS-111 (GVS-111/DVD111/Noopet) exerts nootropic properties in models of brain damage that are associated with excessive release of glutamate, intracellular calcium levels, or free radical production. Chronic treatment with SGS-111 in DS human cortical neurons *in vitro* enhances neuronal survival and prevents the accumulation of intracellular free radicals, peroxidative damage, and neurodegenerative changes (Pelsman et al., 2003). As oxidative stress is documented as early as the fetal stage in DS, SGS-111 was administered to pregnant Ts65Dn females from the day of conception throughout pregnancy, and to their pups for five months (Rueda et al., 2008b). The effects of adult-onset SGS-111 treatment were also assessed, by administering SGS-111 for six weeks to 4–6-month-old Ts65Dn mice. SGS-111 treatment reduced hyperactivity in Ts65Dn mice. However, regardless of when the onset of treatment was administered, SGS-111 failed to improve behavior and cognition in Ts65Dn mice in the MWM and the passive avoidance test, suggesting that this therapeutic intervention does not confer promnesic effects.

α-Tocopherol

The primary component of vitamin E is α-tocopherol, which is a potent lipophilic chain-breaking antioxidant that inhibits lipid peroxidation and protects the organism from free radical–mediated injury. Decreased levels of α-tocopherol are observed in individuals with AD (Jimenez-Jimenez et al., 1997). Many trials have attempted to establish whether vitamin E treatment is an efficacious intervention in AD, with mixed results biased towards an absence of therapeutic efficacy (Dysken et al., 2014, Farina et al., 2012).

Ts65Dn mice show a 40% increase in oxidative stress levels relative to controls. Ts65Dn mice supplemented with a vitamin E–enriched diet show normalized ROS levels and demonstrate a higher working memory load and improved spatial reference learning and memory in the radial arm maze (Lockrow et al., 2009). Significantly, vitamin E–treated Ts65Dn mice showed a delay in BFCN degeneration and normalized levels of calbindin D-28k (CB), a protein that is reduced in aging brain and may sensitize neurons to oxidative damage.

The concentration of lipid peroxidation is reported to be nine-fold higher in the amniotic fluid of mothers who are pregnant with DS fetuses than in those with normal fetuses (Perrone et al., 2007). Prenatal α-tocopherol was administered to pregnant Ts65Dn females from the day of conception throughout the pregnancy, and to their pups for 12 weeks (Shichiri et al., 2011). Chronic supplementation with α-tocopherol rescued anxiety and spatial learning in an elevated plus maze and MWM in Ts65Dn mice. Additionally, α-tocopherol intervention normalized the increased lipid peroxidation products in the plasma, cortex, and hippocampus of Ts65Dn mice. Treatment with α-tocopherol increased granule cell density in the DG, and improved hypocellularity in the DG and cortex.

A trial that supplemented folinic acid with antioxidants, including vitamin E, was administered to infants with DS under the age of seven months. No improvements in psychomotor activity and language development were evident a year later (Ellis et al., 2008). Recently, a trial was conducted to determine the feasibility, tolerability, safety, and efficacy of receiving a daily antioxidant pill (containing α-tocopherol, ascorbic acid, and α-lipoic acid) for two years, to treat dementia in adults with DS (Lott et al., 2011). No improvements in cognitive functioning or stabilization of cognitive decline were observed. A three-year international Phase III trial for α-tocopherol is currently nearing completion, with the aim of delaying cognitive and functional decline in adults with DS (clinical trial #NCT 00056329). Despite strong evidence from animal studies showing amelioration of oxidative stress and improved cognitive performance, clinical trials in DS and AD have, thus far, been disappointing. This may reflect the possibility that the antioxidants that were used were ineffective at the doses and combinations used. Additional trials might still be successful. The safety of developmental exposures to high doses of α-tocopherol in pregnant women also needs to be investigated before recommending this course of action.

THERAPEUTIC STRATEGY III: EXPLORING AND TREATING GENE-DOSAGE EFFECTS ON COGNITION IN DOWN SYNDROME

App

Ts65Dn mice do not exhibit Aβ plaque deposits or NFTs, but they do demonstrate a loss of BFCNs. Ts1Cje mice show no evidence of BFCN degeneration, suggesting that the contribution of one or more of the ~55 extra trisomic genes in Ts65Dn mice are necessary for BFCN degeneration (Sago et al., 1998). Degeneration of BFCN is suggested to be caused, at least in part, by deficits in retrograde axonal transport of nerve growth factor (NGF) (Cooper et al., 2001). Indeed, Ts65Dn mice display a severe impairment of NGF retrograde transport that is six times greater than in Ts1Cje mice (Salehi et al., 2006).

To understand the contribution of specific genes in causing this phenotype, *App* was identified as a candidate gene present in Ts65Dn, but not in Ts1Cje mice. The third copy of *App* in Ts65Dn mice was knocked down to render its expression comparable to disomic levels. Interestingly, in Ts65Dn^{App++-} mice, NGF retrograde transport was restored to that of Ts1Cje mice. Significantly, normalizing APP levels prevented the loss of BFCNs in Ts65Dn mice (Salehi et al., 2006). *APP* gene-dosage imbalance has also been linked to the degeneration of LC neurons, which predates BFCN neuronal loss (Salehi et al., 2009).

BFCN terminal ends in Ts65Dn mice display enlarged early endosomes that contain markers for both NGF and APP, suggesting that the overexpression of *App* causes enlarged early endosomes with disrupted retrograde NGF transport and, consequently, neurodegeneration (Salehi et al., 2006). Interestingly, Ts1Cje mice do not display enlarged early endosomes, and normalizing *App* gene dosage in Ts65Dn^{App++-} mice rescued the enlarged early endosome phenotype (Cataldo et al., 2003). These studies suggest a gene-dosage effect of *APP* in causing enlarged early endosomes and subsequently, neurotrophin axonal transport deficits (Figure 11.1).

The role for *APP* in causing endocytic deficits was further examined by studying key APP proteolytic enzymes (BACE-1 and γ-secretase) and various APP proteolytic fragments (Aβ and βCTF) in DS fibroblasts (Jiang et al., 2010). Morphological and functional endocytic abnormalities in DS fibroblasts were reversed when the expression of *APP* or BACE-1 was lowered. Overexpression of wild-type *APP* was sufficient to induce endosomal pathology in control fibroblasts, which were unaltered when transfected with a mutant form of *APP* that lacked the amino acid sequence required for the β-site cleavage, thus establishing an importance of the βCTF. Reduced

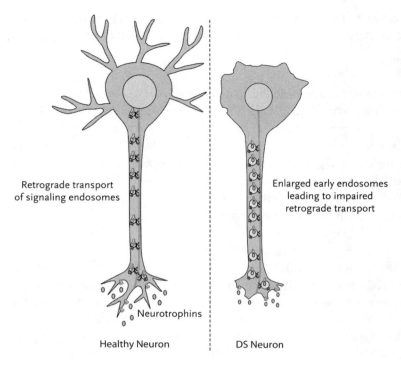

Retrograde transport
of signaling endosomes

Enlarged early endosomes
leading to impaired
retrograde transport

Neurotrophins

Healthy Neuron

DS Neuron

Figure 11.1:
Retrograde axonal transport of neurotrophins in normal and DS neurons. Healthy neurons demonstrate normal retrograde transport of neurotrophin signaling in endosomes that move from the synapse to the cell body along axons. Transport along microtubules is facilitated by regulatory, scaffolding, accessory, and motor proteins, including Rab5 and the dynein/dynactin complex. Neurotrophin signals are essential to maintaining the function and survival of neurons. DS neurons demonstrate impaired axonal transport. The overexpression of APP is postulated to cause enlarged early endosomes and impeded transport of neurotrophin signals, leading to neuronal dysfunction and degeneration.

BACE-1 expression, and thus lowered βCTF production, rescued endosomal pathology in DS fibroblasts. This suggests that endocytic dysfunction, and retrograde axonal transport deficits, are dependent on *APP* gene-dose and processing. Support for this comes from recently halted clinical trials using inhibitors of the γ-secretase enzyme complex. These compounds increase βCTF levels and were shown to negatively impact cognition in people with AD (Hopkins, 2011, Lily, 2010).

Going forward, it will be essential to devise therapeutic strategies focused on *APP*. At least three can be suggested:

1) Agents that act to reduce *APP* gene expression: Here the goal would be to impair the synthesis of APP mRNA or the translation of APP mRNA into the APP protein. One approach envisions the use of antisense

oligonucleotides (ASOs) specific for APP mRNA. ASOs are being tested preclinically and clinically at this time for other disorders, including those affecting children (Rigo et al., 2012).

2) Agents that act to enhance processing of APP to reduce βCTF and Aβ$_{42}$ levels: The former is clearly linked to endosomal defects, while the latter is widely viewed, and extensively suggested, as neurotoxic. One approach is to enhance the processing of the γ-secretase enzyme complex through the use of γ-secretase modulators (GSM) (Kounnas et al., 2010). In essence, GSMs act in the opposite way to γ-secretase inhibitors (GSIs). It is noteworthy that CTF levels are increased in neurons from people with DS (Busciglio & Yankner, 1995) and in the Ts65Dn model and would be expected to be reduced using GSMs.

3) Agents that reduce Aβ levels in the brain: One approach is to employ antibodies to Aβ. In recently completed studies in the Ts65Dn mouse, vaccination against DS, which employs a novel technology to present the Aβ peptide to the immune system, resulted in good antibody titers, reduced levels of Aβ peptides, and cognitive improvement in the NOR and contextual fear-conditioning paradigm (Belichenko et al., submitted).

In the future, using one or more of these approaches, as carefully tested in rigorous clinical trials, may prove effective in enhancing or preserving cognition in people with DS.

DYRK1A

The *dual-specificity tyrosine phosphorylation-regulated kinase (DYRK1A)* gene is strongly expressed during embryonic neurogenesis, particularly in neural precursor cells, and is implicated in dorsal telencephalic ventricular zone proliferation (Guimera et al., 1996). *DYRK1A* overexpression has been proposed to lead to premature neuronal differentiation, depletion of neural precursor cells available during neurogenesis, and inhibition of cell proliferation, presumably through deregulated NOTCH signaling (Hammerle et al., 2002). Furthermore, *DYRK1A* is involved in neuronal differentiation, and increased levels have been reported to perturb a chromatin-remodeling complex, leading to impaired dendritic growth and deregulated pluripotency and embryonic stem cell fate (Canzonetta et al., 2008). *DYRK1A* functionally interacts with and phosphorylates APP, and may thus contribute to the extracellular Aβ plaques seen in AD and DS (Ryoo et al., 2008). Interestingly, *DYRK1A* also phosphorylates Tau at a key priming site (Ryoo et al., 2007).

Normalizing *Dyrk1A* expression to disomic levels in *Ts65Dn* mice had the effect of normalizing signaling cascades, leading to neuronal transcription changes required for LTP establishment, attenuating synaptic plasticity deficits, and recovering thigmotactic behavior in the MWM, suggesting a partial improvement in their hippocampal-dependent search strategy (Altafaj et al., 2013).

Olig1/Olig2

During medial ganglionic eminence (MGE) neurogenesis, transcription factors induce MGE precursor cells to differentiate into either inhibitory interneurons or oligodendrocytes. Transcription factors oligodendrocyte transcription factor 1 (*Olig1*) and lineage factor 2 (*Olig2*) are highly expressed during this process. Both these genes are encoded on HSA21 and have been implicated in the ventral telencephalon inhibitory neuronal phenotype in Ts65Dn mice. Interestingly, normalizing expression of these genes to disomic levels in Ts65Dn mice restored MGE neurogenesis and inhibitory neuron production to normal levels (Chakrabarti et al., 2010). Moreover, the overinhibition phenotype was rescued, implicating a pathological gene-dosage role of these genes in causing the E-I imbalance (Chakrabarti et al., 2010).

Other HSA21 Genes of Interest

Additional key HSA21 genes that may play roles DS-associated neurodevelopment and neurodegeneration are listed in Table 11.1. As with any other case of a gene whose dose negatively impacts cognition function, approaches that reduce gene expression or that reduce the activity of a gene product may serve as treatment targets. Although these genes have not been studied as extensively as those discussed above, some intriguing results have been obtained.

KCNJ6/Girk2 (G-protein-coupled inward rectifying potassium channel) encodes the protein Girk2, which is a subunit of a channel that modulates postsynaptic GABA$_B$ receptors (Kleschevnikov et al., 2012). Increased *Kcnj6* gene-dosage is associated with increased channel density, current, and inhibitory GABA$_B$ signaling, suggesting a functional role for this gene in the excitatory–inhibitory imbalance and neuronal transmission. Down syndrome cell adhesion molecule (*DSCAM*) plays a critical role in facilitating dendritic morphology and neuronal wiring during

Table 11.1 PHYSIOLOGICAL AND PATHOLOGICAL ROLE OF KEY HSA21
GENES IN DS-ASSOCIATED NEURODEVELOPMENT AND
NEURODEGENERATION

HSA21 Gene	Physiological Role	Pathogenic Role
APP	Cell surface receptor and transmembrane glycoprotein that promotes transcriptional activation. Also implicated in synapse formation and neurite outgrowth.	*Neurodevelopment* • Leads to the overexpression of SHH receptor Ptch1, which inhibits SHH signaling pathway, leading to impaired cerebellar neurogenesis. • Loss of dendritic spines and synaptic plasticity. *Neurodegeneration* • Forms the protein basis of Aβ plaques in AD and DS. • Leads to enlarged early endosomes and a deficit in NGF retrograde axonal transport.
DSCAM	Cell adhesion molecule with a crucial role in dendrite morphology and neuronal wiring.	*Neurodevelopment* • Inhibits dendritic branching and causes perturbed synaptic plasticity. • May lead to aberrant NMDA-mediated regulation of DSCAM local translation.
DYRK1A	Kinase involved in regulating several signaling and cell proliferation mechanisms. Also involved in neurogenesis, particularly of neural precursor cells.	*Neurodevelopment* • Leads to premature neuronal differentiation, depletion of neural precursor cells, and inhibition of cell proliferation. • Deregulates genes implicated in dendritic growth, cell pluripotency and embryonic stem cell fate. • Reduces dendritic growth and complexity. *Neurodegeneration* • Phosphorylates APP and may contribute to extracellular Aβ phenotype. • Phosphorylates Tau at a key priming site and therefore can lead to NTFs. • Perturbs recruitment of endocytic proteins to clathrin-coated pits. • Slows retrieval of synaptic vesicle proteins in clathrin-mediated endocytosis. • Affects synaptic vesicle fusion kinetics.
KCNJ6/GIRK2	Effector protein for GABA$_B$ receptors, which modulates potassium channel current and density.	*Neurodevelopment* • Causes GABAergic excitatory-inhibitory imbalance through increased channel density, current and GABA$_B$ signaling. • Reduces membrane potential and neuronal excitability, thereby impeding NMDA-dependent plasticity.

(continued)

Table 11.1 CONTINUED

HSA21 Gene	Physiological Role	Pathogenic Role
OLIG1/OLIG2	Transcription factors implicated in oligodendrogenesis and neurogenesis.	*Neurodevelopment* • Induces perturbed MGE neurogenesis and inhibitory neuron production. • Causes GABAergic excitatory-inhibitory imbalance through an overinhibition phenotype.
SIM2	Transcriptional repressor implicated in synaptic plasticity and morphology.	*Neurodevelopment* • Reduces DBN1 levels, causing morphological cytoskeletal changes at postsynaptic terminals in dendritic spines.
SOD1	Cytoplasmic protein involved in oxidative stress.	*Neurodevelopment* • Decreases hippocampal neuronal progenitors and LTP. • Increases sensitivity to degeneration and apoptosis. • Upregulates GABAergic neurotransmission.
SYNJ1	Nerve terminal protein implicated in membrane trafficking and synaptic transmission. Also catalyzes dephosphorylation of PI(4,5)P$_2$.	*Neurodevelopment* • Inability to maintain stable GABAergic neurotransmission. *Neurodegeneration* • Perturbed dephosphorylation of PI(4,5)P$_2$ and phospholipids during clathrin-dependent endocytosis. • Formation of enlarged early endosomes.

Adapted from Ruparelia et al., 2012, p. 881.

neurodevelopment, and contributes to efficient synaptic plasticity in adulthood. Overexpression of *DSCAM* in hippocampal neurons of a DS mouse model was found to inhibit dendritic branching, which may possibly be caused by a loss of NMDA-mediated regulation of DSCAM local mRNA translation (Alves-Sampaio et al., 2010). Synaptojanin 1 (*SYNJ1*), a presynaptic polyphosphoinositide phosphatase important for membrane trafficking and normal synaptic vesicle recycling, also plays a significant role in maintaining stability of GABAergic neurotransmission (Luthi et al., 2001). Overexpression of the transcriptional repressor SIM2 (single-minded homolog 2) dramatically reduces expression of *DBN1* (*Drebrin 1*) by directly binding to its promoter. *DBN1* is a neuronally expressed gene that affects dendritic spine structure and neuritogenesis and is involved in modulating dendritic spine-cytoskeleton dynamics at postsynaptic terminals (Weitzdoerfer et al., 2001). Significantly, decreased DBN1 levels have been observed in cortices of people with AD and DS (Ooe et al., 2004, Shim & Lubec, 2002).

CONCLUSION

The trisomy of chromosome 21, and the resulting overexpression of many of its 350–500 genes, once encouraged the view that DS would be intractable to understand and treat. However, significant conceptual and technical advances and an increasing body of research encourage the view that the pathogenesis of DS can be defined and treatments discovered. Intellectual disability in children and cognitive decline in the elderly are the most significant challenges to be addressed at this time. A large number of laboratories and industrial efforts are attempting to define and develop therapeutic targets that confer promnesic treatment effects and enhance cognition in DS. To date, approved drugs for alleviating cognitive decline in AD have informed these attempts, but as yet these therapeutic effects in DS clinical trials have been limited and disappointing. It is evident that while aspects of the pathogenesis of AD and DS may be very similar, therapies effective in AD may not necessarily confer the same benefits in DS. Indeed, the additional genetically driven mechanisms and circuits in DS, as well as the multi-system involvement, may act to confound therapeutic benefits of interventions approved for AD. However, the closer we get to understanding and targeting the underlying genes and mechanisms in AD, the better we will be able to devise therapeutic strategies that focus on interrelated genes and mechanisms that also inform DS. In this regard, *APP* is an ideal candidate gene that needs to be further investigated to carefully define its physiological and pathological function, to then target it as a therapeutic intervention for DS.

Insights from the Ts65Dn mouse model of DS have been crucial in the understanding and development of therapeutic targets of cognitive functioning in DS. However, despite promising results in mouse studies, the translational effects in clinical trials are frequently not mirrored. This is not surprising, as translation from mouse to human is limited by differences in genetic content and circuits. However, the closer we get to discovering identical or, at the least, very similar mechanisms and genes, the better we will be able to devise approaches that target underlying processes that lead to the clinical manifestation of DS. An ideal example of this would be the identification of genes and mechanisms that explain the over-inhibition phenotype in mouse models that could then be explored and targeted in DS. Similarly, by further elucidating the cellular, molecular, and neurobiological mechanisms that underlie cognition and memory processes during neurodevelopmental and neurodegeneration in DS, it should be possible to develop and validate pharmacotherapy interventions. This would lead to the emergence of drug targets that are specifically tailored for DS, and could markedly enhance the chance of success in the large, well-designed clinical trials needed to assess the acute and chronic effects of treatments on cognition in children and adults with DS.

DISCLOSURES

Grant sponsors: National Institutes of Health (NS06672, NS24054, PN2EY016525), Down Syndrome Research and Treatment Foundation, Alzheimer's Association, Thrasher Research Fund, the Larry L. Hillblom Foundation, the Lowe Fund of the Denver Foundation, and the Itkin Family Foundation.

The authors declare no conflicts of interest.

Corresponding author: Dr. William Mobley, Department of Neurosciences, University of California–San Diego, 9500 Gilman Drive, CNCB Building, Room 100, La Jolla, California 92093-0752; email: wmobley@ucsd.edu; telephone: 858-534-9434; fax: 858-534-8980.

REFERENCES

Altafaj, X., Martin, E. D., Ortiz-Abalia, J., Valderrama, A., Lao-Peregrin, C., Dierssen, M., & Fillat, C. (2013). Normalization of Dyrk1A expression by AAV2/1-shDyrk1A attenuates hippocampal-dependent defects in the Ts65Dn mouse model of Down syndrome. *Neurobiology of Disease, 52,* 117–127.

Alves-Sampaio, A., Troca-Marin, J. A., & Montesinos, M. L. (2010). NMDA-mediated regulation of DSCAM dendritic local translation is lost in a mouse model of Down's syndrome. *Journal of Neuroscience, 30,* 13537–13548.

Bairy, K. L., Madhyastha, S., Ashok, K. P., Bairy, I., & Malini, S. (2007). Developmental and behavioral consequences of prenatal fluoxetine. *Pharmacology, 79,* 1–11.

Ballard, T. M., Knoflach, F., Prinssen, E., Borroni, E., Vivian, J. A., Basile, J., Gasser, R., et al. (2009). RO4938581, a novel cognitive enhancer acting at GABAA alpha5 subunit-containing receptors. *Psychopharmacology (Berlin), 202,* 207–223.

Banasr, M., Hery, M., Printemps, R., & Daszuta, A. (2004). Serotonin-induced increases in adult cell proliferation and neurogenesis are mediated through different and common 5-HT receptor subtypes in the dentate gyrus and the subventricular zone. *Neuropsychopharmacology, 29,* 450–460.

Belichenko, P. V., Masliah, E., Kleschevnikov, A. M., Villar, A. J., Epstein, C. J., Salehi, A., & Mobley, W. C. (2004). Synaptic structural abnormalities in the Ts65Dn mouse model of Down Syndrome. *Journal of Comparative Neurology, 480,* 281–298.

Bianchi, P., Ciani, E., Contestabile, A., Guidi, S., & Bartesaghi, R. (2010a). Lithium restores neurogenesis in the subventricular zone of the Ts65Dn mouse, a model for Down syndrome. *Brain Pathology, 20,* 106–118.

Bianchi, P., Ciani, E., Guidi, S., Trazzi, S., Felice, D., Grossi, G., Fernandez, M., et al. (2010b). Early pharmacotherapy restores neurogenesis and cognitive performance in the Ts65Dn mouse model for Down syndrome. *Journal of Neuroscience, 30*, 8769–8779.

Bittles, A. H., Bower, C., Hussain, R., & Glasson, E. J. (2007). The four ages of Down syndrome. *The European Journal of Public Health, 17*, 221–225.

Boada, R., Hutaff-Lee, C., Schrader, A., Weitzenkamp, D., Benke, T. A., Goldson, E. J., & Costa, A. C. (2012). Antagonism of NMDA receptors as a potential treatment for Down syndrome: a pilot randomized controlled trial. *Translational Psychiatry, 2*, e141.

Braudeau, J., Dauphinot, L., Duchon, A., Loistron, A., Dodd, R. H., Herault, Y., Delatour, B., et al. (2011a). Chronic treatment with a promnesiant GABA-A alpha5-selective inverse agonist increases immediate early genes expression during memory processing in mice and rectifies their expression levels in a Down syndrome mouse model. *Advances in Pharmacological Sciences, 2011*, 153218.

Braudeau, J., Delatour, B., Duchon, A., Pereira, P. L., Dauphinot, L., de Chaumont, F., Olivo-Marin, J. C., et al. (2011b). Specific targeting of the GABA-A receptor alpha5 subtype by a selective inverse agonist restores cognitive deficits in Down syndrome mice. *Journal of Psychopharmacology, 25*, 1030–1042.

Busciglio, J., Pelsman, A., Helguera, P., Ashur-Fabian, O., Pinhasov, A., Brenneman, D. E., & Gozes, I. (2007). NAP and ADNF-9 protect normal and Down's syndrome cortical neurons from oxidative damage and apoptosis. *Current Pharmaceutical Design, 13*, 1091–1098.

Busciglio, J., & Yankner, B. A. (1995). Apoptosis and increased generation of reactive oxygen species in Down's syndrome neurons in vitro. *Nature, 378*, 776–779.

Canzonetta, C., Mulligan, C., Deutsch, S., Ruf, S., O'Doherty, A., Lyle, R., Borel, C., et al. (2008). DYRK1A-dosage imbalance perturbs NRSF/REST levels, deregulating pluripotency and embryonic stem cell fate in Down syndrome. *American Journal of Human Genetics, 83*, 388–400.

Cataldo, A. M., Petanceska, S., Peterhoff, C. M., Terio, N. B., Epstein, C. J., Villar, A., Carlson, E. J., et al. (2003). App gene dosage modulates endosomal abnormalities of Alzheimer's disease in a segmental trisomy 16 mouse model of down syndrome. *Journal of Neuroscience, 23*, 6788–6792.

Chakrabarti, L., Best, T. K., Cramer, N. P., Carney, R. S., Isaac, J. T., Galdzicki, Z., & Haydar, T. F. (2010). Olig1 and Olig2 triplication causes developmental brain defects in Down syndrome. *Nature Neuroscience, 13*, 927–934.

Clark, S., Schwalbe, J., Stasko, M. R., Yarowsky, P. J., & Costa, A. C. (2006). Fluoxetine rescues deficient neurogenesis in hippocampus of the Ts65Dn mouse model for Down syndrome. *Experimental Neurology, 200*, 256–261.

Collinson, N., Atack, J. R., Laughton, P., Dawson, G. R., & Stephens, D. N. (2006). An inverse agonist selective for alpha5 subunit-containing GABAA receptors improves encoding and recall but not consolidation in the Morris water maze. *Psychopharmacology (Berlin), 188*, 619–628.

Connor, B., Young, D., Yan, Q., Faull, R. L., Synek, B., & Dragunow, M. (1997). Brain-derived neurotrophic factor is reduced in Alzheimer's disease. *Brain Research: Molecular Brain Research, 49*, 71–81.

Contestabile, A., Greco, B., Ghezzi, D., Tucci, V., Benfenati, F., & Gasparini, L. (2013). Lithium rescues synaptic plasticity and memory in Down syndrome mice. *Journal of Clinical Investigation, 123*, 348–361.

Cooper, J. D., Salehi, A., Delcroix, J. D., Howe, C. L., Belichenko, P. V., Chua-Couzens, J., Kilbridge, J. F., et al. (2001). Failed retrograde transport of NGF in a mouse model of Down's syndrome: reversal of cholinergic neurodegenerative phenotypes following NGF infusion. *Proceedings of the National Academy of Science, USA, 98*, 10439–10444.

Costa, A. C., Scott-McKean, J. J., & Stasko, M. R. (2008). Acute injections of the NMDA receptor antagonist memantine rescue performance deficits of the Ts65Dn mouse model of Down syndrome on a fear conditioning test. *Neuropsychopharmacology, 33*, 1624–1632.

Dang, V., Medina, B., Das, D., Moghadam, S., Martin, K. J., Lin, B., Naik, P., et al. (2013). Formoterol, a long-acting beta2 adrenergic agonist, improves cognitive function and promotes dendritic complexity in a mouse model of Down syndrome. *Biological Psychiatry, 75*, 179–188.

Davisson, M. T., Schmidt, C., Reeves, R. H., Irving, N. G., Akeson, E. C., Harris, B. S., & Bronson, R. T. (1993). Segmental trisomy as a mouse model for Down syndrome. *Progress in Clinical & Biological Research, 384*, 117–133.

de Souza, F. M., Busquet, N., Blatner, M., Maclean, K. N., & Restrepo, D. (2011). Galantamine improves olfactory learning in the Ts65Dn mouse model of Down syndrome. *Scientific Reports, 1*, 137.

Dysken, M. W., Guarino, P. D., Vertrees, J. E., Asthana, S., Sano, M., Llorente, M., Pallaki, M., et al. (2014) Vitamin E and memantine in Alzheimer's disease: Clinical trial methods and baseline data. *Alzheimer's & Dementia, 10*, 36–44.

Ellis, J. M., Tan, H. K., Gilbert, R. E., Muller, D. P., Henley, W., Moy, R., Pumphrey, R., et al. (2008). Supplementation with antioxidants and folinic acid for children with Down's syndrome: randomised controlled trial. *British Medical Journal, 336*, 594–597.

Faizi, M., Bader, P. L., Tun, C., Encarnacion, A., Kleschevnikov, A., Belichenko, P., Saw, N., et al. (2011). Comprehensive behavioral phenotyping of Ts65Dn mouse model of Down syndrome: activation of beta1-adrenergic receptor by xamoterol as a potential cognitive enhancer. *Neurobiology of Disease, 43*, 397–413.

Farina, N., Isaac, M. G., Clark, A. R., Rusted, J., & Tabet, N. (2012). Vitamin E for Alzheimer's dementia and mild cognitive impairment. *Cochrane Database of Systematic Reviews, 11*, CD002854.

Fernandez, F., Morishita, W., Zuniga, E., Nguyen, J., Blank, M., Malenka, R. C., & Garner, C. C. (2007). Pharmacotherapy for cognitive impairment in a mouse model of Down syndrome. *Nature Neuroscience, 10*, 411–413.

Grudzien, A., Shaw, P., Weintraub, S., Bigio, E., Mash, D. C., & Mesulam, M. M. (2007). Locus coeruleus neurofibrillary degeneration in aging, mild cognitive impairment and early Alzheimer's disease. *Neurobiology of Aging, 28*, 327–335.

Guidi, S., Stagni, F., Bianchi, P., Ciani, E., Ragazzi, E., Trazzi, S., Grossi, G., et al. (2013). Early pharmacotherapy with fluoxetine rescues dendritic pathology in the Ts65Dn mouse model of down syndrome. *Brain Pathology, 23*, 129–143.

Guimera, J., Casas, C., Pucharcos, C., Solans, A., Domenech, A., Planas, A. M., Ashley, J., et al. (1996). A human homologue of Drosophila minibrain (MNB) is expressed in the neuronal regions affected in Down syndrome and maps to the critical region. *Human Molecular Genetics, 5*, 1305–1310.

Hammerle, B., Vera-Samper, E., Speicher, S., Arencibia, R., Martinez, S., & Tejedor, F. J. (2002). Mnb/Dyrk1A is transiently expressed and asymmetrically segregated in neural progenitor cells at the transition to neurogenic divisions. *Developmental Biology, 246*, 259–273.

Hanney, M., Prasher, V., Williams, N., Jones, E. L., Aarsland, D., Corbett, A., Lawrence, D., et al. (2012). Memantine for dementia in adults older than 40 years with Down's syndrome (MEADOWS): a randomised, double-blind, placebo-controlled trial. *Lancet, 379*, 528–536.

Hanson, J. E., Blank, M., Valenzuela, R. A., Garner, C. C., & Madison, D. V. (2007). The functional nature of synaptic circuitry is altered in area CA3 of the hippocampus in a mouse model of Down's syndrome. *Journal of Physiology, 579*, 53–67.

Hattori, M., Fujiyama, A., Taylor, T. D., Watanabe, H., Yada, T., Park, H. S., Toyoda, A., et al. (2000). The DNA sequence of human chromosome 21. *Nature, 405*, 311–319.

Heinen, M., Hettich, M. M., Ryan, D. P., Schnell, S., Paesler, K., & Ehninger, D. (2012). Adult-onset fluoxetine treatment does not improve behavioral impairments and may have adverse effects on the Ts65Dn mouse model of Down syndrome. *Neural Plasticity, 2012*, 467251.

Heller, J. H., Spiridigliozzi, G. A., Doraiswamy, P. M., Sullivan, J. A., Crissman, B. G., & Kishnani, P. S. (2004). Donepezil effects on language in children with Down syndrome: results of the first 22-week pilot clinical trial. *American Journal of Medical Genetics A, 130A*, 325–326.

Heller, J. H., Spiridigliozzi, G. A., Sullivan, J. A., Doraiswamy, P. M., Krishnan, R. R., & Kishnani, P. S. (2003). Donepezil for the treatment of language deficits in adults with Down syndrome: a preliminary 24-week open trial. *American Journal of Medical Genetics A, 116A*, 111–116.

Hill, J. M., Ades, A. M., McCune, S. K., Sahir, N., Moody, E. M., Abebe, D. T., Crnic, L. S., & Brenneman, D. E. (2003). Vasoactive intestinal peptide in the brain of a mouse model for Down syndrome. *Experimental Neurology, 183*, 56–65.

Hopkins, C. R. (2011). ACS chemical neuroscience molecule spotlight on ELND006: another gamma-secretase inhibitor fails in the clinic. *ACS Chemical Neuroscience, 2*, 279–280.

Incerti, M., Horowitz, K., Roberson, R., Abebe, D., Toso, L., Caballero, M., & Spong, C. Y. (2012). Prenatal treatment prevents learning deficit in Down syndrome model. *PLoS One, 7*, e50724.

Jiang, Y., Mullaney, K. A., Peterhoff, C. M., Che, S., Schmidt, S. D., Boyer-Boiteau, A., Ginsberg, S. D., et al. (2010). Alzheimer's-related endosome dysfunction in Down syndrome is Abeta-independent but requires APP and is reversed by BACE-1 inhibition. *Proceedings of the National Academy of Science, USA, 107*, 1630–1635.

Jimenez-Jimenez, F. J., de Bustos, F., Molina, J. A., Benito-Leon, J., Tallon-Barranco, A., Gasalla, T., Orti-Pareja, M., et al. (1997). Cerebrospinal fluid levels of alpha-tocopherol (vitamin E) in Alzheimer's disease. *Journal of Neural Transmission, 104*, 703–710.

Jovanovic, S. V., Clements, D., & MacLeod, K. (1998). Biomarkers of oxidative stress are significantly elevated in Down syndrome. *Free Radical Biology & Medicine, 25*, 1044–1048.

Kaufmann, H. (2008). L-dihydroxyphenylserine (Droxidopa): a new therapy for neurogenic orthostatic hypotension: the US experience. *Clinical Autonomic Research, 18*(Suppl 1), 19–24.

Kishnani, P. S., Heller, J. H., Spiridigliozzi, G. A., Lott, I., Escobar, L., Richardson, S., Zhang, R., et al. (2010). Donepezil for treatment of cognitive dysfunction in children with Down syndrome aged 10–17. *American Journal of Medical Genetics A, 152A*, 3028–3035.

Kishnani, P. S., Sommer, B. R., Handen, B. L., Seltzer, B., Capone, G. T., Spiridigliozzi, G. A., Heller, J. H., et al. (2009). The efficacy, safety, and tolerability of donepezil for the treatment of young adults with Down syndrome. *American Journal of Medical Genetics A, 149A*, 1641–1654.

Kleschevnikov, A. M., Belichenko, P. V., Gall, J., George, L., Nosheny, R., Maloney, M. T., et al. (2012). Increased efficiency of the GABAA and GABAB receptor-mediated neurotransmission in the Ts65Dn mouse model of Down syndrome. *Neurobiology of Disease, 45*, 683–691.

Kleschevnikov, A. M., Belichenko, P. V., Villar, A. J., Epstein, C. J., Malenka, R. C., & Mobley, W. C. (2004). Hippocampal long-term potentiation suppressed by increased inhibition in the Ts65Dn mouse, a genetic model of Down syndrome. *Journal of Neuroscience, 24*, 8153–8160.

Kounnas, M. Z., Danks, A. M., Cheng, S., Tyree, C., Ackerman, E., Zhang, X., Ahn, K., et al. (2010). Modulation of gamma-secretase reduces beta-amyloid deposition in a transgenic mouse model of Alzheimer's disease. *Neuron, 67*, 769–780.

Li, S., Jin, M., Zhang, D., Yang, T., Koeglsperger, T., Fu, H., & Selkoe, D. J. (2013). Environmental novelty activates beta2-adrenergic signaling to prevent the impairment of hippocampal LTP by Abeta oligomers. *Neuron, 77*, 929–941.

Lily (2010). Lilly halts development of Semagacestat for Alzheimer's disease based on preliminary results of Phase III clinical trials. https://investor.lilly.com/releasedetail.cfm?ReleaseID=499794. Accessed July 29, 2013.

Lockrow, J., Boger, H., Bimonte-Nelson, H., & Granholm, A. C. (2011). Effects of long-term memantine on memory and neuropathology in Ts65Dn mice, a model for Down syndrome. *Behavioural Brain Research, 221*, 610–622.

Lockrow, J., Prakasam, A., Huang, P., Bimonte-Nelson, H., Sambamurti, K., & Granholm, A. C. (2009). Cholinergic degeneration and memory loss delayed by vitamin E in a Down syndrome mouse model. *Experimental Neurology, 216*, 278–289.

Lott, I. T., Doran, E., Nguyen, V. Q., Tournay, A., Head, E., & Gillen, D. L. (2011). Down syndrome and dementia: a randomized, controlled trial of antioxidant supplementation. *American Journal of Medical Genetics A, 155A*, 1939–1948.

Luthi, A., Di Paolo, G., Cremona, O., Daniell, L., De Camilli, P., & McCormick, D. A. (2001). Synaptojanin 1 contributes to maintaining the stability of GABAergic transmission in primary cultures of cortical neurons. *Journal of Neuroscience, 21*, 9101–9111.

Malberg, J. E., Eisch, A. J., Nestler, E. J., & Duman, R. S. (2000). Chronic antidepressant treatment increases neurogenesis in adult rat hippocampus. *Journal of Neuroscience, 20*, 9104–9110.

Mann, D. M., & Esiri, M. M. (1989). The pattern of acquisition of plaques and tangles in the brains of patients under 50 years of age with Down's syndrome. *Journal of the Neurological Sciences, 89*, 169–179.

Marin-Padilla, M. (1976). Pyramidal cell abnormalities in the motor cortex of a child with Down's syndrome. A Golgi study. *Journal of Comparative Neurology, 167*, 63–81.

Martinez-Cue, C., Martinez, P., Rueda, N., Vidal, R., Garcia, S., Vidal, V., Corrales, A., et al. (2013). Reducing GABAA alpha5 receptor-mediated inhibition rescues functional and neuromorphological deficits in a mouse model of down syndrome. *Journal of Neuroscience, 33*, 3953–3966.

Masters, C. L., Simms, G., Weinman, N. A., Multhaup, G., McDonald, B. L., & Beyreuther, K. (1985). Amyloid plaque core protein in Alzheimer disease and Down syndrome. *Proceedings of the National Academy of Science, USA, 82*, 4245–4249.

Mathias, C. J., Senard, J. M., Braune, S., Watson, L., Aragishi, A., Keeling, J. E., & Taylor, M. D. (2001). L-threo-dihydroxyphenylserine (L-threo-DOPS; droxidopa) in the management of neurogenic orthostatic hypotension: a multi-national, multi-center, dose-ranging study in multiple system atrophy and pure autonomic failure. *Clinical Autonomic Research*, *11*, 235–242.

Menendez, M. (2005). Down syndrome, Alzheimer's disease and seizures. *Brain Development*, *27*, 246–252.

Mitra, A., Blank, M., & Madison, D. V. (2012). Developmentally altered inhibition in Ts65Dn, a mouse model of Down syndrome. *Brain Research*, *1440*, 1–8.

Murphy, C. (1999). Loss of olfactory function in dementing disease. *Physiology & Behavior*, *66*, 177–182.

Nelson, P. G., Kuddo, T., Song, E. Y., Dambrosia, J. M., Kohler, S., Satyanarayana, G., Vandunk, C., et al. (2006). Selected neurotrophins, neuropeptides, and cytokines: developmental trajectory and concentrations in neonatal blood of children with autism or Down syndrome. *International Journal of Developmental Neuroscience*, *24*, 73–80.

Nutt, D. J., Besson, M., Wilson, S. J., Dawson, G. R., & Lingford-Hughes, A. R. (2007). Blockade of alcohol's amnestic activity in humans by an alpha5 subtype benzodiazepine receptor inverse agonist. *Neuropharmacology*, *53*, 810–820.

Ooe, N., Saito, K., Mikami, N., Nakatuka, I., & Kaneko, H. (2004). Identification of a novel basic helix-loop-helix-PAS factor, NXF, reveals a Sim2 competitive, positive regulatory role in dendritic-cytoskeleton modulator drebrin gene expression. *Molecular Cell Biology*, *24*, 608–616.

Pelsman, A., Hoyo-Vadillo, C., Gudasheva, T. A., Seredenin, S. B., Ostrovskaya, R. U., & Busciglio, J. (2003). GVS-111 prevents oxidative damage and apoptosis in normal and Down's syndrome human cortical neurons. *International Journal of Developmental Neuroscience*, *21*, 117–124.

Perrone, S., Longini, M., Bellieni, C. V., Centini, G., Kenanidis, A., De Marco, L., Petraglia, F., et al. (2007). Early oxidative stress in amniotic fluid of pregnancies with Down syndrome. *Clinical Biochemistry*, *40*, 177–180.

Prasher, V. P., Adams, C., Holder, R., & Down Syndrome Research, G. (2003). Long term safety and efficacy of donepezil in the treatment of dementia in Alzheimer's disease in adults with Down syndrome: open label study. *International Journal of Geriatric Psychiatry*, *18*, 549–551.

Prasher, V. P., Farrer, M. J., Kessling, A. M., Fisher, E. M., West, R. J., Barber, P. C., & Butler, A. C. (1998). Molecular mapping of Alzheimer-type dementia in Down's syndrome. *Annals of Neurology*, *43*, 380–383.

Reisberg, B., Doody, R., Stoffler, A., Schmitt, F., Ferris, S., Mobius, H. J., & Memantine Study, G. (2003). Memantine in moderate-to-severe Alzheimer's disease. *New England Journal of Medicine*, *348*, 1333–1341.

Rigo, F., Hua, Y., Krainer, A. R., & Bennett, C. F. (2012). Antisense-based therapy for the treatment of spinal muscular atrophy. *Journal of Cell Biology*, *199*, 21–25.

Roche (2011). Roche starts early stage clinical trial in Down syndrome. Roche USA. http://www.rocheusa.com/portal/usa/press_releases_nutley?siteUuid=re7180004&paf_gear_id=38400020&pageId=re7425113&synergyaction=show&paf_dm=full&nodeId=1415-fbfa4d37db2611e0953b3d6bec9c2782&currentPage=0. Accessed July 29, 2013.

Rueda, N., Florez, J., & Martinez-Cue, C. (2008a). Chronic pentylenetetrazole but not donepezil treatment rescues spatial cognition in Ts65Dn mice, a model for Down syndrome. *Neuroscience Letters*, *433*, 22–27.

Rueda, N., Florez, J., & Martinez-Cue, C. (2008b). Effects of chronic administration of SGS-111 during adulthood and during the pre- and post-natal periods on the cognitive deficits of Ts65Dn mice, a model of Down syndrome. *Behavioural Brain Research, 188,* 355–367.

Rueda, N., Llorens-Martin, M., Florez, J., Valdizan, E., Banerjee, P., Trejo, J. L., & Martinez-Cue, C. (2010). Memantine normalizes several phenotypic features in the Ts65Dn mouse model of Down syndrome. *Journal of Alzheimer's Disease, 21,* 277–290.

Ruparelia, A., Pearn, M. L., & Mobley, W. C. (2012). Cognitive and pharmacological insights from the Ts65Dn mouse model of Down syndrome. *Current Opinion in Neurobiology, 22,* 880–886.

Ryoo, S. R., Cho, H. J., Lee, H. W., Jeong, H. K., Radnaabazar, C., Kim, Y. S., Kim, M. J., et al. (2008). Dual-specificity tyrosine(Y)-phosphorylation regulated kinase 1A-mediated phosphorylation of amyloid precursor protein: evidence for a functional link between Down syndrome and Alzheimer's disease. *Journal of Neurochemistry, 104,* 1333–1344.

Ryoo, S. R., Jeong, H. K., Radnaabazar, C., Yoo, J. J., Cho, H. J., Lee, H. W., Kim, I. S., et al. (2007). DYRK1A-mediated hyperphosphorylation of Tau. A functional link between Down syndrome and Alzheimer disease. *Journal of Biological Chemistry, 282,* 34850–34857.

Sago, H., Carlson, E. J., Smith, D. J., Kilbridge, J., Rubin, E. M., Mobley, W. C., Epstein, C. J., &et al. (1998). Ts1Cje, a partial trisomy 16 mouse model for Down syndrome, exhibits learning and behavioral abnormalities. *Proceedings of the National Academy of Science, USA, 95,* 6256–6261.

Salehi, A., Delcroix, J. D., Belichenko, P. V., Zhan, K., Wu, C., Valletta, J. S., Takimoto-Kimura, R., et al. (2006). Increased App expression in a mouse model of Down's syndrome disrupts NGF transport and causes cholinergic neuron degeneration. *Neuron, 51,* 29–42.

Salehi, A., Faizi, M., Colas, D., Valletta, J., Laguna, J., Takimoto-Kimura, R., Kleschevnikov, A., et al. (2009). Restoration of norepinephrine-modulated contextual memory in a mouse model of Down syndrome. *Science Translational Medicine, 1,* 7ra17.

Santarelli, L., Saxe, M., Gross, C., Surget, A., Battaglia, F., Dulawa, S., Weisstaub, N., et al. (2003). Requirement of hippocampal neurogenesis for the behavioral effects of antidepressants. *Science, 301,* 805–809.

Sayre, L. M., Zelasko, D. A., Harris, P. L., Perry, G., Salomon, R. G., & Smith, M. A. (1997). 4-Hydroxynonenal-derived advanced lipid peroxidation end products are increased in Alzheimer's disease. *Journal of Neurochemistry, 68,* 2092–2097.

Scott-McKean, J. J., & Costa, A. C. (2011). Exaggerated NMDA mediated LTD in a mouse model of Down syndrome and pharmacological rescuing by memantine. *Learning & Memory, 18,* 774–778.

Shichiri, M., Yoshida, Y., Ishida, N., Hagihara, Y., Iwahashi, H., Tamai, H., & Niki, E. (2011). Alpha-Tocopherol suppresses lipid peroxidation and behavioral and cognitive impairments in the Ts65Dn mouse model of Down syndrome. *Free Radical Biology & Medicine, 50,* 1801–1811.

Shim, K. S., & Lubec, G. (2002). Drebrin, a dendritic spine protein, is manifold decreased in brains of patients with Alzheimer's disease and Down syndrome. *Neuroscience Letters, 324,* 209–212.

Stagni, F., Magistretti, J., Guidi, S., Ciani, E., Mangano, C., Calza, L., & Bartesaghi, R. (2013). Pharmacotherapy with fluoxetine restores functional connectivity from the dentate gyrus to field CA3 in the Ts65Dn mouse model of down syndrome. *PLoS One, 8,* e61689.

Takashima, S., Ieshima, A., Nakamura, H., & Becker, L. E. (1989). Dendrites, dementia and the Down syndrome. *Brain Development, 11,* 131–133.

Tariot, P. N., Solomon, P. R., Morris, J. C., Kershaw, P., Lilienfeld, S., & Ding, C. (2000). A 5-month, randomized, placebo-controlled trial of galantamine in AD. The Galantamine USA-10 Study Group. *Neurology, 54,* 2269–2276.

Toso, L., Cameroni, I., Roberson, R., Abebe, D., Bissell, S., & Spong, C. Y. (2008). Prevention of developmental delays in a Down syndrome mouse model. *Obstetrics & Gynecology, 112,* 1242–1251.

Wang, J. W., David, D. J., Monckton, J. E., Battaglia, F., & Hen, R. (2008). Chronic fluoxetine stimulates maturation and synaptic plasticity of adult-born hippocampal granule cells. *Journal of Neuroscience, 28,* 1374–1384.

Weitzdoerfer, R., Dierssen, M., Fountoulakis, M., & Lubec, G. (2001). Fetal life in Down syndrome starts with normal neuronal density but impaired dendritic spines and synaptosomal structure. *Journal of Neural Transmission, Suppl,* 59–70.

Winblad, B., Kilander, L., Eriksson, S., Minthon, L., Batsman, S., Wetterholm, A. L., Jansson-Blixt, C., et al. (2006). Donepezil in patients with severe Alzheimer's disease: double-blind, parallel-group, placebo-controlled study. *Lancet, 367,* 1057–1065.

Wisniewski, K. E. (1990). Down syndrome children often have brain with maturation delay, retardation of growth, and cortical dysgenesis. *American Journal of Medical Genetics, Supplement, 7,* 274–281.

CHAPTER 12

Targeted Treatments for Phenylketonuria

BILLUR MOGHADDAM

INTRODUCTION

Phenylalanine hydroxylase deficiency (PKU) is one of best-known inborn errors of metabolism, resulting in intolerance to the dietary intake of the essential amino acid phenylalanine, and it can cause a spectrum of effects varying from classic PKU to non-PKU hyperphenylalaninemia. This disorder has been called the epitome of biochemical genetics. In 1934, Asjbørn Følling was the first physician who noted that severe intellectual disability was observed in children with elevated phenylalanine levels in their bodily fluids. It was not until the mid-1950s that the hepatic deficiency of the enzyme phenylalanine hydroxylase was recognized as the etiology of this disorder. By the 1960s, mass screening of newborns by Guthrie microbial inhibition assays provided early diagnosis. Shortly thereafter, it was shown that affected individuals could be treated with dietary restriction of phenylalanine, and their prognosis was excellent. It was not until the 1970s that the hyperphenylalaninemia related to cofactor tetrahydrobiopterin, BH4 recycling, or synthesis defects became known. Since then, a lot more information became available on various PAH alleles and their impact on the enzyme production, and dietary breakthroughs have been made in the dietary management of this autosomal recessive genetic disorder.

PKU has an annual incidence of 1:16,000 births in the United States.

CLINICAL FEATURES OF PKU/HYPERPHENYLALANINEMIA

Newborns with PKU show no physical symptoms of the disorder. If untreated, patients develop microcephaly, seizure disorders, decreased skin pigmentation, a musty body odor, severe intellectual disability, and behavioral abnormalities.

These clinical characteristics are hardly ever seen in infants born in countries administering the population newborn screening programs. However, untreated children are known to show impaired brain development, both functionally and structurally. The excretion of phenylalanine and its metabolites, phenylpyruvic and phenylacetic acids, results in the body odor and skin manifestations, most typically, eczema. These metabolites are neurotoxic. The inhibition of tyrosinase is responsible for decreased skin and hair pigmentation.

Affected individuals show decreased myelin formation and also decreased production of neurotransmitters such as dopamine, norepinephrine, and serotonin.

Later in life, positive neurological findings emerge, and these are a broad range of abnormalities varying from increased deep tendon reflexes to tremors, seizures, and paraplegia and hemiplegias. Additional features include severe psychiatric and behavioral manifestations (Pietz et al., 1997; Williams, 1998; Hanley, 2004).

Studies show that even children with strict adherence to diet and neonatal identification of the diagnosis may have suboptimal cognitive outcomes (Burton et al., 2013). The incidence of psychological problems in this population is increased when compared with siblings and the general population (Waisbren et al., 2007).

Adults who abandon the diet have slow information processing, decreased attention span, and slow motor reaction time (Moyle et al., 2007). These adults are also at risk of positive neurological findings such as tremors and brisk deep tendon reflexes. The incidence of depression, panic attacks, anxiety, and phobias is increased in individuals who quit the diet in the second decade of life (Koch et al., 2002).

Chronic effects of dietary noncompliance include EEG abnormalities and structural changes in the brain MRI. Sudden psychiatric deterioration has been reported (Weglage et al., 2000). Finally, osteopenia and vitamin B12 deficiency can be cited among other complications of this disorder (Modan-Moses et al., 2007).

BIOLOGY OF PHENYLKETONURIA

Phenylalanine hydroxylase (PAH) is predominantly expressed in the liver (but also in the kidneys and the pancreas) and catalyzes the irreversible hydroxylation of phenylalanine, an essential amino acid, to tyrosine.

PAH is a homotetramer that requires iron and molecular oxygen as well as the unconjugated pterin cofactor, BH4, for catalytic activity. BH4 is synthesized *de novo* from guanosine triphosphate in several tissues, including liver, but it is also recycled after phenylalanine hydroxylation through enzymatically catalyzed reduction. Inherited deficiency of BH4 synthesis or recycling enzymes is the cause of hyperphenylalaninemia in approximately 2% of infants detected through newborn screening. Treatment of these children frequently requires chronic oral or parenteral BH4 administration in addition to dietary phenylalanine restriction.

DIAGNOSIS AND TESTING

The diagnosis of phenylalanine hydroxylase deficiency is based on an elevated phenylalanine (Phe) concentration, which is identifiable by quantitative plasma amino acid analysis. Individuals with PHA deficiency show consistently elevated Phe concentrations higher than 120 mmol/L (2 mg/dl), when untreated (Schriver & Kauffman, 2001). Patients with these

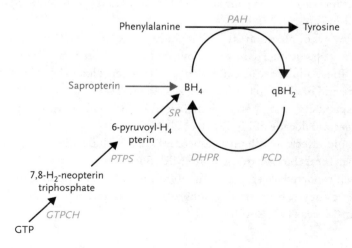

Figure 12.1:
The schematic role of Saptopterin in the activation of Phenylalanine Hydroxylase

elevated levels should get urine pterin studies by liquid chromatography and dihidropterin reductase measurement.

PAH deficiency is routinely identified in the newborn screening programs using dried blood spots by Guthrie bacterial inhibition assay, flourimetric analysis, or tandem mass spectrometry (MS/MS). The MS/MS method is the one that is most commonly used in the United States' newborn screening programs. Enzyme studies are typically not used because PAH is a hepatic enzyme.

The initial newborn screening test yields a significant number of false positive results. This is because of liver immaturity, thick blood sample, and possible heterozygosity in premature infants (Hennerman et al., 2004). These infants are tested a second time, and those who are positive go through the urine pterin test to distinguish the 2% who have BH4 synthesis or recycling defects. Red blood cell dihydropterin reductase measurement is typically added to this study (Blau et al., 2011). The low phenylalanine diet should be initiated prior to the completion of the studies.

Molecular Genetic Testing

Genotyping, though not necessary for diagnosis, can help better anticipate dietary needs of the infant and severity of the disorder. Genotyping may also aid in determining BH4 responsiveness, which is a treatment modality that will be addressed in the next section.

PAH deficiency is an autosomal recessive disorder, and genotyping may also help with the genetic counseling questions and prenatal diagnosis of families that are interested in this aspect of evaluation.

CLASSIFICATION OF PHENLYALANINE HYDROXYLASE DEFICIENCY (GULDBERG ET AL., 1998)

- Classic PKU is caused by a complete or near-complete deficiency of PAH activity. Affected individuals tolerate less than 250–350 mg of dietary phenylalanine per day to keep plasma concentration of Phe at a safe level of no more than 300 μmol/L (5 mg/dL). Without dietary treatment, most individuals develop profound, irreversible intellectual disability.
- Moderate PKU: Affected individuals tolerate 350–400 mg of dietary phenylalanine per day.
- Mild PKU: Affected individuals tolerate 400–600 mg of dietary phenylalanine per day.

- Mild hyperphenylalaninemia (MHP): Affected infants have plasma Phe concentrations lower than 600 µmol/L (10 mg/dL) on a normal diet.

TRADITIONAL MANAGEMENT OF PHENYLALANINE HYDROXYLASE DEFICIENCY

Dietary restriction of phenylalanine has been the mainstay of therapy for phenylketonuria. To establish the extent of the disease, the initial studies, including blood phenylalanine concentration and phenylalanine tolerance, as well as the BH4 loading tests, are performed. The phenylalanine tolerance of the affected individual is determined by dietary adjustments and frequent phenylalanine evaluations based on the individuals' needs.

The generally accepted goal of the treatment is to keep the plasma phenylalanine and tyrosine levels normal. The Phe levels of 120–360 mmol/l (2–6 mg/dl) are considered safe, and the diet that is restricted in Phe should be started soon after birth. It is generally accepted that the diet should be administered lifelong. It should be continued at least into adolescence.

A meta-analysis by Weisbren et al. in 2007 showed a reduction of IQ of 1.9 to 3.8 points for every 100 µmol/L increase in lifetime blood phenylalanine level. In addition, despite normal IQ, children and adolescents treated early have a higher frequency of ADHD, decreased autonomy, and school problems compared to either healthy controls or chronically ill peers (Simon et al., 2008; Antshel, 2010; Brumm et al., 2010).

The patients are followed closely by metabolic dietitians who monitor the phenylalanine intake and plasma amino acid profiles of patients to customize the diet to each patient's needs. The goal is for the patient to maintain normal growth and intake of essential nutrients in this process. This requires the use of a Phe-free formula. These formulas and multiple other products are available. Breastfeeding is encouraged in infants along with the formula, with careful monitoring of the analytes. Intake of tyrosine and the other amino acids is monitored via regular measurements of quantitative plasma amino acid profiles as well as measurement of other nutritional parameters such as prealbumin, calcium, vitamin D, ferritin, etc.

TARGETED TREATMENTS IN PHENYLALANINE HYDROXYLASE DEFICIENCY

Despite the increase in the number and variety of phenylalanine-free products, the PAH diet is difficult, especially during the teenage years, and physicians dealing with the care of children with PKU know very well that most patients have problems with compliance. This led to the development of multiple treatment modalities.

Large Neutral Amino Acid (LNAA) Transporters

Although PAH deficiency occurs at the hepatic level, the clinical effects of hyperphenylalaninemia are on brain development and function. The blood–brain barrier is formed by the brain capillary endothelial cells with tight junctions between them. The barrier prevents the exchange of intrinsic proteins and lipids between the luminal and abluminal domains. At the blood–brain barrier, phenylalanine shares a transporter with other large neutral amino acids (leucine, tyrosine, tryptophan, threonine, isoleucine, valine, methionine, and histidine). Phe has the highest affinity for the transport system; therefore, high Phe levels impair uptake of the other large neutral amino acids into the brain.

As early as 1953, Christensen proposed that high concentrations of Phe could interfere with the transport of the other LNAA into the brain (Christensen, 1952). About 30 years later, branched-chain amino acid supplementation was shown to result in a 21% reduction of cerebrospinal/serum ratio of Phe with no reported amino acid imbalances (Berry et al., 1982). Subsequent proton resonance spectroscopy studies provided a way to quantify the influx of Phe into the cerebrum in adult patients with PKU (Kreis et al., 1995).

Some individuals exclude excess phenylalanine efficiently because of the variation in the transport of LNAA across the blood–brain barrier (Weglage et al., 2002). The LNAA administration has decreased the transport of phenylalanine by competing for the transporter. This may benefit the patients' brains by decreasing the toxicity that may occur due to high levels of phenylalanine exposure in noncompliant adults. Clinical benefit was seen with significant improvement in ability to focus and decreased self-injurious behaviors in clinical trials (Kalkanoglu, 2005).

A similar transporter exists in the intestines, and another compound of LNAA decreased the blood Phe concentration by 40–50% in a small number of individuals with PKU (Matalon et al., 2006). These supplements would not replace the phenylalanine restricted diet especially in younger patients; however, they may help partially liberalize the diet of already treated patients.

Sapropterin Treatment

Individuals with PAH deficiency have normal biopterin content in the blood and the urine; however, oral administration of additional BH4 to some patients with hyperphenylalaninemia showed some reduction in the blood phenylalanine content without altering the dietary phenylalanine intake (Kure et al., 1999). This was replicated by several other investigators (Lindner et al., 2001; Bernegger et al., 2002; Shintaku et al., 2004; Matalon et al., 2005; Blau et al., 2004).

The basis of BH4 responsiveness may be related to different molecular mechanisms. The increase in the liver BH4 content may stimulate the activity of mutant, partially active PAH enzyme, or it may act as a chemical chaperone to stabilize the mutant PAH monomers (Dobrowolski et al., 2009). Some specific PAH mutations are known to affect the affinity of the PAH enzyme for its biopterin cofactor, and, in these patients, oral biopterin administration may overcome the block and at least partially restore the enzyme activity. Studies have shown that BH4 responsiveness in an individual with PKU cannot always be accurately predicted from their PAH genotype (Karacic et al., 2009; Trefz et al., 2009).

Several protocols have been investigated in the determination process for BH4 responsiveness. These protocols have included varying doses, durations, and percentage decreases in the average blood phenylalanine levels, all in an effort to develop a standardized trial protocol. A rational algorithm for testing BH4 responsiveness in a routine clinical trial setting has been proposed and endorsed by clinicians in Europe and the United States. The protocol involves evaluation of both short-term response and the long-term efficacy of the BH4 treatment. In this protocol, the blood phenylalanine level is measured prior to the sapropterin administration, and on days 1, 7, 14, and 28 following daily sapropterin administration at 20 mg/kg.

One school of thought characterizes 20–30% reduction in the phenylalanine level as "responsiveness." Another approach is to not define responsiveness by a percentage level reduction but instead by whether the decrease in the phenylalanine is thought by the clinician and the patient to be clinically meaningful.

The cost of the sapropterin treatment versus the PKU diet should also be taken into consideration. The cost of the sapropterin treatment is about 6–7 times that of dietary treatment, including the medical foods.

In summary, the systematic evaluation of BH4 responsiveness in the PKU population and the availability of a validated, commercial form of the medication have provided a new therapeutic option for patients with phenylketonuria. The relatively mild adverse-effect profile has been another positive aspect for patients who are interested in the trials. Continuance of a strict diet is still recommended lifelong, though practically difficult and often associated with poor compliance in adolescent and adult patients with this disorder. The introduction of sapropterin treatment has been a means for improving the quality of life in a select patient population (Harding, 2010). Sapropterin hydrochloride has been approved for use by the U.S. Food and Drug Administration.

Phenylalanine Ammonia Lyase Treatment

The classic PKU diet requires a major alteration in lifestyle, and compliance has historically been challenging. Moreover, dietary therapy can be associated with deficiencies in several nutrients. Most dietary products are not palatable. A combination of enzyme therapy with phenylalanine ammonia lyase and controlled low-protein diet may be a possibility in the future. Cristineh et al. (1953) have published their initial studies using mouse orthologues of human PKU and non-PKU hyperphenylaninemia.

The PAL enzyme derived from the yeast *Rhodospiridium tiruloides* can degrade phenylalanine by converting it to a harmless metabolite derivative that is cleared from the body by the kidneys. Oral administration has shown benefit; however, it is subject to proteolysis. Intravenous administration of PAL triggers immune recognition and reactions. Current work and clinical trials involve PEGylation (conjugation with polyethylene glycol) in order to reduce this effect (Wang et al., 2009). There is evidence suggesting that PEGylation may be successful in decreasing the immune response of the patients to the enzymes.

Investigations and Clinical Trials Are Under Way

In recent years, new approaches for the treatment of PKU have been proposed. Gene therapy, suggesting the replacement of the mutant gene by the wild-type sequence encoding the normal PAH gene, has successfully been tested on mice and can eventually be used as the ultimate therapy. Unfortunately, this mode of therapy is still not applicable to humans, due to technical problems that have yet to be resolved.

Enzyme replacement therapy involves the administration of the wild-type PAH enzyme; however, for the enzyme to be delivered to the bloodstream and to have the desired effect, it must be delivered to the site of action, the liver. Use of an adequate targeting moiety for this function will probably have the potential for great benefits (Eavri & Lorberboum-Galski, 2010).

The past decade has been highly productive in the development of new dietary products, potential medications, and prospective enzyme treatments, and phenylketonuria will potentially be a pioneer disorder for the development of novel treatment modalities for other inborn errors of metabolism with similar mechanisms.

DISCLOSURES

The author has no conflicts of interest to disclose.

REFERENCES

Antshel, K. M. (2010). ADHD, learning, and academic performance in phenylketonuria. *Molecular Genetics & Metabolism, 99*(Suppl 1), S52–S58.

Bernegger, C., & Blau, N. (2002). High frequency of tetrahydrobiopterin-responsiveness among hyperphenylalaninemias: A study of 1,919 patients observed from 1988 to 2002. *Molecular Genetics & Metabolism, 77*, 304–313.

Berry, H. K., Bofinger, M. K., Hunt, M. M., Philipps, P. J., & Guilfoile, M. B. (1982). Reduction of cerebrospinal fluid phenylalanine after oral administration of valine, isoleucine and leucine. *Pediatric Research, 16*, 751–755.

Blau, N. (2006). Nomenclature and laboratory diagnosis of tetrahydrobiopterin deficiencies. *Advances in Phenylketonuria and Tetrahydrobiopterin*. Accessed Jan. 23, 1013.

Blau, N., Bélanger-Quintana, A., Demirkol, M., Feillet, F., Giovannini, M., MacDonald, A., et al. (2009). Optimizing the use of sapropterin (BH(4)) in the management of phenylketonuria. *Molecular Genetics & Metabolism, 96*, 158–163.

Blau, N., & Erlandsen, H. (2004). The metabolic and molecular bases of tetrahydrobiopterin-responsive phenylalanine hydroxylase deficiency. *Molecular Genetics & Metabolism, 82*, 101–111.

Blau, N., Hennermann, J. B., Langenbeck, U., & Lichter-Konecki, U. (2011). Diagnosis, classification, and genetics of phenylketonuria and tetrahydrobiopterin (BH4) deficiencies. *Molecular Genetics & Metabolism, 104*(Suppl), S2–S9.

Brumm, V. L., Bilder, D., & Waisbren, S. E. (2010). Psychiatric symptoms and disorders in phenylketonuria. *Molecular Genetics & Metabolism, 99*(Suppl 1), S59–S63.

Burton, B. K., Adams, D. J., Grange, D. K., Malone, J. I., Jurecki, E., Bausell, H., et al. (2011). Tetrahydrobiopterin therapy for phenylketonuria in infants and young children. *Journal of Pediatrics, 158*, 410–415.

Burton, B. K., Leviton, L., Vespa, H., Coon, H., Longo, N., Lundy, B. D., et al. (2013). A diversified approach for PKU treatment: Routine screening yields high incidence of psychiatric distress in phenylketonuria clinics. *Molecular Genetics & Metabolism, 108*, 8–12.

Christensen, H. N. (1953). Metabolism of amino acids and proteins. *Annual Review of Biochemistry, 22*, 233–260.

Eavri, R., & Lorberboum-Galski, H. (2010). Annales Nestle. 68/2:70–77.

Fiege, B., Bonafé, L., Ballhausen, D., Baumgartner, M., Thöny, B., Meili, D., et al. (2005). Extended tetrahydrobiopterin loading test in the diagnosis of cofactor-responsive phenylketonuria: A pilot study. *Molecular Genetics & Metabolism, 86*(Suppl 1), S91–S95.

Guldberg, P., Rey, F., Zschocke, J., Romano, V., François, B., Michiels, L., et al. (1998). A European multicenter study of phenylalanine hydroxylase deficiency: Classification of 105 mutations and a general system for genotype-based prediction of metabolic phenotype. *American Journal of Human Genetics*, *63*, 71–79.

Güttler, F., & Guldberg, P. (2006). Genotype/phenotype correlations in phenylalanine hydroxylase deficiency. In: Blau, N. (ed.), *PKU and BH4—Advances in Phenylketonuria and Tetrahydrobiopterin* (pp. 211–320). Heilbronn, Germany: SPS Verlagsgesellschaft.

Hanley, W. B. (2004). Adult phenylketonuria. *American Journal of Medicine*, *117*, 590–595.

Harding, C. (2010). New era in treatment for phenylketonuria: Pharmacologic therapy with sapropterin. *Biologics*, *4*, 231–236.

Hennermann, J. B., Loui, A., Weber, A., & Mönch, E. (2004). Hyperphenylalaninemia in a premature infant with heterozygosity for phenylketonuria. *Journal of Perinatal Medicine*, *32*, 383–385.

Kalkanoğlu, H. S., Ahring, K. K., Sertkaya, D., Møller, L. B., Romstad, A., Mikkelsen, I., et al. (2005). Behavioural effects of phenylalanine-free amino acid tablet supplementation in intellectually disabled adults with untreated phenylketonuria. *Acta Paediatrica*, *94*, 1218–1222.

Karacic, I., Meili, D., Sarnavka, V., et al. (2009). Genotype-predicted tetrahydrobiopterin (BH4)-responsiveness and molecular genetics in Croatian patients with phenylalanine hydroxylase (PAH) deficiency. *Molecular Genetics & Metabolism*, *97*(3), 165–171.

Koch, R., Burton, B., Hoganson, G., Peterson, R., Rhead, W., Rouse, B., et al. (2002). Phenylketonuria in adulthood: a collaborative study. *Journal of Inherited Metabolic Disease*, *25*, 333–346.

Kreis, R., Pietz, J., Penzien, J., Herschkowitz, N., & Boesch, C. (1995). Identification and quantitation of phenylalanine in the brain of patients with phenylketonuria by means of localized in vivo 1H magnetic-resonance spectroscopy. *Journal of Magnetic Resonance*, *B107*, 242–251.

Kure, S., Hou, D. C., Ohura, T., Iwamoto, H., Suzuki, S., Sugiyama, N., et al. (1999). Tetrahydrobiopterin-responsive phenylalanine hydroxylase deficiency. *Journal of Pediatrics*, *135*, 375–378.

Levy, H. L. (1999). Phenylketonuria: Old disease, new approach to treatment. *Proceedings of the National Academy of Sciences, USA.*, *96*, 1811–1813.

Lindner, M., Steinfeld, R., Burgard, P., Schulze, A., Mayatepek, E., & Zschocke, J. (2003). Tetrahydrobiopterin sensitivity in German patients with mild phenylalanine hydroxylase deficiency. *Human Mutation: Mutation in Brief*, *588*, 1–4.

Matalon, R., Koch, R., Michals-Matalon, K., Moseley, K., Surendran, S., Tyring, S., et al. (2004). Biopterin responsive phenylalanine hydroxylase deficiency. *Genetics in Medicine*, *6*, 27–32.

Matalon, R., Michals-Matalon, K., Bhatia, G., Grechanina, E., Novikov, P., McDonald, J. D., et al. (2006). Large neutral amino acids in the treatment of phenylketonuria (PKU). *Journal of Inherited Metabolic Disease*, *29*, 732–738.

Modan-Moses, D., Vered, I., Schwartz, G., Anikster, Y., Abraham, S., Segev, R., et al. (2007). Peak bone mass in patients with phenylketonuria. *Journal of Inherited Metabolic Disease*, *30*, 202–208.

Moyle, J. J., Fox, A. M., Arthur, M., Bynevelt, M., & Burnett, J. R. (2007). Meta-analysis of neuropsychological symptoms of adolescents and adults with PKU. *Neuropsychology Review*, *17*, 91–101.

National Institutes of Health Consensus Development Panel (2001). National Institutes of Health Consensus Development Conference Statement: Phenylketonuria: screening and management. October 16–18, 2000. *Pediatrics, 108*, 972–982.

Pietz, J., Fätkenheuer, B., Burgard, P., Armbruster, M., Esser, G., & Schmidt, H. (1997). Psychiatric disorders in adult patients with early-treated phenylketonuria. *Pediatrics, 99*(3), 345–350.

Rocha, J. C., & Martel, F. (2009). Large neutral amino acid supplementation in phenyl-ketonuric patients. *Journal of Inherited Metabolic Disease, 32*, 472–480.

Sarkissian, C. N., & Gámez, A. (2005). Phenylalanine ammonia lyase, enzyme substitution therapy for phenylketonuria, where are we now? *Molecular Genetics & Metabolism, 86*(Suppl 1), S22–S26.

Sarkissian, C. N., Shao, Z., Blain, F., Peevers, R., Su, H., Heft, R., et al. (1999). A different approach to treatment of phenylketonuria: Phenylalanine degradation with recombinant phenylalanine ammonia lyase. *Proceedings of the National Academy of Sciences, USA, 96*, 2339–2344.

Shintaku, H., Kure, S., Ohura, T., Okano, Y., Ohwada, M., Sugiyama, N., et al. (2004). Long-term treatment and diagnosis of tetrahydrobiopterin-responsive hyper-phenylalaninemia with a mutant phenylalanine hydroxylase gene. *Pediatric Research, 55*, 425–430.

Scriver, C. R., & Kaufman, S. (2001). Hyperphenylalaninemia: Phenylalanine hydroxy-lase deficiency. In: Scriver, C. R., Beaudet al., Sly, S. W., Valle, D. (eds.); Childs, B., Kinzler, K. W., Vogelstein, B. (assoc. eds.), *The Metabolic and Molecular Bases of Inherited Disease*, 8th ed. (pp. 1667–1724). New York: McGraw-Hill:.

Simon, E., Schwarz, M., Roos, J., Dragano, N., Geraedts, M., Siegrist, J., et al. (2008). Evaluation of quality of life and description of the sociodemographic state in adolescent and young adult patients with phenylketonuria (PKU). *Health & Quality of Life Outcomes, 6*, 25.

Trefz, F. K., & Blau, N. (2003). Potential role of tetrahydrobiopterin in the treatment of maternal phenylketonuria. *Pediatrics, 112*, 1566–1569.

Trefz, F. K., Scheible, D., Götz, H., & Frauendienst-Egger, G. (2009). Significance of genotype in tetrahydrobiopterin-responsive phenylketonuria. *Journal of Inherited Metabolic Disease, 32*, 22–26.

Waisbren, S. E., Noel, K., Fahrbach, K., Cella, C., Frame, D., Dorenbaum, A., et al. (2007). Phenylalanine blood levels and clinical outcomes in phenylketonuria: A systematic literature review and meta-analysis. *Molecular Genetics & Metabolism, 92*, 63–70.

Weglage et al., (2000).

Weglage, J., Oberwittler, C., Marquardt, T., Schellscheidt, J., von Teeffelen-Heithoff, A., Koch, G., et al. (2000). Neurological deterioration in adult phenylketonuria. *Journal of Inherited Metabolic Disease, 23*, 83–84

Weglage, J., Wiedermann, D., Denecke, J., Feldmann, R., Koch, H. G., Ullrich, K., et al. (2002). Individual blood-brain barrier phenylalanine transport in siblings with classical phenylketonuria. *Journal of Inherited Metabolic Disease, 25*, 431–436.

Williams, K. (1998). Benefits of normalizing plasma phenylalanine: impact on behaviour and health. A case report. *Journal of Inherited Metabolic Disease*, Dec; *21*(8), 785–790.

CHAPTER 13

Muscular Dystrophies

Diagnosis and New Treatments

BETHANY M. LIPA, QUE T. NGUYEN, AND JAY J. HAN

INTRODUCTION

Muscular dystrophy is a heterogeneous group of acquired or inherited genetic disorders with progressive muscle weakness, often leading to functional impairments such as problems ambulating or difficulties with performing the activities of daily living. Cardiopulmonary dysfunctions are often found in this population. The list of muscular dystrophies is extensive, and the clinical findings, diagnostic workup, and treatment options for all types cannot be fully covered in a single chapter. As such, this chapter will only present the most common muscular dystrophies, which include dystrophinopathies, myotonic dystrophies, facioscapulohumeral dystrophy, and the most common types of limb-girdle muscular dystrophies, as well as new targeted treatments for each.

DYSTROPHINOPATHIES

Dystrophin is a large cytoskeletal protein commonly found in the inner surface of the sarcolemma of skeletal muscles (Figure 13.1). A missense, nonsense, or point mutation in the dystrophin gene results in either an absent or reduced amount of dystrophin protein produced, leading to membrane instability. When the amount of dystrophin produced is markedly reduced (<3% of normal levels) or absent, the condition is categorized as *Duchenne muscular dystrophy* (DMD) (Hoffman, 1988). When it is reduced by 10–60% or is lower in molecular weight than normal, a *Becker muscular dystrophy*

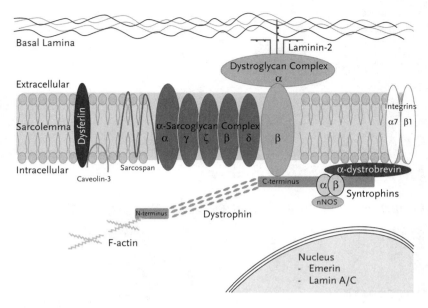

Figure 13.1:
This simplified figure of the dystrophin-associated glycoprotein complex (DGC) demonstrates the role of dystrophin as a membrane-stabilizing protein.

(BMD) phenotype is seen. An intermediate phenotype would show variable dystrophin expression with a quantity somewhere in between.

The incidence of DMD has been estimated at 1 in 5,000 male births with a prevalence of approximately 1 in 18,000 males (CDC, MMWR, 2009). Symptoms of DMD are often first noticed before the age of four. When learning to walk, the affected child is noted to exhibit an abnormal gait, experiences frequent falls, and has difficulties climbing stairs and keeping up with his peers when running or walking. In these children, the hip and knee extensors are often weak, leading to the compensatory toe-walking pattern observed. With progression of the disease process, the chronic muscle damage leads to muscle fibrosis, impairing muscle function. Clinical findings include progressive generalized muscle weakness that is predominantly proximal early on, calf pseudohypertrophy, posterior axillary depression sign due to atrophy of the posterior axillary fold with relative preservation of bordering infraspinatus and deltoid muscles (Figure 13.2) (Pradhan, 1994), positive Gower's sign (Figure 13.3), tight heel cords and hamstrings, and decreased or absent muscle stretch reflexes. Sensation is not commonly affected. On average, untreated DMD children transition to a wheelchair between 8 and 13 years of age, depending on the severity of genetic defect, with death occurring between 15 and 25 years of age.

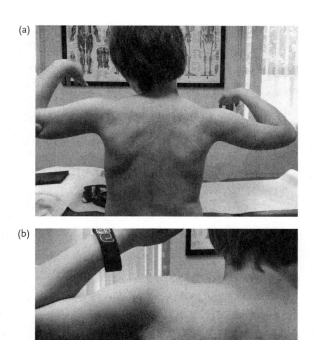

Figure 13.2:
(a) Posterior axillary depression sign in an eight-year-old boy with Duchenne muscular dystrophy. (b) The posterior axillary depression sign is most remarkable in patients with Duchenne muscular dystrophy between the ages of 8 and 11. Note the oval depression due to atrophy of the posterior axillary fold with relative preservation of bordering muscles, including infraspinatus and deltoid.

The Becker muscular dystrophy (BMD) phenotype is similar to DMD's, however, symptoms are not as severe and disease progression is typically slower. The incidence of BMD is about one-fifth that of Duchenne muscular dystrophy, and the prevalence is approximately 14×10^{-6} (Emery, 1991). In the severe BMD phenotype, symptoms may initially present between four to twelve years of age. In milder cases, symptoms may not be apparent until adulthood. Gait abnormalities, frequent falls, calf pseudohypertrophy, and difficulties getting up from the floor or navigating stairs are commonly noted in affected children. In adult-onset, common presentation includes proximal muscle weakness, muscle cramps or pain with exercise, or cardiopulmonary complaints. Affected individuals can often ambulate

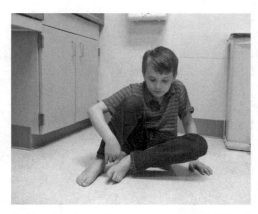

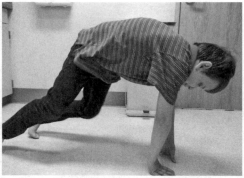

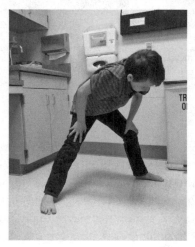

Figure 13.3:
The Gower's sign describes a patient that has to use his hands and arms to "walk" up his own body from a squatting position due proximal lower-limb weakness. It is classically seen in DMD, but is also seen in various other conditions associated with proximal muscle weakness.

into their twenties and beyond, depending on the severity. The most common cause of death in BMD is heart failure due to dilated cardiomyopathy.

The dystrophin protein is present in cardiac muscles of healthy individuals. In those with DMD or BMD, the lack of dystrophin increases the risk of cardiac arrhythmias, dilated cardiomyopathies, and congestive heart failure. The absence of dystrophin in brain tissues also leads to cognitive delay and intellectual disability in most individuals with DMD. As progressive weakness of skeletal and respiratory muscles ensues, joint contractures, scoliosis, and restrictive lung disease may develop.

Diagnostic Testing

The presence of a dystrophinopathy should be suspected when serum creatine kinase level is significantly elevated. Individuals with Duchenne muscular dystrophy could have levels 10–100 times that of normal, while those with Becker muscular dystrophy could have levels as high as 20 times that of normal. Molecular genetic testing of the DMD gene can aid in determining the type and site of the mutation. A negative test, however, does not necessarily rule out this disease process, as a small percentage of affected individuals may have an unidentifiable mutation. A muscle biopsy with dystrophin staining may also be considered. Individuals with DMD often have absent or severely reduced levels of dystrophin, and those with BMD have levels between 10% and 60% of normal, or dystrophin proteins with lower molecular weight. The diagnosis of DMD and BMD should take into account the individual's clinical history, physical exam findings, family history, serum creatine kinase level, molecular genetic testing, and/or muscle biopsy result with dystrophin staining (Table 13.1).

Treatment

The administration of corticosteroids is currently the standard of care in the treatment of DMD (Bushby, 2009). It has been found to prolong ambulation by 2–5 years, delay the need for noninvasive ventilation, aid in cardiovascular protection, reduce the incidence of scoliosis, and maintain upper-body strength (Mendell, 1989; Moxley, 2010; King, 2007). The most common side effects include weight gain, behavioral issues, increased risk of cataracts, adrenal suppression, increased fracture risk of the spine and long bones, and hypertension. Efficacy has been found to be dose-dependent, with the minimum effective dose being 0.30mg/kg/day. Aggressive treatment is recommended, however, with a starting oral prednisone dose of

Table 13.1 SUMMARY OF SELECTED FINDINGS IN DUCHENNE AND
BECKER MUSCULAR DYSTROPHY

	Duchenne Muscular Dystrophy	Becker Muscular Dystrophy
Onset	2–6 years of age	As early as 4 years of age and may present in adulthood
Clinical presentation	Abnormal gait/toe-walking Frequent falling Difficulties climbing stairs Calf pseudohypertrophy Hyperlordotic gait Joint contractures	Variable, but may include: Abnormal gait/toe-walking Frequent falling Proximal muscle weakness Calf pseudohypertrophy Muscle cramps/pain after exercise
Creatine kinase (CK)	10–100 times normal	5–20 times normal
Muscle biopsy pathology	Variable fiber size Myopathic grouping Endomysial fibrosis and fatty infiltration Dystrophin staining: absent/severely reduced	Variable fiber size Myopathic grouping Endomysial fibrosis and fatty infiltration Dystrophin staining: reduced (10–60% of normal)
Genetic testing	Sequencing of the dystrophin gene: deletion, duplication, or point mutation Out-of-frame mutation: severe phenotype	Sequencing of the dystrophin gene: deletion, duplication, or point mutation In-frame mutation: mild phenotype

0.75mg/kg/day, up to the maximum dose of 30–40mg/day. This can be adjusted as needed based upon side effects. Weekend dosing at 10mg/kg/week divided over two days has been shown to be equally effective (Escolar, 2011); therefore, it is a good alternative option for those with significant side effects on daily dosing. In addition, prednisolone sodium phosphate disintegrating tablets are available for those who cannot swallow pills. Deflazacort, a sodium-sparing corticosteroid, is also available and has been found to be as efficacious as prednisone (Biggar, 2006); however, this corticosteroid is not FDA-approved in the United States at this time. The starting dose is recommended to be 0.9mg/kg/day, up to a maximum of 36–39mg/day. With deflazacort, the incidence of weight gain is lower than with prednisone; however, the risk of cataracts is higher.

Additional treatments options include the use of ACE inhibitors, angiotensin II-receptor blockers or beta-blockers for cardiovascular protection, and the use of noninvasive positive-pressure ventilation for respiratory support in those with restrictive lung disease. Idebenone has been recommended for its strong antioxidant properties, and vitamin D supplementation has been prescribed to replenish low vitamin D level, a condition that may affect muscle and bone health.

At the present time, there is no known cure for dystrophinopathies. In general, the current research goal is to prevent disease progression, increase strength, prolong ambulation time, and improve quality of life. At the time of this writing, clinical trials are being conducted to explore the efficacy of exon skipping in certain mutations using antisense oligonucleotides (AONs) (Cirak, 2011; Aartsma-Rus, 2007). With this approach, AONs target specific exons at the pre-mRNA level, allowing certain axons to be omitted in order to restore an open reading frame from an out-of-frame mutation. Smaller and partially functional dystrophin proteins would be produced, altering a severe DMD into a milder phenotype such as that of Becker muscular dystrophy. Phase II clinical trial data obtained thus far have shown a modest increase of sarcolemmal dystrophin using this approach (Cirak, 2011) (Figures 13.4 and 13.5).

Another molecular approach focuses on stop codon read-through in approximately 10–15% of DMD patients with premature stop codons (Figure 13.6). In the mdx mouse model, PTC 124 or Ataluren has been found to modestly increase dystrophin production by binding to the 60S ribosomal subunit and allowing premature stop codon read-through. Preliminary data of the Phase IIb trial provides evidence of a strong safety profile; however, the primary outcome measurement did not reach statistical significance. Additional analysis is being conducted to demonstrate its clinical efficacy in DMD.

Additional therapies being researched include the use of myostatin inhibitors, which have been found in the animal model to increase strength and size of muscle fibers, and trials of epicatechin, a compound in dark chocolate that may improve skeletal musculature and decrease muscle fatigue. Utrophin upregulators, which share 80% of the dystrophin sequence, have been found to be well tolerated in healthy individuals. However, due to their pharmacokinetics during the phase I clinical trial, further development has been halted in order to improve on current formulations (Pichavant, 2011).

Neuromuscular conditions often present with similar symptoms. In assessing dystrophinopathies, it is important to consider *limb-girdle muscular dystrophy*, *Emery-Dreifuss muscular dystrophy*, and spinal muscular atrophy in the list of differential diagnoses. *Facioscapulohumeral dystrophy*, congenital myopathies, and Lambert-Eaton myasthenic syndrome may be considered as well. Adults with proximal muscle weakness should also be

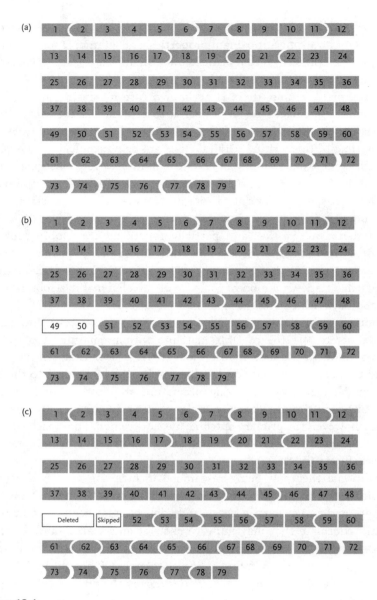

Figure 13.4:
(a) The dystrophin gene has 79 exons. (b) Deletion of exons 49–50 creates an out-of-frame mutation. (c) Exon 51 skipping restores the reading frame.

evaluated for Pompe disease and immune or inflammatory myopathies, as these are conditions with available treatments.

Tremendous advances have taken place in elucidating the molecular basis and disease mechanism of dystrophinopathies over the past two decades. Largely based on this growing body of knowledge, several clinical safety

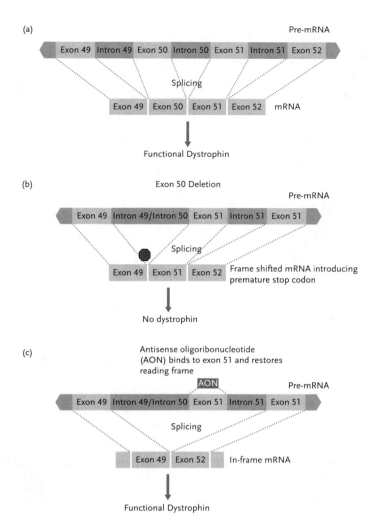

Figure 13.5:
(a) Splicing of mRNA in normal dystrophin gene. (b) Splicing of mRNA in Exon 50 deletion results in a frame shift and premature stop codon. (c) Exon 51 skipping restores reading frame.

and efficacy trials evaluating novel therapeutic agents have recently taken place, and more are planned for the future. With clinical trials targeting specific genetic mutations in DMD, it is becoming more important to determine the genetic characterization of dystrophin gene mutations in patients who are considering participation in clinical trials. Information-sharing and updating the patients and families regarding upcoming clinical studies are important parts of the neuromuscular clinic visits. Information about the U.S. clinical trials website (http://clinicaltrials.gov/) should also

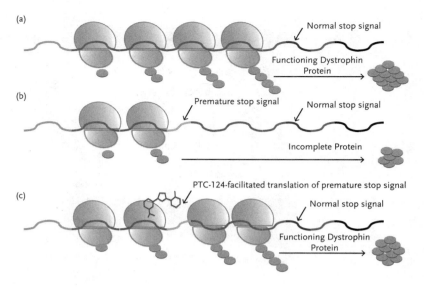

Figure 13.6:
(a) Normal translation; (b) Incomplete translation; (c) PTC-124-facilitated translation.

be shared with patients for them to learn about potential studies that are recruiting subjects.

MYOTONIC MUSCULAR DYSTROPHY, TYPES 1 AND 2

Myotonic dystrophy is the most common form of muscular dystrophy in adults, affecting 5–20 people per 100,000 worldwide (Harper, 2001). It is an autosomal dominant, slowly progressive multisystemic disease that affects both males and females in equal distribution. In the following sections, the pathophysiology, physical exam findings, diagnostic workup, and available treatment options for myotonic dystrophy types 1 and 2 will be discussed.

Myotonic dystrophy type 1 (DM1), also known as *Steinert disease*, is caused by an expanded CTG repeat in the dystrophia myotonica protein kinase gene (*DMPK*) on gene map locus 19q13.32 (Harley, 1991). Normal number of repeats is between 5 and 35. Those with 50 or more CTG repeats are often symptomatic, while those with repeats between 36 and 49 are often asymptomatic, but are at risk of having symptomatic children due to a phenomenon known as *anticipation* (Martorell, 2001). With anticipation, the age of onset decreases with each successive generation, and the disease severity increases. As such, affected individuals tend to have more severe symptoms, with signs showing up earlier in life than their affected parent's.

Symptoms of myotonic dystrophy type 1 include grip myotonia, distal extremity weakness, muscle pain, stiffness, fatigue, and hypersomnia. Weakness of the neck and facial muscles, such as eyelids, mouth, and jaw muscles, are also common. Individuals with symptoms during childhood may exhibit motor delays, as well as mild to severe intellectual impairments. On physical examination, affected individuals often have a long, thin face with temporal and masseter wasting as well as tented mouth. Frontal balding and gonadal atrophy may be observed in males. Special maneuvers can elicit percussion and grip myotonia, both of which are common findings in myotonic dystrophy due to sustained muscle contraction (Figure 13.7). Weakness and atrophy in DM1 predominantly affects distal muscles, such as those in the hands and distal lower limbs, affecting gait and the ability to perform activities of daily living. Posterior capsular cataracts with green

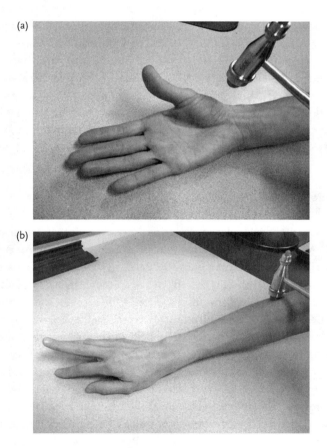

Figure 13.7:
Percussion myotonia of the abductor pollicis brevis (a) and extensor digitorum communis muscles (b).

and red iridescent opacities on slit lamp test, insulin insensitivity, dysphagia, and cardiac conduction defects are common findings in this patient population. Myotonic dystrophy type 1 should be suspected in infants with hypotonia, generalized weakness, respiratory insufficiency, facial weakness, and deformities such as clubfoot.

Myotonic dystrophy type 2 (DM2), also known as *proximal myotonic myopathy* (PROMM) is caused by a heterozygous expansion of CCTG repeat in zinc finger protein 9 (*ZNF9*) in intron 1 of chromosome 3 (Liquori, 2001). Pathogenic alleles could have anywhere from 75–11,000 repeats (Liquori, 2001; Day, 2003; Todd & Paulson, 2010). Symptoms typically present in the third decade of life; however, childhood cases have been reported. Similar to DM1, typical findings of PROMM include myotonia, muscle weakness, pain, and stiffness. Cataracts, cardiac conduction defects, insulin insensitivity, and testicular failure may be present, but are less common. Unlike DM1, developmental defects, intellectual impairment, and facial weakness are less common in PROMM. The distribution of weakness is more proximal, and most prominent in the shoulders, hips, and neck muscles. Finger flexion weakness may still be present; however, distal lower limb weakness is rare. Calf hypertrophy is a hallmark of this disease process (McDonald, 2012). Respiratory insufficiency, hypotonia, congenital clubfoot, and craniofacial abnormalities have not been reported in individuals with PROMM.

Diagnostic Testing

In myotonic dystrophy, serum creatine kinase is often normal or mildly elevated. An EMG may show myopathic units that are more prominent distally in DM1 and proximally in PROMM, as well as myotonia that may not be present in all muscles tested. Nerve conduction study of an affected PROMM individual may show mild to modest increase in compound muscle action potential (CMAP) amplitude after exercise with progressive reduction by 40% during rest (McDonald, 2012). MRI of the brain reveals abnormalities in the gray and white matter, and MRI of the limbs may assist in determining the pattern of muscle involvement. In DM1, muscle biopsy exhibits variation in fiber size, ring fibers, sarcoplasmic masses, and increased number of intrafusal fibers, as well as internal nuclei that are often organized in longitudinal chains. Type 1 fiber predominance with atrophy is often seen, which distinguishes it from PROMM. In PROMM, pyknotic nuclear clumps, cytoplasmic granules, type 2 muscle atrophy, and internal nuclei that are predominantly in type 2 muscle fibers are often found.

Definitive diagnosis of myotonic dystrophy type 1 and 2 can be obtained by molecular genetic testing, which identifies the exact number of repeats in DMPK or ZNF9, respectively. Prenatal testing is available via chorionic villus sampling and amniocentesis. Obtaining an individual's complete history, including family history; performing a thorough physical examination, including neurological, cardiac, and vision exams; and obtaining appropriate diagnostic testing may assist in determining the appropriate genetic test to order. Once myotonic dystrophy has been confirmed, additional laboratory tests to consider include testosterone, FSH and TSH levels, as well as tests such as hemoglobin A1C and fasting serum glucose level to assess for insulin insensitivity. Affected individuals are strongly recommended to obtain surveillance eye exams to screen for cataracts every two years and cardiac exams along with ECGs and 24-hour Holter monitors yearly to assess for cardiac dysfunction.

Treatment

In myotonic dystrophy, individuals experience muscle stiffness and difficulties relaxing their muscles. This leads to significant discomfort and, when coupled with patient's underlying weakness, may become disabling. Therapy and management are geared towards supportive care of clinical manifestations, as no curative treatment exists at this time. Pharmacological treatments include the use of mexiletine and carbamazepine for myotonia, nonsteroidal anti-inflammatory drugs or tricyclic antidepressants for musculoskeletal pain, and gabapentin for neuropathic pain. Low-dose steroids may be considered as well, and have been found to be effective in some patients. If detected, any thyroid dysfunction, insulin insensitivity, or hypogonadism issues should be treated accordingly. In addition, cataracts or cardiac dysfunctions should be carefully monitored and managed by specialists in the respective specialties. Cholesterol-lowering medications should be avoided as they can worsen muscle pain and weakness. Adaptive equipment and assistive devices should be considered to ensure safety and aid with mobility and activities of daily living.

FACIOSCAPULOHUMERAL MUSCULAR DYSTROPHY

Facioscapulohumeral muscular dystrophy (FSHD) is the third most common form of muscular dystrophy, affecting 1–5 in 100,000 (Emery1991). The inheritance pattern is autosomal dominant; however, spontaneous *de novo* mutations can occur in up to 30% of affected individuals (Kohler, 1996). The age of FSHD initial symptom onset is variable. While some affected individuals remain asymptomatic throughout their lifetime, most individuals show some sign of the disease process during childhood or teenage years. The prognosis is typically worse with earlier onset; however, life expectancy is often similar to that of the general population. The most common clinical feature of facioscapulohumeral muscular dystrophy is facial and limb-girdle weakness. Affected individuals often have symptoms before 20 years of age, though severity is variable and may not affect function until late into adulthood. Symptoms are often asymmetrical and may include involvement of the orbicularis oris, orbicularis oculi, zygomaticus, shoulder external rotators, scapular stabilizers, and shoulder abductors. Affected individuals often have difficulties whistling, using straws, closing their eyes completely, puckering their lips, smiling, or raising their arms above shoulder level. Dysarthria may be present, and foot extensor as well as abdominal muscle weakness (positive Beevor's sign) are not uncommon. Additional findings include posterior and lateral scapular winging (Figure 13.8), and muscle atrophy of the biceps, latissimus dorsi, lower trapezius, rhomboids, and serratus anterior. With disease progression, weakness of proximal lower limb muscles and hyperlordosis may develop. Approximately twenty percent of affected individuals become wheelchair-dependent. The deltoid,

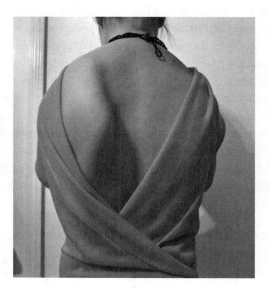

Figure 13.8:
Asymmetrical scapular winging.

masseter, temporalis, extraocular, and bulbar muscles are often spared (McDonald, 2012).

Individuals with FSHD may exhibit progressive sensorineural hearing loss (Padberg, 1995), intellectual impairment, cardiovascular abnormalities such as arrhythmias and conduction block (Laforet, 1998), and retinal diseases such as telangiectasia and retinal detachment (Coats disease) (Fitzsimons, 1987). Respiratory complications such as restrictive lung disease may present in individuals with moderate to severe disease severity. As such, careful monitoring through routinely scheduled specialist visits is highly encouraged.

Diagnostic Testing

Definitive diagnosis of facioscapulohumeral dystrophy is by genetic testing showing abnormalities in the D4Z4 DNA fragment. Two different mutations are possible in the D4Z4 DNA segment leading to FSHD1 and FSHD2. Sporadic mutation of the D4Z4 DNA segment may occur in 10% to 30% of cases in FSHD1 and 67% of cases in FSHD2 (Lemmers, 2012), leading to a mild phenotype of FSHD or asymptomatic individuals due to somatic mosaicism. Disease severity has been linked to the repeat size of D4Z4 segment, with larger deletions, smaller number of D4Z4 repeats resulting in a more severe phenotype with earlier onset in FSHD1 (Zatz, 1995). In FSHD2, symptom onset occurs later, and the disease severity is the same in both males and females.

EMGs may show myopathic changes such as low amplitude, short-duration motor unit action potentials. Findings on MRI of the proximal lower extremity include increased T2 signals in the semimembranosus, semitendinosus, adductor magnus, and/or biceps femoris, suggestive of edema in a specific pattern that is not present in unaffected individuals (Friedman, 2012). Muscle biopsy may reveal myopathic changes such as variation in fiber size, round and angulated fibers, endomysial and perivascular inflammation, and hypertrophic muscle fibers with few internal nuclei. Creatine kinase is normal or mildly elevated in affected individuals, levels of which are at most five times the upper limit of normal.

Treatment

There is no curative treatment for facioscapulohumeral dystrophy available at this time. Management is by supportive care to prevent disease complications, maximize function, and improve quality of life. Functional impairments such as decreased mobility and difficulties in performing activities of daily living secondary to muscle weakness can be managed by providing appropriate orthosis, special adaptive equipments, and/or mobility devices. Affected individuals should obtain regular screening vision exams, including dilated ophthalmoscopy, to assess for retinal telangiectasias and detachment, both of which are treatable. Due to the increased incidence of high-frequency hearing loss in this patient population, surveillance audiograms should be performed on a regular basis as well. This is particularly important for infantile-onset FSHD, as delayed treatment may interfere with language development.

Individuals with facioscapulohumeral dystrophy may experience musculoskeletal pain of the joints or surrounding structures due to muscle weakness and imbalance. In this population, low- to moderate-intensity aerobic exercises, stretching programs, and low-intensity resistive strengthening exercises over several months for muscles with at least antigravity strength have been found to be greatly beneficial at improving overall endurance, energy level, and strength in atrophied and disused muscles (Fowler, 2002). For pain control, anti-inflammatory medication is recommended. Hypoventilation due to restrictive lung disease may be treated with nighttime use of noninvasive positive pressure ventilation for respiratory support. Surgical options that have been employed include scapula fixation to the chest wall to improve arm mobility, upper eyelid implant with gold weights to aid in eye closure, and tendon transfer to assist with ankle dorsiflexion weakness. Pharmacological interventions have been explored with limited success, since studies thus far have yielded negative or inconclusive results when trying corticosteroids, β2 agonists, myostatin inhibitors, and creatine monohydrate for treatment of facioscapulohumeral muscular dystrophy symptoms (Tawil, 2008).

Many conditions may present with symptoms similar to that of facioscapulohumeral dystrophy. It is important to also consider scapuloperoneal muscular dystrophy syndromes, limb-girdle muscular dystrophy, myotonic dystrophy types 1 and 2, congenital myopathies, Becker muscular dystrophy, Emery-Dreifuss muscular dystrophy, and mitochondrial myopathy in the list of differential diagnosis. Various genetically confirmed phenotypes of FSHD also exist, which include, among others, focal monomelic lower-limb atrophy, distal myopathy, and facial-sparing scapulohumeral dystrophy. A detailed history, including family history, and a thorough physical examination may assist in guiding diagnostic workup. Treatment strategies involving the myostatin inhibition is currently being considered for FSHD.

LIMB-GIRDLE MUSCULAR DYSTROPHY

Limb-girdle muscular dystrophy (LGMD) is a term used for a group of highly heterogeneous disorders that are similar to but distinct from X-linked dystrophinopathies. Symptoms are symmetrical, and the disease progression is slow. Proximal muscle weakness is common on initial presentation. With certain genetic mutations or with disease progression, distal muscle involvement can be found. Initial symptoms can present anywhere from childhood to adulthood, with the average onset being between 10 to 30 years of age. Early onset is often associated with more rapid progression and worse prognosis.

As of 2012, mutations at over 50 loci have been identified and associated with limb-girdle muscular dystrophy. The phenotype for each is variable, with diverse clinical presentations. The overall prevalence of limb-girdle muscular dystrophy is difficult to determine due to the extent of heterogeneity; however, the range is estimated to be between 1 in 14,500 to 1 in 123,000 (van der Kooi, 1996; Urtasun, 1998). Inheritance pattern can either be autosomal dominant, autosomal recessive, or X-linked. Autosomal dominant forms are referred to as *LGMD1* and autosomal recessive forms are *LGMD2*, with various lettered types established to indicate the order of gene mapping. At this time, there have been 7 types of *LGMD1* (lettered A–C and E–H) and 17 types of *LGMD2* (lettered A–Q) identified, with new mutations continually detected and added to the list (Pegoraro, 2012). These mutations lead to defects in the respective proteins needed to directly or indirectly stabilize the muscle membrane. Additional information on selected LGMDs is available in Table 13.2. Individuals with limb-girdle muscular dystrophy present with variable progressive signs and symptoms that may include shoulder and hip-girdle weakness, muscle atrophy, waddling gait, hypotonia, pain, and joint contractures. Distal muscles are usually stronger compared to proximal muscles in the extremities; however, this can vary among individuals and types of LGMD. Calf hypertrophy, scapular winging, and myoglobinuria may be present, and facial weakness as well as bulbar symptoms, though rare, have been reported in certain LGMDs. Symptoms are often symmetrical, a clinical feature that differentiates LGMD from facioscapulohumeral dystrophy. Extramuscular involvement is uncommon, but the disease may affect cognitive function and cardiopulmonary processes such as restrictive lung disease, cardiomyopathy, and congestive heart failure.

Diagnostic Testing

Advances in science now offer genetic testing for definitive diagnosis of twenty individual types of LGMD mutations at the time of this writing.

Table 13.2 SUMMARY OF AUTOSOMAL DOMINANT (A) AND AUTOSOMAL RECESSIVE (B) SUBTYPES OF LIMB GIRDLE MUSCULAR DYSTROPHIES

(a)

	LGMD1A	LGMD1B	LGMD1C	LGMD1D	LGMD1E
Inheritance	AD	AD	AD	AD	AD
Gene location	5q31	1q11-q21	3p25	7q36.3	2q35
Protein	Myotillin	Lamin A/C	Caveolin	Member 6 (DNAJB6)	Desmin
Onset	Variable Third to seventh decade Anticipation	<20 yrs	5 yrs to adulthood	3rd to 6th decade	2nd decade or later
Severity and course	Slow progression Rare: late-onset, rapidly progressive, loss of ambulation and respiratory failure	Slow progression Upper limbs involved by the third or fourth decade	Moderate severity and progression Adults with Gower's maneuver	Slow progression	Slow progression; all retain ambulation
Weakness	Legs and arms Symmetrical Proximal at onset Early foot-drop Distal with disease progression Wrist and finger extensors + deltoid Dysarthria (30%) Facial (17%) Neck extensors in some patients	Lower limb Symmetrical Proximal Variant: quadriceps weakness with Arg 377His mutation	Proximal	Variable Proximal>distal or Distal>proximal Legs>arms Dysphagia (20%)	Proximal
Ambulation status	Late loss of ambulation (>10 yrs after onset)		Mild: adults continue to ambulate	Wheelchair after 20 to 30 years	

Cardiac	Cardiomyopathy (50%) Onset sixth or seventh decade	Cardiomyopathy 62%	No cardiomyopathy	Arrhythmia (early feature); CHF with 4-chamber enlargement in 3rd to 5th decades; Sudden death without prior symptoms
Respiratory	Mild restrictive lung disease	Mild restrictive lung disease	Mild restrictive lung disease	
Muscle size				
Musculoskeletal	Ankle contractures (30%)	No contractures	Calf hypertrophy Cramps after exercise	Occasional calf hypertrophy
Central nervous system	No intellectual defect reported	No intellectual defect reported	No intellectual defect reported	
Muscle pathology	Myopathic Variable fiber size Fiber degeneration and regeneration Rimmed vacuoles Normal levels of myotilin or increased immunostaining Reduced laminin-γ1 Type 1 predominance with increasing vacuoles Normal dystrophin and sarcoglycan	Laminin A subcellular localization: Normal: nucleus: colocalizes with emerin Mutated: Can aggregate in nucleus and be present in cytoplasm	Myopathic Reduced caveolin-3 staining: no 21k-D band on Western blot	Myopathic Small muscle fibers Rounded Angulated Endomysial fibrosis Rimmed vacuoles Eosinophilic cytoplasmic bodies Aggregates: Contain SMI-31, TDP-43 & DNAJB6 Small fibers express neonatal & fetal myosin
Blood chemistry	CK: 1–15 times normal; commonly twice normal	CK: Normal to mildly elevated	CK: 4–25 times normal	Normal to 5x elevated

(continued)

Table 13.2 CONTINUED

(b)

	LGMD2A	LGMD2B	LGMD2C	LGMD2D	LGMD2E	LGMD2F	LGMD2G	LGMD2I
Inheritance	AR	AR	AR	AR	AR	AR	AR	AR
Gene location	4p21	2p12-14	13q12	17q21	4q12	5q33	17q12	19q13.3
Protein	Calpain-3	Dysferlin	γ-Sarcoglycan	α-Sarcoglycan	β-Sarcoglycan	δ-Sarcoglycan	Telethonin	Fukutin-related protein
Onset	*Early:* <12 yrs *Leyden-Mobius type:* 13–29 yrs *Late:* >30 yrs	12–39 yrs Mean 19 ± 3	Mean 5–6 yrs C283Y mutation: <2 yrs	2–15 hrs	3 yrs–teens Intrafamilial variability	2–10 yrs	Mean 12.5 yrs Range 9–15 yrs	0.5–27 yrs 61% <5 yrs
Severity and course	Variable Mild in majority Early-onset has more severe progression	Slow progression Mild weakness	Variable progression (some like DMD; others like BMD) Death common in second decade	Variable Absent adhalin: rapid progression Reduced adhalin: later onset and milder weakness	Moderate progression and severity	Rapid progression Death in second decade	Slow progression Mild weakness	Variable Early onset: nonambulant by teens Later onset: slowly progressive
Weakness	Scapula Pelvis Girdle and trunk weakness Proximal legs>arms	Weakness in gastrocnemius, quadriceps, and psoas muscle Weakness in biceps after legs	Proximal> distal Patchy distribution with some mutations Quadriceps spared	Proximal> distal Symmetrical Quadriceps weakness	Proximal	Proximal Symmetrical	Arms: proximal Legs: proximal and distal (foot drop)	Proximal> distal Legs: proximal Arms: proximal Face: mild weakness in older patients

Ambulation status	Loss of ambulation 10–30 yrs after onset	Loss of ambulation 10–30 yrs after onset Most walk until their fourth decade	Loss of ambulation: 10–37 yrs (mean 16 yrs)	Early onset: loss of adhalin Later onset: reduced adhalin	Often in wheelchair by 10–15 yrs; usually by 25 yrs	Loss of ambulation 9–16 yrs	40% nonambulatory in 3rd to 4th decades	30% nonambulatory by 4th to 6th decades
Cardiac	No involvement	No involvement	Occasional: especially late in disease course	Dilated cardiomyopathy	Occasional cardiomyopathy	Dilated cardiomyopathy described; may occur without myopathy	Cardiac involvement in 55%	Dilated cardiomyopathy in 30–50% of patients
Respiratory	Rarely involved Pulmonary Function Test (PFTs) rarely <80% predicted	Rarely involved	Forced Vital Capacity (FVC) ranges from normal to severe	FVC ranges from normal to severe	Variable respiratory involvement	Variable respiratory involvement		Variable respiratory involvement; some severe
Muscle size	Limbs, pelvic & shoulder Atrophy of Posterior compartments	Hypertrophy uncommon	Hypertrophy of calf & tongue in some patients	Calf hypertrophy in some patients	Prominent muscle hypertrophy	Calf hypertrophy Cramps	Calf hypertrophy 50% Calf atrophy 50%	Calf, tongue and thigh hypertrophy Wasting in regions of weakness
Musculo-skeletal	Contractures: calf (toe walking may be present)	Contractures: calf (toe walking may be presenting sign)	Lumbar hyperlordosis Scapular winging	Scapular winging	Shoulders: scapular winging & muscle wasting	Scapular winging		Contractures in ankles (especially in nonambulant) Scoliosis
Central nervous system	Intelligence: normal to mild mental retardation	No intellectual defect reported	No intellectual defect reported Hearing loss	No intellectual defect reported	No intellectual defect reported	No intellectual defect reported	No intellectual defect reported	No intellectual defect reported
Blood chemistry	CK: 7–80 times normal	CK: 10–72 times normal	CK: very high	CK: very high (often >5000)	CK: very high (often >5000)	CK: 10–50 times normal	CK: 3–30 times normal	CK: very high (1000–8000)

Genetic testing technique is expected to improve with time, which will increase the number of genetically detectable LGMD mutations in the future. Prenatal testing is also available at this time via chorionic villus sampling and amniocentesis as early as the tenth to twelfth weeks of gestation. There are risks to prenatal testing, and no curative treatment is available at this time for LGMD, so individuals are strongly encouraged to discuss the risks and benefits of this option with a neuromuscular specialist and/or obstetrician prior to getting tested.

Additional tests to consider in the diagnostic workup of LGMD include checking creatine kinase level, which is usually elevated in certain types. Muscle biopsy may be performed, which shows dystrophic features such as variation in fiber size, rounded atrophic fibers, split fibers, increased central nuclei, and endomysial fibrosis. These findings are nonspecific and present in similar processes. As such, when available, studies to assess certain protein expressions are of great value in assessing suspected LGMD genetic defects. These include immunostaining or immunoblotting to evaluate for sarcoglycanopathy, calpainopathy, dysferlinopathy, and dystroglycanopathy. A nerve conduction study/EMG may assist by ruling out other processes or by keeping LGMD as a consideration if myopathic units are found. MRI of the extremities may be helpful in assessing the pattern of muscle involvement and to assist in determining the severity of the disease process (Wattjes, 2010). A 2006 study looked at the distribution of LGMD subtypes among patients in the United States at six medical centers. Muscle biopsies provided histopathology and immunodiagnostic testing, and their protein abnormalities along with clinical parameters directed mutation screening. The diagnosis in 23 patients was a disorder other than LGMD. 266 out of 289 unrelated patients had muscle biopsies sufficient for complete microscopic evaluation; 121 also underwent Western blotting. From this combined evaluation, the distribution of immunophenotypes was 12% calpainopathy, 18% dysferlinopathy, 15% sarcoglycanopathy, 15% dystroglycanopathy, and 1.5% caveolinopathy. The study indicates that establishing a putative subtype is possible more than half the time, using available diagnostic testing during that timeframe. An efficient approach to genotypical diagnosis is muscle biopsy immunophenotyping, followed by directed mutational analysis. The most common LGMDs in the United States are calpainopathies, dysferlinopathies, sarcoglycanopathies, and dystroglycanopathies. (Moore, 2006) The differential diagnosis for limb-girdle muscular dystrophy includes, but is not limited to: FSHD, myotonic dystrophy, X-linked dystrophinopathies, metabolic myopathies, congenital muscular dystrophy, and Emery-Dreifuss muscular dystrophy.

Treatment

There is no curative treatment available at this time. Those with limb-girdle muscular dystrophy are encouraged to participate in aerobic exercises to maintain their strength, improve their energy and endurance, and sustain their general health and well-being. Aquatic therapies, stretching, brisk walks, resistant therapy-band exercises, and recumbent cycling are highly encouraged as tolerated. Bracing may be required to prevent contractures and to aid with ambulation. In severe cases, walkers or wheelchairs may be needed to assist with mobility and ensure safety. Steroids have been tried with positive responses in several cases of LGMD, including LGMD2D (Angelini, 1998), LGMD2I (Darin, 2007) and LGMD2M (Godfrey, 2006). If an extramusculoskeletal manifestation such as cardiomyopathy is present, affected individuals are recommended to follow up with specialists for care and management. Current options for gene therapy are being explored with the goal of decreasing disease progression and improving strength as well as quality of life. Gene therapy through local injection into muscles using the adeno-associated virus (AAV) as the vector has been tried in the past with little success; however, there are renewed efforts to optimize the delivery and reduce immune reactions that may be limiting the efficacy of gene delivery strategies (Mendell, 2012).

CONCLUSION

The growing knowledge of neuromuscular disorders and muscular dystrophies presents new opportunities and strategies for pharmacological interventions. Although there are no cures, there are many interventions that can improve the natural history of the various conditions. Many of the neuromuscular diseases and muscular dystrophies affect not only the musculoskeletal system but also other organ systems. In addition, there are significant needs of this population regarding their education, vocational training, psychological support, as well as community integration needs. A multidisciplinary approach to taking care of individuals with various neuromuscular disorders and muscular dystrophies is recommended, which includes specialists in neuromuscular medicine, neurology, physical medicine and rehabilitation, genetics, pulmonology, cardiology, physical and occupational therapy, speech therapy, rehabilitation psychology, medical equipment specialist, and social work, to name a few. At this time, no significant dietary regimen, antioxidant, or supplement (such as creatine) has shown to impact the natural history of the various muscular dystrophies or to improve muscle function significantly. However, appropriate therapy intervention as well as equipment prescriptions (for improving activities of daily living and mobility) and prevention of comorbidities will improve the functioning and increase the quality of life of those suffering from neuromuscular disorders. The continued advances in therapeutic strategies for neuromuscular diseases and muscular dystrophies are encouraging, and the future remains optimistic for significant pharmacological interventions and, possibly, cures.

DISCLOSURES

Conflicts: Dr. Lipa: none. Dr. Nguyen: none. Dr. Han serves on the Speaker's Bureau for Genzyme/Sanofi.

REFERENCES
Aartsma-Rus, A., Janson, A. A., van Ommen, G. J., & van Deutekom, J. C. (2007). Antisense-induced exon skipping for duplications in Duchenne muscular dystrophy. *BMC Medical Genetics*, *Jul 5*, 8, 43.

Angelini, C., Fanin, M., Menegazzo, E., et al. (1998). Homozygous alpha-sarcoglycan mutation in two siblings: One asymptomatic and one steroid-responsive mild limb-girdle muscular dystrophy patient. *Muscle & Nerve*, *21*, 769–775.

Biggar, W. D., Harris, V. A., Eliasoph, L., & Alman, B. (2006). Long-term benefits of deflazacort treatment for boys with Duchenne muscular dystrophy in their second decade. *Neuromuscular Disorders*, *16*(4), 249–255.

Bushby, K., Finkel, R., Birnkrant, D. J., et al., & Care Considerations Working Group. (2010). Diagnosis and management of Duchenne muscular dystrophy, Part 1: Diagnosis, and pharmacological and psychosocial management. *Lancet Neurology*, *9*(1), 77–93.

Centers for Disease Control and Prevention (CDC). (2009). Prevalence of Duchenne/Becker muscular dystrophy among males aged 5–24 years—four states, 2007. *MMWR Morbidity & Mortality Weekly Report*, *58*(40), 1119–1122.

Cirak, S., Arechavala-Gomeza, V., Guglieri, M., et al. (2011). Exon skipping and dystrophin restoration in patients with Duchenne muscular dystrophy after systemic phosphorodiamidate morpholino oligomer treatment: An open-label, phase 2, dose-escalation study. *Lancet*, *378*(9791), 595–605.

Darin, N., Kroksmark, A. K., Ahlander, A. C., et al. (2007). Inflammation and response to steroid treatment in limb-girdle muscular dystrophy 2I. *European Journal of Paediatric Neurology*, *11*, 353–357.

Day, J. W., Ricker, K., Jacobsen, J. F., et al. (2003). Myotonic dystrophy type 2: molecular, diagnostic and clinical spectrum. *Neurology*, *60*(4), 657–664.

Emery, A. E. (1991). Population frequencies of inherited neuromuscular diseases—A world survey. *Neuromuscular Disorders*, *1*, 19–29.

Escolar, D. M., Hache, L. P., Clemens, P. R., et al. (2011). Randomized, blinded trial of weekend vs. daily prednisone in Duchenne muscular dystrophy. *Neurology*, *77*, 444–452.

Fitzsimons, R. B., Burwin, E. B., & Bird, A. C. (1987). Retinal vascular abnormalities in facioscapulohumeral muscular dystrophy: A general association with genetic and therapeutic implications. *Brain*, *110*, 631–648.

Fowler, W. M. (2002). Role of physical activity and exercise training in neuromuscular diseases. *American Journal of Physical Medicine & Rehabilitation*, *81*(11 Suppl), S187–S195.

Friedman, S. D., Poliachik, S. L., Carter, G. T., et al. (2012). The magnetic resonance imaging spectrum of facioscapulohumeral muscular dystrophy. *Muscle & Nerve*, *45*, 500–506.

Godfrey, C., Escolar, D., Brockington, M., et al. (2006). Fukutin gene mutations in steroid-responsive limb-girdle muscular dystrophy. *Annals of Neurology*, *60*, 603–610.

Harley, H. G., Walsh, K. V., Rundle, S., et al. (1991). Localisation of the myotonic dystrophy locus to 19q13.2-19q13.3 and its relationship to twelve polymorphic loci on 19q. *Human Genetics*, *87*, 73–80.

Harper, P. S. (2001). *Major Problems in Neurology: Myotonic Dystrophy*. London: WB Saunders.

Hoffman, E. P., Fischbeck, K. H., Brown, R. H., et al. (1988). Characterization of dystrophin in muscle-biopsy specimens from patients with Duchenne's or Becker's muscular dystrophy. *New England Journal of Medicine*, *318*, 1363–1368.

King, W. M., Ruttencutter, R., Nagaraja, H. N., et al. (2007). Orthopedic outcomes of long-term daily corticosteroid treatment in Duchenne muscular dystrophy. *Neurology*, *68*, 1607–1613.

Kohler, J., Rupilius, B., Otto, M., et al. (1996). Germline mosaicism in 4q35 facioscapulohumeral muscular dystrophy (FSHD1A) occurring predominantly in oogenesis. *Human Genetics*, *98*(4), 485–490.

Laforêt, P., de Toma, C., Eymard, B., et al. (1998). Cardiac involvement in genetically confirmed facioscapulohumeral muscular dystrophy. *Neurology*, *51*(5), 1454–1456.

Lemmers, R. J. L. F., Miller, D. G., & van der Maarel, S. M. (1999). Facioscapulohumeral muscular dystrophy. Mar 8 (Updated 2012 Jun 21). *GeneReviews*™ (Internet). University of Washington, Seattle; 1993–2013. Available from: http://www.ncbi.nlm.nih.gov/books/NBK1443/.

Liquori, C. L., Ricker, K., Moseley, M. L., et al. (2001). Myotonic dystrophy type 2 caused by a CCTG expansion in intron 1 of ZNF9. *Science*, *293*, 864–867.

Martorell, L., Monckton, D. G., Sanchez, A., et al. (2001). Frequency and stability of the myotonic dystrophy type 1 premutation. *Neurology 56*, 328–335.

McDonald, C. M. (2012). Clinical approach to the diagnostic evaluation of hereditary and acquired neuromuscular diseases. *Physical Medicine & Rehabilitation Clinics of North America*, *23*(3), 495–563.

Mendell, J. R., Moxley, R. T., Griggs, R. C., et al. (1989). Randomized, double-blind six-month trial of prednisone in Duchenne's muscular dystrophy. *New England Journal of Medicine*, *320*, 1592–1597.

Mendell, J. R., Rodino-Klapac, L., Sahenk, Z., Malik, V., Kaspar, B. K., Walker, C. M., & Clark, K. R. (2012). Gene therapy for muscular dystrophy: Lessons learned and path forward. *Neuroscience Letters*, *527*(2), 90–99.

Moore, S. A., Shilling, C. J., Westra, S., et al. (2006). Limb-girdle muscular dystrophy in the United States. *Journal of Neuropathology & Experimental Neurology*, *10*, 995–1003.

Moxley, R. T., Pandya, S., Ciafoli, E., et al. (2010). Change in natural history of Duchenne muscular dystrophy with long-term corticosteroids treatment: Implications for management. *Journal of Child Neurology, 25,* 1116–1129.

Padberg, G. W., Brouwer, O. F., de Keizer, R. F., et al. (1995). On the significance of retinal vascular disease and hearing loss in facioscapulohumeral muscular dystrophy. *Muscle & Nerve,* S73–S80.

Pegoraro, E., & Hoffman, E. P. (2000). Limb-girdle muscular dystrophy overview. Jun 8 (Updated 2012 Aug 30). *GeneReviews™* (Internet). University of Washington, Seattle; 1993-. Available from: http://www.ncbi.nlm.nih.gov/books/NBK1408/.

Pichavant, C., Aartsma-Rus, A., Clemens, P. R., et al. (2011). Current status of pharmaceutical and genetic therapeutic approaches to treat DMD. *Molecular Therapy, 19*(5), 830–840.

Pradhan, S. (1994). New clinical sign in Duchenne muscular dystrophy. *Pediatric Neurology, 11*(4), 298–300.

Tawil, R. (2008). Facioscapulohumeral muscular dystrophy. *Neurotherapeutics, 5*(4), 601–606.

Todd, P. K., & Paulson, H. L. (2010). RNA-mediated neurodegeneration in repeat expansion disorders. *Annals of Neurology, 67,* 291–300.

Urtasun, M., Saenz, A., Roudaut, C., et al. (1998). Limb-girdle muscular dystrophy in Guipuzcoa (Basque Country, Spain). *Brain, 121*(Pt 9), 1735–1747.

van der Kooi, A. J., Barth, P. G., Busch, H. F., et al. (1996). The clinical spectrum of limb-girdle muscular dystrophy. A survey in the Netherlands. *Brain, 119,* 1471–1480.

Wattjes, M. P., Kley, R. A., & Fisher, D. (2010). Neuromuscular imaging in inherited muscle disease. *European Radiology, 20*(10), 2447–2460.

Zatz, M., Marie, S. K., Passos-Bueno, M. R., et al. (1995). High proportion of new mutations and possible anticipation in Brazilian facioscapulohumeral muscular dystrophy families. *American Journal of Human Genetics, 56,* 99–105.

CHAPTER 14

Translating Treatments from the Laboratory to the Clinic

RANDI JENSSEN HAGERMAN, BILLUR MOGHADDAM, JAN NOLTA, MARIA DIEZ-JUAN, AND ROBERT L. HENDREN

INTRODUCTION

This book is meant to stimulate a new way of thinking about the treatment of neurodevelopmental disorders (ND). We have chosen disorders where there are exciting advances in understanding the molecular foundation that are facilitating new treatments in animal models and human studies. The number of common mechanisms of molecular dysfunction across disorders is remarkable, including oxidative stress, mitochondrial dysfunction, and GABA/glutamate imbalances, and the final common pathway is usually the synapse and how it responds to environmental stimuli. As we discuss new pharmacological treatments that have the potential to reverse the neurobiological dysregulation caused by a mutation, we must not forget that the long-term strengthening of a synapse requires environmental input and learning paradigms to keep it strong (as described next).

Parallel to the advances in molecular biology and targeted treatments are the advances in educational technology and the digital age, particularly with the use of iPADs and other tablets for which a variety of applications for academic, social, and language learning abound. Most clinicians have seen their patients applying these digital aids to learning, sometimes with remarkable progress in language and academic skills, but other times with obsessive utilization to the detriment of their behavior when the aids are taken away. How to use these tools to enhance learning in an individualized and interactive way is also reviewed in this chapter because these are interventions that can be currently recommended by clinicians.

We hope that clinicians will utilize the advances in treatment and educational technology now so that the children with ND can benefit as soon as possible from these new interventions. Many families wait months for an appointment with a specialist for a diagnosis or treatment recommendations. However, there is much that the primary care doctor in pediatrics or family medicine can do, in ordering the appropriate genetic and other laboratory testing to make the diagnosis, understanding the mechanism of the disturbed function, and developing targeted treatments for the patient. Advances in newborn screening will facilitate the identification of many more genetic disorders so that early intervention can be initiated. The further development of biomarkers will enhance our ability to identify children at risk for autism spectrum disorders (ASD) and other ND and to uncover which pathways may be dysregulated so that the treatments can be targeted to specific pathways.

COMMONALITIES ACROSS DISORDERS

Seizures and FMRP Dysregulation

There are a number of problems that occur across multiple disorders, and seizures come to mind first, because they occur in ASD, Rett syndrome, fragile X syndrome, fragile X premutation disorders, tuberous sclerosis (TS), Angelman syndrome, and many other disorders not covered in this book, such as neurofibromatosis and fetal alcohol syndrome. A recent study demonstrated that the prevalence of seizures in a variety of ND, including TS, idiopathic ASD, and neurofibromatosis, correlated with the severity of ASD symptoms and overall IQ (Hagerman, 2013; van Eeghen, Pulsifer et al., 2013). The presence of seizures, particularly early-life seizures, further disrupts development (Marsh, Freeman, et al., 2006). Expression of miRNAs changes with seizures, and these changes can influence the expression of many genes involved in autism and other ND, such as *CNTNAP2*, *GABRB3*, *FMR1*, *MeCP2*, *RELN*, *TSC1*, and *TSC2* (Abu-Elneel, Liu, et al., 2008; Nudelman, Rebibo-Sabbah, et al., 2009; Qureshi, Mattick, et al., 2010). Matrix metalloproteinase 9 (MMP9) is upregulated with seizures, and this protein is probably involved with seizure-induced dendritic spine pruning, and is also upregulated in fragile X syndrome (Chapter 9). Seizures also increase aberrant synaptogenesis and mossy fiber sprouting, and these activities also involve MMP9 (Wilczynski, Konopacki, et al., 2008).

The work of the Benke Laboratory at the University of Colorado gives insight into why these changes occur with seizures. They have demonstrated that, in a rat, without any mutations, early-life seizures dysregulate

FMRP by disrupting the FMRP/Akt complex and pulling FMRP away from the dendritic spines and into the cell body (Bernard, Castano, et al., 2013). This FMRP dysfunction has significant consequences for the development of synaptic plasticity, thereby leading to worsening of autistic symptoms and overall cognition in this rat model. Therefore early intervention for seizures is an important component of treatment for all NDs that have a seizure component.

For many individuals with neurodevelopmental disorders, there is often a history of "staring spells" that are questionable seizures, and the EEG may show spike wave discharges. Although the tradition in neurology has been not to treat spike wave discharges when there is not a clear seizure, when there are questionable seizures in the neurodevelopmental disorders described here, it is worthwhile to give the patient a trial of anticonvulsants to see if development and behavior improve on anticonvulsants. Although there are side effects of anticonvulsants that must be taken into consideration, there may be additional benefits besides the stopping of seizures that impact the subsequent development of the child. One example is the change in gene expression that can occur with valproate treatment because gene expression, including the expression of *FMR1,* may improve with this treatment (Marsh, Freeman, et al., 2006; Bagni, Tassone, et al., 2012). Limited studies have shown benefit of valproate treatment in autism (see Chapter 2) and in fragile X syndrome (see Chapter 9).

Another commonality that is emerging across several neurodevelopmental disorders is a deficit of FMRP, the protein produced by the *FMR1* gene that is missing in fragile X syndrome (Chapter 9). Studies from the Fatemi Laboratory first reported deficits of FMRP in the brains of patients who had depression, schizophrenia, or bipolar disorder but without an *FMR1* mutation (Fatemi & Folsom, 2011a). These researchers also reported deficits of FMRP and upregulation of the mGluR5 pathway in the brains of adults with autism compared to controls (Fatemi & Folsom, 2011b). Their most recent studies have assessed downstream proteins, including homer1, amyloid beta A 4 precursor protein (APP), Ras-related C3 botulinum toxin substrate 1 (Rac 1), striated enriched protein tyrosine phosphatase (STEP), all linked to changes in FMRP levels and are dysregulated in the brains of individuals with autism who do not have an *FMR1* mutation (Fatemi, Folsom, et al., 2013). They postulate that deficiency of FMRP can lead to these downstream protein effects in autism.

The Fatemi lab had previously reported on downregulation of $GABA_A$ and $GABA_B$ receptor subunits in the cerebellum, parietal cortex, and BA9 in the brains of those with autism (Fatemi, Reutiman, et al., 2009; Fatemi, Reutiman, et al., 2010) in addition to downregulation of Reelin in the blood, cerebellum, and BA8 in adults with autism compared to controls (Fatemi, Snow, et al., 2005). These findings, in addition to the other abnormalities previously reported, are thought to all stem from an FMRP deficit, although what is downregulating FMRP is not known. FMRP is upregulated with learning and with sensory stimulation (Chapter 9) and miRNA dysregulation will also impact the expression of FMRP, as described below.

Another research group has reported on FMRP deficits in blood and in the brain of those with schizophrenia but without an *FMR1* mutation. In their study of 36 adults with schizophrenia (mean age 35.5, SD 6.9) compared to 30 controls age-matched, FMRP was significantly reduced as measured by enzyme-linked immunosorbent assay (ELISA) in blood compared to controls. Lower FMRP was associated with reduced IQ and an earlier onset of schizophrenia (Kovács, Kelemen, et al., 2013). Kelemen et al. (Kelemen, Kovács, et al., 2013) carried out neuropsychological testing in those with schizophrenia and found that the level of FMRP correlated with visual perceptual abilities, including contrast sensitivity of low spatial and high temporal frequencies, perceptual integration, and motion perception. This is reminiscent of the studies of young children with fragile X syndrome and premutation involvement where the metabotropic (M) pathway important for motion perception is more significantly affected by the lack or deficiency of FMRP than the parvocellular (P) pathway important for static visual processing (Farzin, Rivera, et al., 2011). Kelemen and colleagues (Kelemen, Kovács, et al., 2013) also found that an attention test correlated significantly with FMRP levels, such that the lower the FMRP, the greater the attention problems. Similar findings were previously reported in the general population (Kéri & Benedek, 2011). Neuroimaging studies also have demonstrated correlations between brain size and FMRP in the general population, especially involving the frontal regions, which are important for attention (Wang, Hessl, et al., 2013).

Glutamate and GABA Abnormalities

The balance between glutamate (stimulatory) and GABA (inhibitory) systems is mentioned in just about every chapter in this volume. For most disorders, the GABA system is downregulated: including in ASD, fragile X syndrome, Angelman syndrome, ADHD, schizophrenia, and PKU, with the exception of Down syndrome, where there is enhanced GABA activity, and a $GABA_A$ inverse antagonist is currently being studied as a targeted treatment. The development of $GABA_A$ agonists is likely to be helpful for several disorders, and ganaxolone is currently being studied in fragile X syndrome.

Another agonist, allopregnanolone, a natural neurosteroid GABA$_A$ agonist, is being utilized in traumatic brain injury and shows promise in the treatment of Alzheimer disease and in the fragile X-associated tremor ataxia syndrome (FXTAS) (Cao, Hulsizer, et al., 2013).

The upregulation of the mTOR system is also seen in many disorders, including RASopathies (Chapter 7), tuberous sclerosis (Chapter 8), fragile X syndrome (Chapter 9), ASD (Chapter 2), and perhaps others. mGluR5 antagonists are currently undergoing trials in fragile X syndrome, and they will subsequently be started in ASD. If efficacy is shown, then these medications can be utilized by the practicing clinician, perhaps within one or two years after the publication of this book.

Currently, there are a couple of medications that can be prescribed that will downregulate the mTOR system. Lithium will inhibit the enzyme glycogen synthase kinase 3β (GSK3β), and downstream effects will reduce both tau protein phosphorylation and amyloid B$_{42}$ production. Lithium also reduces proinflammatory status and decreases oxidative stress. Chronic use of lithium increases cortical thickening and leads to a larger hippocampal and amygdala volume in patients with bipolar disorder. Lithium also inhibits inositol monophosphatase (IMP) and stimulates gene expression and release of neurotrophic factors, including brain-derived neurotropic factor (BDNF) and vascular endothelial growth factor (VEGF) (Gervain & Mehler, 2010; Diniz, Machado-Vieira, et al., 2013).

Lithium has been used for years in patients with bipolar disorder, who also have elevation of mTOR, perhaps through a mechanism of reduced FMRP (Folsom & Fatemi, 2012). Lithium is also a targeted treatment for Down syndrome (Chapter 11) and fragile X syndrome (Chapter 9) (Berry-Kravis, Sumis, et al., 2008). Patients with ASD who have evidence of upregulation of mTOR through biomarkers (Hoeffer, Sanchez, et al., 2012) would also be expected to benefit from lithium. Lovastatin is also considered a targeted treatment for fragile X syndrome (Osterweil, Chuang, et al., 2013) and perhaps for several RASopathies who have upregulation of extracellular signal regulated kinase (ERK) phosphorylation.

Neurodevelopmental and Neurodegenerative Disorders

Throughout several chapters in this book, there is evidence of commonalities between neurodevelopmental and neurodegenerative disorders. Perhaps the most obvious is in the development of Alzheimer disease in aging individuals with Down syndrome (Chapter 11). However, other disorders have also been documented to have aging problems associated with them, including Parkinson disease in fragile X syndrome (Utari, Adams, et al., 2010), in Angelman syndrome (Chapter 10), and *FMR1* premutation involvement leading to the fragile X-associated tremor ataxia syndrome (FXTAS) (Hagerman & Hagerman, 2013). The commonalities across disorders relate to a number of mechanisms, including increased APP production in Down syndrome, fragile X syndrome and *FMR1* premutation involvement; mitochondrial dysfunction in all of the neurodevelopmental and neurodegenerative disorders; and enhanced reactive oxygen species (ROS) leading to oxidative stress in multiple disorders and in aging.

There is an emerging knowledge regarding microRNA (miRNA) dysregulation in neurodevelopmental disorders described in this volume and neurodegenerative disorders also mentioned (Martino, di Girolamo, et al., 2009; Im & Kenny, 2012). There are many commonalities across disorders because miRNAs regulate so many processes, including transcription, translation, neuronal migration, differentiation, synaptic plasticity, and neurogenesis, throughout life (Miller, Zeier, et al., 2012; Ji, Lv, et al., 2013). For instance, miR-132 expression in the dorsolateral prefrontal cortex regulates the expression of the schizophrenia phenotype and controls development-associated genes such as *DNMT3A*, *GATA2*, and *DPYSL3*; controls genes associated with synaptic plasticity, including *MECP2* and *P250GAP*; and the NMDAR dependent synaptic pruning that takes place in adolescence and young adulthood (Miller, Zeier, et al., 2012). miR-132 also controls Dnmt3a, a DNA methyltransferase that appears to be important for hypermethylation of schizophrenia-risk genes, including *GAD1* and *Reelin*, which are also important for reduced expression of GABA and neuronal migration, respectively.

In the Down syndrome mouse model Ts65DN, both miR-155 and miR-802 are over-expressed, and these miRNAs target migration of neurons, differentiation of microglia, the mTOR pathway, and *MECP2* expression (Keck-Wherley, Grover, et al., 2011). For each of the neurodevelopmental disorders, there are emerging miRNA signatures. Even in ASD that is heterogeneous in etiology, the multiple copy number variants (CNVs) associated with ASD harbor miRNAs that regulate transcription factors, many of which are involved in synapse formation (Vaishnavi, Manikandan, et al., 2013). In depression there is significant dysregulation of many miRNAs, including miR-16 which targets the serotonin transporter SERT, and miR-30e, which also regulates tumor-suppression and is associated with schizophrenia also (Hansen & Obrietan, 2013). The use of antidepressants will upregulate BDNF, which will then influence a number of regulatory feedback loops within neurons, including enhancing the expression of miR-132, which couples synaptic activity to dendritic morphogenesis. miR-132 is also induced by light within the SCN and regulates a number of clock genes that modulate the capacity of light to entrain circadian rhythmicity (Hansen & Obrietan, 2013). Thus miR-132 is important in regulating neuroplasticity and modulating sleep/wake cycles, which affect depressive neurophysiology.

Perhaps most importantly, the use of drugs of abuse, including alcohol, opioids, and others, significantly impacts miRNAs (Tal & Tanguay, 2012). For instance, cocaine leads to upregulation of miR-212, which inhibits *MECP2* gene expression and activates the mTOR pathway. In addition, neurotoxicants such as heavy metals, organophosphates, and others are mediators, effectors, and adaptive agents of neurotoxicants (Tal & Tanguay, 2012). Although the clinician will not be measuring miRNA levels currently, these data help us understand some of the mechanisms of environmental toxicity and problems associated with substance abuse.

The development of therapeutics that treat dysregulation of miRNAs include the use of antagomirs (cholesterol conjugated 2-O methyl RNA antisense oligonucleotides) that can lower excessive miRNAs. These interventions are being developed for a number of disease models associated with miRNA dysregulation (Hansen & Obrietan, 2013).

LESSONS LEARNED TO TRANSLATE INTO CLINICAL PRACTICE

The Earlier the Intervention, the Better

The studies so far have shown that the earlier the intervention starts, the better for the child. This was demonstrated in ASD, where the Early Start Denver Model (ESDM) utilized with toddlers not only improved their developmental scores and socialization but also normalized the EEG abnormalities of those with ASD, whereas community intervention, including applied behavioral analysis (ABA), did not (Rogers, Estes, et al., 2012; Dawson, 2013). Although the ESDM is designed specifically for autism, it is likely that most neurodevelopmental disorders will benefit from such intensive and early intervention, particularly those that are associated with ASD, including those covered in this book.

The animal models for most neurodevelopmental disorders show significant benefits from early intervention with a targeted treatment (Dansie, Phommahaxay, et al., 2013), although the use of targeted treatments can be helpful even for many adults with neurodevelopmental disorders (Jacquemont, Curie, et al., 2011; Barichello, Santos, et al., 2012; Michalon, Sidorov, et al., 2012; Dansie, Phommahaxay, et al., 2013). Most studies of animal models show more dramatic benefits than what has been seen so far in patients, however.

Combination Treatment

It appears that for most disorders there needs to be a combination of interventions, even of targeted treatments, because a mutation in even one gene affecting a single protein, such as MeCP2 or FMRP, has ramifications for many neurotransmitters and many pathways that influence brain development, including synaptic plasticity. The complexity of each of the neurodevelopmental disorders discussed in this volume is significant, and the list of current and future targeted treatments is long. The benefit to the clinician is that some of the interventions can be started now in the patients who are seen regularly.

Individual Variability in Response and the Need for Biomarkers

Although some of the targeted treatments described are undergoing randomized controlled trials (RTC) in humans to demonstrate efficacy, there is significant variability in the response that is related to environmental differences and background genetic effects. For instance, in the recently discontinued trials of Arbaclofen, a GABA$_B$ agonist for fragile X syndrome and ASD, there was a subgroup of definite responders (Chapters 9 and 2), but the overall efficacy data was not significant enough to continue the trials. It will take more research to find a biomarker that can identify those who will have a good response to this and other targeted treatments. What the clinician is faced with is considering a medication or intervention that will influence a pathway known to be dysfunctional in a given neurodevelopmental disorder when there are few or no efficacy data or no currently available biomarker that could predict efficacy. For many medications, individual trials are carried out, often off-label, to see if there is a benefit. This book is written to help clinicians guide these individual trials and to also become knowledgeable about even newer targeted treatments where efficacy data is (or will be) available. Parents are often desperate for guidance in what may be helpful, and the astute psychopharmacologist will consider a variety of interventions, even dietary changes. Choosing among antipsychotics, mood stabilizers, antidepressants, and alpha-adrenergic agonists for the management of irritability is now based on symptoms and educated guessing. Biomarker targets will be helpful in selecting the treatment most likely to be of benefit and adjusting the approach when one strategy is not successful.

Nutrition and Sleep Are Important Issues for Treatment

Nutrition, particularly in early childhood, is very important because of the widespread evidence of mitochondrial problems and oxidative stress in cells with a mutation leading to neurodevelopmental disorders. Although the research is limited for the benefit of antioxidants, there are a few studies in animals (de Diego-Otero, Romero-Zerbo, et al., 2009; Romero-Zerbo, Decara, et al., 2009) and in patients (Wirojanan, Jacquemont, et al., 2009; Hardan, Fung, et al., 2012) regarding the benefits of antioxidants such as N-acetylcysteine (NAC) or melatonin, also an antioxidant besides a sleep hormone. The benefits of uninterrupted sleep are also clear for behavior, in addition to solidifying the synaptic changes that occur during the day related to the stimulation received. Physicians can prescribe melatonin and other sleep-inducing medication to facilitate sleep, which is beneficial for brain development (and also parental sanity).

Antioxidants and Mitochondrial Dysfunction

The use of antioxidants has been essential for those with mitochondrial disorders caused by mutations either in the mitochondrial DNA or in the nuclear genes that produce a protein utilized in the mitochondria. However, the neurodevelopmental disorders discussed in this volume do not have a primary mitochondrial disorder, but instead mitochondrial dysfunction that is secondary to the primary genetic disorder. The treatments of mitochondrial disorders are very similar to the treatment principles of the neurodevelopmental disorders described in this volume. The general medical approach includes focusing on maintenance of optimum health; interventions for preventing, or aggressive management of physiological stressors, such as infections, dehydration, and surgeries, and avoidance of toxins. In mitochondrial disorders there is significant evidence regarding the benefit of using antioxidant supplements (Kelley, Frye, Delatorre, et al., 2013).

These treatments are aimed to promote critical enzymatic reactions, reduce sequelae of excess free radicals, and provide alternative energy sources for cell metabolism and energy production. Some supplements are intended to bypass biochemical blocks within the respiratory chain.

The mitochondrial disease patients have unique caloric needs compared to the general population, but perhaps similar to those with neurodevelopmental disorders that also have mitochondrial dysfunction. Optimization of the number and the quality of the calories is known to improve health in these patients. Mitochondrial disorders may manifest with gastrointestinal disturbances such as abnormal gut motility, swallowing dysfunction, and gastro-esophageal reflux, and the treatment of these issues may allow a more optimized caloric intake.

Avoidance of drugs with reported mitochondrial toxicity is also recommended. These include valproic acid, antiretrovirals, statins, aspirin, aminoglycosides, platinum chemotherapeutics, metformin, beta blockers, and steroids in some mitochondrial disorders such as Kearns-Sayre syndrome.

Treatments used with varying degrees of evidence include carnitine, coenzyme Q10, vitamin C, lipoic acid, pantothenate, and vitamin E (see Table 14.1). Coenzyme Q10 is synthesized in mammalian mitochondria and is an integral component of the mitochondrial respiratory electron transport chain, participating in redox shuttling.

Recently, reduced CoQ10 has become commercially available in the form of ubiquinone that has better absorption and efficacy. Recommended Ubiquinol doses are 2-8 mg/kg/day to be used twice daily, and it has been approved by the FDA for treatment of mitochondrial disease. The regimen of antioxidants outlined in Table 14.1 is for patients with mitochondrial disorders, but these can also be considered for neurodevelopmental disorders that have mitochondrial dysfunction. Mitochondrial dysfunction in children with ASD has been reviewed in detail, and mitochondrial dysfunction is the most common metabolic abnormality in these children (Giulivi, Zhang, et al., 2010). Several studies suggested that treatment with mitochondria cofactor supplementation, including antioxidants (vitamin C, carnosine, and glutathione), Coenzyme Q10, and B vitamins, may improve behavior in children with autism (Rossignol & Frye, 2012).

Avoidance of Toxins

An important aspect of nutrition and basic health is the avoidance of toxins. Since neurons with the mutations described in this volume are more vulnerable to cell death, they are generally considered to be more vulnerable to environmental toxins (discussed in Chapters 2 and 9). Since environmental neurotoxicants are common, the clinician should talk to the family regarding the avoidance of pesticides (consider the use of organic

Table 14.1 ANTIOXIDANTS TO USE IN TREATMENT OF
MITOCHONDRIAL DYSFUNCTION

First-Tier Supplements	
Supplement	Dose Range
CoQ10	5–15 mg/kg/day
Levo-carnitine	Variable, starting dose of 30 mg/kg/day, typical maximum of 100 mg/kg/day
Riboflavin (B2)	100–400 mg a day

Second-Tier Supplements	
Supplement	Dose Range
Acetyl-L-carnitine	250–1000 mg a day
Thiamine (B1)	50–100 mg a day
Nicotinamide (B3)	50–100 mg a day
Vitamin E	200–400 IU; 1–3 times a day
Vitamin C	100–500 mg; 1–3 times a day
Lipoic acid (a-lipoate)	60–200 mg; 3 times a day
Selenium	25–50 micrograms a day
b-carotene	10,000 IU; every other day to daily
Biotin	2.5–10 mg a day
Folic acid	1–10 mg a day

products), avoidance of top-carnivore fish that have high mercury levels (such as sharks, swordfish, dolphins), avoidance of flame retardants that are now in some types of furniture, to name a few. The avoidance of substances of abuse is also important to discuss with the family and with the patient directly. This is mainly an issue in those who are high-functioning or have normal cognitive abilities but are at risk for neuropsychiatric problems or neurodegeneration, such as premutation carriers who are at risk for FXTAS. Upregulation of the mGluR5 system is also associated with drug abuse (Blednov & Adron Harris, 2008; Schumann, Johann, et al., 2008), and this is common in teenage premutation carriers but less common in those with ASD who are high-functioning.

A recent report from Westmark (Westmark, 2014) has demonstrated that the use of soy infant formula is associated with an increased risk of seizures in those with ASD. She found that 17.5% of children with ASD in the Simons data base of several hundred patients used soy formulas. Soy has a protein, daidzein, which is a phytoestrogen that upregulates the mGluR5 pathway and increases seizure risk. There is a 2.6-fold higher rate of febrile seizures, 2.1-fold higher rate of epilepsy comorbidity, and a 4-fold higher rate of simple partial seizures in autistic children fed a soy-based formula compared to those who did not receive soy. Therefore it is recommended that children with ASD and also children with fragile X syndrome avoid soy formulas and perhaps soy products in general.

Currently Available Targeted Treatments

The use of currently available targeted treatments is recommended, including the use of minocycline or lithium in fragile X syndrome (Chapter 9); and the use of SSRIs when depression, anxiety, or obsessive compulsive behavior are present clinically in psychiatric disorders, *FMR1* premutation carriers, those with a full mutation, and in selected cases of ASD as outlined in Chapter 2. Minocycline also appears to be beneficial in Angelman syndrome from preliminary reports (Chapter 10).

The use of SSRIs to stimulate neurogenesis in Down syndrome and perhaps other disorders has not been investigated, but these medications are beginning to show promise in stimulating language in fragile X syndrome (Winarni, Schneider, et al., 2012) and perhaps in young children with ASD (DeLong, Ritch, et al., 2002; Chugani, 2005). Because they stimulate the expression of BDNF in addition to neurogenesis, which are both beneficial to many neurodevelopmental disorders, SSRIs are perhaps underutilized currently. Exercise can also stimulate neurogenesis, and this can be prescribed not only for children, but also for their parents and aging individuals in the family, particularly if they are at risk for neurodegeneration. It is essential that the clinician inquire about and perhaps suggests treatment of health/psychiatric problems of the parents of children with neurodevelopmental disorders, since depression, anxiety, and significant stress are common problems that impact the health of the child with a neurodevelopmental disorder and the whole family.

DIGITAL TECHNOLOGY

Currently the new generation of digital technology called *touch-screen* devices is valuable in the psycho-educational approach to treating neurodevelopmental disorders. However, implementation is limited by the paucity of clinical studies demonstrating its efficacy, and by the lack of a therapeutic consensus of good practices in the use of these appliances for intervention (Maglione, Gans, et al., 2012).

Touch-screen technologies such as the iPAD and other tablets are used by children and young adults with developmental difficulties in the academic setting, and it is also common to see families carrying several devices for their children's entertainment and even for managing unwanted behaviors. Parents intuitively learn how to provide their child with striking applications, cartoons, movies, books, etc.; however, not always within a framework of education and learning.

The great majority of existing literature reveals that touch-screen devices can be successfully utilized within educational programs targeting academic, communication, employment, and leisure skills for individuals with neurodevelopmental disorders (Kagohara, van der Meer, et al., 2013). Success relies on the use of well-established instructional procedures based on the principles of applied behavioral analysis or other specific models integrated in the community and/or the family.

Some studies generally describe children with typical development as "encountering" technologies in the home, because this suggests fleeting or unplanned practices rather than a predictable pattern of use (Plowman et al., 2012; Plowman & McPake, 2013). In our clinical practice with families of children with neurodevelopmental disorders, we also found that ownership does not guarantee parental engagement in supporting their child's use for educational purposes. This is the main reason why we offered advice to parents so they could make a difference in their child's development through the use of an iPAD program at home.

There are more than 26,000 applications in Education at the App Store from the iphone (Shen, Zhang, et al., 2012) with an extraordinary increase in the last three years. Clinicians need to review them and advise parents on which are the more suitable applications for their child's profile and needs. Parents need to identify how technology can support their children to accomplish learning objectives (Weiqin, 2012). The iPads or tablets, when coupled with effective applications such as Proloquo2Go or PiktoPlus, can also be augmentative communication devices.

The MIND APPs project is an emerging model that integrates technology at home for enhancing language development, social communication skills, and learning strategies in children with neurodevelopmental disorders. The model provides active psycho-educational guidance to parents about touch-screen technology and generates a list of applications fully adjusted and individualized to their needs and the goals they aim to achieve with their child. It is also important to assess the level of expertise and the motor control skills of the child before implementing the program so we know their competence.

Clinicians are called to acquire expertise in this area of intervention and guide parents and school professionals to be coordinated under the same "digital umbrella" by sharing apps that contain joint behavioral strategies, academic goals, social skills, language competences, and daily life activities.

Below are some interesting links, an explanatory picture of the psycho-educational approach used in the model (Figure 14.1), and a list of the main applications utilized by children with a variety of neurodevelopmental disorders such as ASD and fragile X syndrome (Table 14.2). This list will give preliminary guidance for the family, and it is recommended that children with neurodevelopmental disorders work with a learning specialist to further incorporate the appropriate apps into their learning curriculum. Speech and language therapists may also utilize these applications in their work with children with neurodevelopmental disorders. The use of a multidisciplinary team that also includes speech and language therapy, physical therapy and occupational therapy, particularly with a sensory integration approach, is critical for the success of the child with neurodevelopmental disorders in school and at home.

LINKS

http://a4cwsn.com/
http://www.iautism.info/en/
http://readingroom.mindspec.org/?page_id=10603

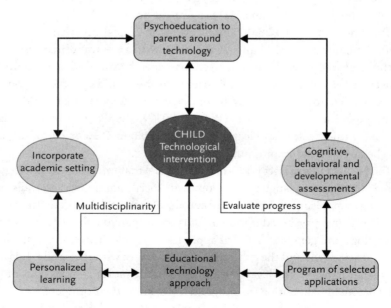

Figure 14.1:
Overview of digital technology use.

Table 14.2 APPLICATIONS BY CATEGORY OF LEARNING

Category	Description	App	Category	Description	App
Social apps	These applications are specifically designed for children and adolescents to improve their social cognition and theory of mind. Acquiring social thinking is critical in their development.	Social Express Social Quest Between the Lines FindMe Full social skillB Happy Geese Feel electric! Social Adventures	Learning apps	There are many applications for promoting learning, mainly writing, spelling, tracing, and reading comprehension. Also for enhancing memory, attention, and first learnings for toddlers.	iWriteWords Touch Write Sorting 1, 2, 3 Endless ABC Articulation PRO iSequences Injini Visual Attention
Sensory apps	Beautiful interactive realtime fluid dynamics simulation, control fluid flow and stunning colors at the tips of children's fingers. Points of light and sensations across the screen.	Somantics Reactickles Magic Balls Happy Bubbles Sound Box Fireworks Arcade Sea Creatures Live Artist	Motor control apps	Apps that promote the coordination of small muscle movements that occur in body parts such as the fingers, usually in coordination with the eyes. Dexterity is the basis of future learnings.	Playmatic play lab Blackboard BeBop Blox Toca Builders Tangrams FingerFun Dexteria Jr.

(continued)

Table 14.2 CONTINUED

Category	Description	App	Category	Description	App
Play apps	Playing is the best framework to encourage social interaction and cooperative skills. These apps provide a dynamic environment for sharing and having fun together.	Pepi Bath Pepi Tree Toca Kitchen Toca Doctor Let's create! Jelly Toons Go Go Games	Parents' apps	These apps help parents better understand and manage their child's behavior. These Apps promote structure and scheduling, & also provide information and tracking resources.	iPrompts PRO Sharing Timer AbaPlanet AutismApps Maily Timbuktu Care Circles
Language apps	Verbal ability is boosted through the use of these applications, specifically designed to stimulate both the receptive and the expressive channel.	Pictello Kit in story Language Empires Seek and Find 100 Words Special Words	Emotion apps	Emotional Intelligence-EQ is part of our well-being. These apps provide strategies for children to properly regulate their mood and self-esteem and increase their self-awareness.	Emotionary Smiling Mind Positive Penguins Be confident! Book Zones of regulation MeMoves

http://www.autismspeaks.org/autism-apps
http://www.dart.ed.ac.uk/wp-content/uploads/2013/07/
  MIND-APPs-guidelines_082013.pdf
http://www.coolmomtech.com/2013/04/tips-for-managing-kids-screen-t
  ime.php

FUTURE THERAPY

Not a day goes by without at least one family wanting to know about the
use of stem cells to treat neurodevelopmental disorders, so the following is
a current response to such questions.

Stem cells are under investigation or being considered to treat many neurodevelopmental disorders and neurodegenerative disorders. An important
distinction when considering different stem and progenitor cell candidates
is that some types may actually replace lost or damaged neurons, while
other types exert their effects by influencing neural cell growth, survival,
and neurite extension through factors that they secrete. In general, neural
stem cells and fetal neural progenitors are thought to be the only cell types
to actually generate neurons, while other cell types such as mesenchymal
stem cells/marrow stromal cells (MSCs) and astrocytes can produce factors
that encourage existing neurons to remain viable or to reconnect.

There is evidence in preclinical models that MSCs or astrocytes can
be used to treat neurodegenerative diseases through providing neurotrophic factors to encourage repair and potentially new growth of neurons. Therapies will capitalize upon the innate trophic support from the
cells or on augmented growth factor support, such as glial-derived neurotrophic factor (GDNF) to go into the brain to support injured neurons,
using genetically engineered stem/progenitor cells as the delivery vehicles
(Suzuki, McHugh, et al., 2007; Ramaswamy, Soderstrom, et al., 2009;
Sadan, Shemesh, et al., 2009; Dey, Bombard, et al., 2010; Olson, Pollock,
et al., 2012; Krakora, Mulcrone, et al., 2013).

For neurodegenerative disorders such as Huntington's disease (HD),
fetal striatal progenitor implantation techniques and protocols have been
well described by Dr. Bachoud-Levi and colleagues in France (Bachoud-Levi,
Gaura, et al., 2006), and by a group led by Rosser and Dunnet in the United
Kingdom (Dunnett & Rosser, 2011). The French group is currently conducting Phase II clinical trials (grants.gov trial #NCT00190450). HD
patients treated with fetal striatal neurons have safely received immuno-
suppression for 6–24 months, and the injections have proven safe (Rosser,
Barker, et al., 2002; Bachoud-Levi, Gaura, et al., 2006). Bachoud-Lévi and

colleagues transplanted human fetal neurons into the brains of five patients with HD (Gaura, Bachoud-Levi, et al., 2004; Bachoud-Levi, Gaura, et al., 2006). Three out of five patients with HD produced motor and cognitive improvements two years after the fetal neural graft. The group obtained convincing evidence that these human fetal striatal grafts were capable of reconnection and activation of the frontal lobes. Clinical improvement plateaued after two years, and then faded off variably four to six years after the implantation (Gaura, Bachoud-Levi, et al., 2004; Bachoud-Levi, Gaura, et al., 2006). These and other studies demonstrate that fetal striatal neurons can be safely implanted into the brain without adverse events, and they appear to have restorative effects in neurodegenerative disease.

Neurodevelopmental disorders are harder to envision treating through stem cell therapy currently, largely due to an incomplete understanding of the causes of some of the disorders, such as ASD. Mesenchymal stem cell (MSC) therapy has been proposed as a treatment for autism (Siniscalco, Sapone, et al., 2012). It is tempting to think that, since MSCs can have a significant positive effect in animal models of neurodegenerative disease (reviewed in Joyce, Annett, et al., 2010; and Olson, Pollock, et al., 2012) that some of these beneficial effects might extend to neurodevelopmental disorders. For instance, in addition to enhancing neural survival and encouraging neurite extension, MSCs have well-documented immunomodulatory effects (Le Blanc, 2006; English & Mahon, 2011). In ASD, innate and adaptive immunity changes have been reported (Gupta, Samra, et al., 2010). Patients with ASD show an imbalance in CD3$^+$, CD4$^+$, and CD8$^+$ T cells, and in natural killer (NK) cells. Long-term immune alterations have been documented (Enstrom, Onore, et al., 2010). However, whether MSC-mediated immunomodulatory activity could restore this immune imbalance, or would result in further deficits, is so far unknown.

There are presently no definitive studies on the use of MSCs in ASD models. There has been, however, one clinical trial (NCT01343511: see http://www.clinicaltrial.gov/) to test the safety and efficacy of human umbilical cord mesenchymal stem cells and human cord-blood mononuclear cell transplantation in patients with autism. The trials were completed in China in May, 2011, and reported recently (Lv, Zhang, et al., 2013). Transplantations included four stem cell infusions through intravenous and intrathecal injections once a week. The Childhood Autism Rating Scale (CARS), Clinical Global Impression (CGI) scale, and Aberrant Behavior Checklist (ABC) were used to evaluate the therapeutic efficacy at baseline (pre-treatment) and following treatment. There were no severe adverse events, and the patients were reported to have some improvement in symptoms (Lv, Zhang, et al., 2013).

In this age of all types of information being readily available on the Internet, parents of children with neurodevelopmental disorders can easily find descriptions of clinics offering unproven stem cell interventions. It is important to keep in mind that these interventions are often characterized by undetermined efficacy and safety. There are many clinics, unfortunately, that offer "stem cell tourism" for therapies that may be currently considered premature by the U.S. Food & Drug Administration. Bell et al. offer advice to clinicians for responding to parents inquiring about stem cell therapy and hyperbaric oxygen chambers in cerebral palsy, a leading cause of pediatric physical disability (Bell, Wallace, et al., 2011). Further discussion on stem cell tourism was covered by the national television show *60 Minutes* in a segment called "21st Century Snakeoil," and it is also available in the literature (Sleeboom-Faulkner, 2013). Mason et al. urge interested parties to beware of "predators disguised as life-saving physicians" (Mason & Manzotti, 2010). Useful information is found on websites hosted by the International Society for Stem Cell Research (http://www.closerlookatstemcells.org/) and the California Institute for Regenerative Medicine (http://www.cirm. ca.gov/about-stem-cells/concerns-about-stem-cell-tourism).

An interesting application of stem cells to research on neurodevelopmental disorders is through the examination of neurons derived from the induced pluripotent stem cell (iPSC) lines developed from patients with different known genetic alterations. These lines are useful tools in developing a better understanding of the disorders and how genetic alterations affect developing neurons. Our group used this technology to examine the fragile X-associated tremor ataxia syndrome (FXTAS) (Chapter 9). FXTAS arises through a toxic gain of function of the expanded CGG-repeat in the premutation range in *FMR1*, leading to excess *FMR1*-mRNA (Garcia-Arocena & Hagerman, 2010). As with many neurodevelopmental disorders, a lack of human neuronal models has impeded the understanding of the exact molecular mechanisms underlying the disease at the cellular level. In part, this is due to the fact that the mouse models do not fully recapitulate the clinical human FXTAS phenotype (Berman & Willemsen, 2009; Hunsaker, Arque, et al., 2012).

We produced iPSC-derived neurons from patients with FXTAS and demonstrated that neurons differentiated from them had reduced PSD95 protein expression, reduced synaptic puncta density, and reduced neurite length (Liu, Koscielska, et al., 2012). Importantly, such neurons are also functionally abnormal, with calcium transients of higher amplitude and increased frequency than for neurons harboring the normal-active allele. Moreover, sustained calcium elevation was found in these neurons after glutamate application. Thus we demonstrated neuronal phenotypes directly linked to the *FMR1* premutation to aid the development of targeted therapeutics for FXTAS, and more broadly as a model for the study of neurodevelopmental and neurodegenerative disorders (Liu, Koscielska, et al., 2012).

Other groups have used similar techniques to examine neurons differentiated from the iPSC lines generated from patients with Rett syndrome (Marchetto, Carromeu, et al., 2010; Kim, Hysolli, et al., 2011), a variety of ASDs (Chailangkarn, Acab, et al., 2012; Kim, Jung, et al., 2012), and additional neurodevelopmental disorders (Juopperi, Song, et al., 2011; Mattis & Svendsen, 2011). The use of patient-derived neurons to examine the molecular basis of disease in the relevant cell type is a powerful new model to better understand the disorders and to inform development of novel therapeutics as described in many of the chapters in this book.

CONCLUSION

This is an exciting time to be in the field of neurodevelopmental disorders with the advent of targeted treatments that will change the lives of many with the disorders that we are now treating. It is difficult for the clinician to keep up with the pace of new developments, and this book is designed to make this easier and exciting for the clinician. We learn every day from the parents and children that we are treating and from the researchers working with the animal models. This book will hopefully be a framework on which one can pin on new developments as they arise.

DISCLOSURES

Conflicts: Dr. Hagerman has received funding from Novartis, Roche, Seaside Therapeutics, Curemark, and Forest for treatment trials in fragile X syndrome and autism. She has also consulted with Genentech, Roche, and Novartis regarding treatment trials.

Dr. Hendren has received research grants from Forest Pharmaceuticals, Inc., Curemark, BioMarin Pharmaceutical, Roche, Shire, Autism Speaks, the Vitamin D Council, and the National Institute of Mental Health, and is on advisory boards for BioMarin, Forest, Coronado, BioZeus, and Janssen. The other authors have nothing to disclose.

Acknowledgments: This work was supported by grants from National Institute of Health: grants HD036071, the Autism Research Training Program grant CASADEVALL; R40MC22641; Department of Defense grant

PR101054, support from the Health and Human Services Administration on Developmental Disabilities grant 90DD05969; and the National Center for Advancing Translational Research UL1 TR000002.

REFERENCES

Abu-Elneel, K., Liu, T., Gazzaniga, F. S., Nishimura, Y., Wall, D. P., Geschwind, D. H., Lao, K., et al. (2008). Heterogeneous dysregulation of microRNAs across the autism spectrum. *Neurogenetics, 9*(3), 153–161.

Bachoud-Levi, A. C., Gaura, V., Brugieres, P., Lefaucheur, J. P., Boisse, M. F., Maison, P., Baudic, S., et al. (2006). Effect of fetal neural transplants in patients with Huntington's disease 6 years after surgery: A long-term follow-up study. *Lancet Neurology, 5*(4), 303–309.

Bagni, C., Tassone, F., Neri, G., & Hagerman, R. (2012). Fragile X syndrome: causes, diagnosis, mechanisms, and therapeutics. *The Journal of Clinical Investigation, 122*(12), 4314–4322.

Barichello, T., Santos, A. L., Savi, G. D., Generoso, J. S., Otaran, P., Michelon, C. M., Steckert, A. V., et al. (2012). Antioxidant treatment prevents cognitive impairment and oxidative damage in pneumococcal meningitis survivor rats. *Metabolic Brain Disease, 27*(4), 587–593.

Bell, E., Wallace, T., Chouinard, I., Shevell, M., & Racine, E. (2011). Responding to requests of families for unproven interventions in neurodevelopmental disorders: Hyperbaric oxygen treatment and stem cell therapy in cerebral palsy. *Developmental Disabilities Research Reviews, 17*(1), 19–26.

Berman, R. F., & Willemsen, R. (2009). Mouse models of fragile X-associated tremor ataxia. *Journal of Investigative Medicine, 57*(8), 837–841.

Bernard, P. B., Castano, A. M., O'Leary, H., Simpson, K., Browning, M. D., & Benke, T. A. (2013). Phosphorylation of FMRP and alterations of FMRP complex underlie enhanced mLTD in adult rats triggered by early life seizures. *Neurobiology of Disease, 59,* 1–17.

Berry-Kravis, E., Sumis, A., Hervey, C., Nelson, M., Porges, S. W., Weng, N., Weiler, I. J., et al. (2008). Open-label treatment trial of lithium to target the underlying defect in fragile X syndrome. *Journal of Developmental & Behavioral Pediatrics, 29*(4), 293–302.

Blednov, Y. A., & Adron Harris, R. (2008). Metabotropic glutamate receptor 5 (mGluR5) regulation of ethanol sedation, dependence and consumption: Relationship to acamprosate actions. *The International Journal of Neuropsychopharmacology, 11*(06), 775–793.

Cao, Z., Hulsizer, S., Cui, Y., Pretto, D. L., Kim, K. H., Hagerman, P. J., Tassone, F., et al. (2013). Enhanced asynchronous Ca(2+) oscillations associated with impaired glutamate transport in cortical astrocytes expressing Fmr1 gene premutation expansion. *Journal of Biological Chemistry, 288*(19), 13831–13841.

CBS's 60 Minutes (U.S.). 2010 segment: 21st Century Snake Oil.

Chailangkarn, T., Acab, A., & Muotri, A. R. (2012). Modeling neurodevelopmental disorders using human neurons. *Current Opinion in Neurobiology, 22*(5), 785–790.

Chugani, D. C. (2005). Pharmacological intervention in autism: Targeting critical periods of brain development. *Clinical Neuropsychiatry, 2,* 346–353.

Dansie, L. E., Phommahaxay, K., Okusanya, A. G., Uwadia, J., Huang, M., Rotschafer, S. E., Razak, K. A., et al. (2013). Long-lasting effects of minocycline on behavior in young but not adult fragile X mice. *Neuroscience, 246,* 186–198.

Dawson, G. (2013). Early intensive behavioral intervention appears beneficial for young children with autism spectrum disorders. *The Journal of Pediatrics, 162*(5), 1080–1081.

de Diego-Otero, Y., Romero-Zerbo, Y., el Bekay, R., Decara, J., Sanchez, L., Rodriguez-de Fonseca, F., & del Arco-Herrera, I. (2009). Alpha-tocopherol protects against oxidative stress in the fragile X knockout mouse: An experimental therapeutic approach for the Fmr1 deficiency. *Neuropsychopharmacology, 34*(4), 1011–1026.

DeLong, G. R., Ritch, C. R., & Burch, S. (2002). Fluoxetine response in children with autistic spectrum disorders: Correlation with familial major affective disorder and intellectual achievement. *Developmental Medicine & Child Neurology, 44*(10), 652–659.

Dey, N. D., Bombard, M. C., Roland, B. P., Davidson, S., Lu, M., Rossignol, J., Sandstrom, M. I., et al. (2010). Genetically engineered mesenchymal stem cells reduce behavioral deficits in the YAC 128 mouse model of Huntington's disease. *Behavioural Brain Research, 214*(2), 193–200.

Diniz, B. S., Machado-Vieira, R., & Forlenza, O. V. (2013). Lithium and neuroprotection: Translational evidence and implications for the treatment of neuropsychiatric disorders. *Neuropsychiatric Disease & Treatment, 9,* 493–500.

Dunnett, S. B., & Rosser, A. E. (2011). Cell-based treatments for Huntington's disease. *International Review of Neurobiology, 98,* 483–508.

Dunnett, S. B., & Rosser, A. E. (2011). Clinical translation of cell transplantation in the brain. *Current Opinion in Organ Transplantation, 16*(6), 632–639.

English, K., & Mahon, B. P. (2011). Allogeneic mesenchymal stem cells: Agents of immune modulation. *Journal of Cellular Biochemistry, 112*(8), 1963–1968.

Enstrom, A. M., Onore, C. E., Van de Water, J. A., & Ashwood, P. (2010). Differential monocyte responses to TLR ligands in children with autism spectrum disorders. *Brain, Behavior, & Immunity, 24*(1), 64–71.

Farzin, F., Rivera, S. M., & Whitney, D. (2011). Resolution of spatial and temporal visual attention in infants with fragile X syndrome. *Brain, 134*(11), 3355–3368.

Fatemi, S. H., & Folsom, T. D. (2011a). The role of fragile x mental retardation protein in major mental disorders. *Neuropharmacology, 60,* 1221–1226.

Fatemi, S. H., & Folsom, T. D. (2011b). Dysregulation of fragile X mental retardation protein and metabotropic glutamate receptor 5 in superior frontal cortex of individuals with autism: A postmortem brain study. *Molecular Autism, 2*(6), 1–11.

Fatemi, S. H., Folsom, T. D., Kneeland, R. E., Yousefi, M. K., Liesch, S. B., & Thuras, P. D. (2013). Impairment of fragile X mental retardation protein-metabotropic glutamate receptor 5 signaling and its downstream cognates Ras-related C3 botulinum toxin substrate 1, amyloid beta A4 precursor protein, striatal-enriched protein tyrosine phosphatase, and homer 1, in autism: A postmortem study in cerebellar vermis and superior frontal cortex. *Molecular Autism, 4*(1), 21.

Fatemi, S. H., Reutiman, T. J., Folsom, T. D., Rooney, R. J., Patel, D. H., & Thuras, P. D. (2010). mRNA and protein levels for GABAAα4, α5, β1 and GABABR1 receptors are altered in brains from subjects with autism. *Journal of Autism and Developmental Disorders, 40*(6), 743–750.

Fatemi, S. H., Reutiman, T. J., Folsom, T. D., & Thuras, P. D. (2009). GABAA receptor downregulation in brains of subjects with autism. *Journal of Autism and Developmental Disorders, 39*(2), 223–230.

Fatemi, S. H., Snow, A. V., Stary, J. M., Araghi-Niknam, M., Reutiman, T. J., Lee, S., Brooks, A. I., et al. (2005). Reelin signaling is impaired in autism. *Biological Psychiatry, 57*(7), 777–787.

Folsom, T. D., & Fatemi, S. H. (2013). The involvement of Reelin in neurodevelopmental disorders. *Neuropharmacology, 68,* 122–135.

Frye, R. E., Delatorre, R., Taylor, H., Slattery, J., Melnyk, S., Chowdhury, N., & James, S. J. (2013). Redox metabolism abnormalities in autistic children associated with mitochondrial disease. *Translational Psychiatry, 3*, e273.

Garcia-Arocena, D., & Hagerman, P. J. (2010). Advances in understanding the molecular basis of FXTAS. *Human Molecular Genetics, 19*(R1), R83–R89.

Gaura, V., Bachoud-Levi, A. C., Ribeiro, M. J., Nguyen, J. P., Frouin, V., Baudic, S., Brugieres, P., et al. (2004). Striatal neural grafting improves cortical metabolism in Huntington's disease patients. *Brain, 127*(Pt 1), 65–72.

Gervain, J., & Mehler, J. (2010). Speech perception and language acquisition in the first year of life. *Annual Review of Psychology, 61,* 191–218.

Giulivi, C., Zhang, Y. F., Omanska-Klusek, A., Ross-Inta, C., Wong, S., Hertz-Picciotto, I., Tassone, F., et al. (2010). Mitochondrial dysfunction in autism. *JAMA: The Journal of the American Medical Association, 304*(21), 2389–2396.

Gupta, S., Samra, D., & Agrawal, S. (2010). Adaptive and innate immune responses in autism: Rationale for therapeutic use of intravenous immunoglobulin. *Journal of Clinical Immunology, 30*(Suppl 1), 90–96.

Hagerman, R., & Hagerman, P. (2013). Advances in clinical and molecular understanding of the FMR1 premutation and fragile X-associated tremor/ataxia syndrome. *Lancet Neurology, 12*(8), 786–798.

Hagerman, R. J. (2013). Epilepsy drives autism in neurodevelopmental disorders. *Developmental Medicine & Child Neurology, 55*(2), 101–102.

Hansen, K. F., & Obrietan, K. (2013). MicroRNA as therapeutic targets for treatment of depression. *Neuropsychiatric Disease & Treatment, 9,* 1011–1021.

Hardan, A. Y., Fung, L. K., Libove, R. A., Obukhanych, T. V., Nair, S., Herzenberg, L. A., Frazier, T. W., et al. (2012). A randomized controlled pilot trial of oral N-acetylcysteine in children with autism. *Biological Psychiatry, 71*(11), 956–961.

Hoeffer, C. A., Sanchez, E., Hagerman, R. J., Mu, Y., Nguyen, D. V., Wong, H., Whelan, A. M., et al. (2012). Altered mTOR signaling and enhanced CYFIP2 expression levels in subjects with fragile X syndrome. *Genes, Brain, and Behavior, 11*(3), 332–341. PMID:22268788 PMCID:PMC23319643.

Hunsaker, M. R., Arque, G., Berman, R. F., Willemsen, R., & Hukema, R. K. (2012). Mouse models of the fragile X premutation and the fragile X associated tremor/ataxia syndrome. *Results & Problems in Cell Differentiation, 54,* 255–269.

Im, H. I., & Kenny, P. J. (2012). MicroRNAs in neuronal function and dysfunction. *Trends in Neuroscience, 35*(5), 325–334.

Jacquemont, S., Curie, A., des Portes, V., Torrioli, M. G., Berry-Kravis, E., Hagerman, R. J., Ramos, F. J., et al. (2011). Epigenetic modification of the FMR1 gene in fragile X syndrome is associated with differential response to the mGluR5 antagonist AFQ056. *Science Translational Medicine, 3*(64), 64ra61.

Ji, F., Lv, X., & Jiao, J. (2013). The role of microRNAs in neural stem cells and neurogenesis. *Journal of Genetics & Genomics, 40*(2), 61–66.

Joyce, N., Annett, G., Wirthlin, L., Olson, S., Bauer, G., & Nolta, J. A. (2010). Mesenchymal stem cells for the treatment of neurodegenerative disease. *Regenerative Medicine, 5*(6), 933–946.

Juopperi, T. A., Song, H., & Ming, G. L. (2011). Modeling neurological diseases using patient-derived induced pluripotent stem cells. *Future Neurology, 6*(3), 363–373.

Kagohara, D. M., van der Meer, L., Ramdoss, S., O'Reilly, M. F., Lancioni, G. E., Davis, T. N., et al. (2013). Using iPods® and iPads® in teaching programs for individuals with developmental disabilities: A systematic review. *Research in Developmental Disabilities, 34*(1), 147–156.

Keck-Wherley, J., Grover, D., Bhattacharyya, S., Xu, X., Holman, D., Lombardini, E. D., Verma, R., et al. (2011). Abnormal microRNA expression in Ts65Dn hippocampus and whole blood: Contributions to Down syndrome phenotypes. *Developmental Neuroscience, 33*(5), 451–467.

Kelemen, O., Kovács, T., & Kéri, S. (2013). Contrast, motion, perceptual integration, and neurocognition in schizophrenia: The role of fragile-X related mechanisms. *Progress in Neuro-Psychopharmacology and Biological Psychiatry, 46*(0), 92–97.

Kelley, R. I. (2009). Evaluation and treatment of patients with autism and mitochondrial disease.

Kéri, S., & Benedek, G. (2011). Fragile X protein expression is linked to visual functions in healthy male volunteers. *Neuroscience, 192,* 345–350.

Kim, K. Y., Hysolli, E., & Park, I. H. (2011). Neuronal maturation defect in induced pluripotent stem cells from patients with Rett syndrome. *Proceedings of the National Academy of Science, USA, 108*(34), 14169–14174.

Kim, K. Y., Jung, Y. W., Sullivan, G. J., Chung, L., & Park, I. H. (2012). Cellular reprogramming: A novel tool for investigating autism spectrum disorders. *Trends in Molecular Medicine, 18*(8), 463–471.

Kovács, T., Kelemen, O., & Kéri, S. (2013). Decreased fragile X mental retardation protein (FMRP) is associated with lower IQ and earlier illness onset in patients with schizophrenia. *Psychiatry Research.*

Krakora, D., Mulcrone, P., Meyer, M., Lewis, C., Bernau, K., Gowing, G., Zimprich, C., et al. (2013). Synergistic effects of GDNF and VEGF on lifespan and disease progression in a familial ALS rat model. *Molecular Therapy, 21*(8), 1602–1610.

Le Blanc, K. (2006). Mesenchymal stromal cells: Tissue repair and immune modulation. *Cytotherapy, 8*(6), 559–561.

Liu, J., Koscielska, K. A., Cao, Z., Hulsizer, S., Grace, N., Mitchell, G., Nacey, C., et al. (2012). Signaling defects in iPSC-derived fragile X premutation neurons. *Human Molecular Genetics, 21*(17), 3795–3805.

Lv, Y. T., Zhang, Y., Liu, M., Qiuwaxi, J. N., Ashwood, P., Cho, S. C., Huan, Y., et al. (2013). Transplantation of human cord blood mononuclear cells and umbilical cord-derived mesenchymal stem cells in autism. *Journal of Translational Medicine, 11*(1), 196.

Maglione, M. A., Gans, D., Das, L., Timbie, J., & Kasari, C. (2012). Nonmedical interventions for children with ASD: Recommended guidelines and further research needs. *Pediatrics, 130* Suppl 2: S169–S178.

Marchetto, M. C., Carromeu, C., Acab, A., Yu, D., Yeo, G. W., Mu, Y., Chen, G., et al. (2010). A model for neural development and treatment of Rett syndrome using human induced pluripotent stem cells. *Cell, 143*(4), 527–539.

Marsh, E. B., Freeman, J. M., Kossoff, E. H., Vining, E. P., Rubenstein, J. E., Pyzik, P. L., et al. (2006). The outcome of children with intractable seizures: A 3- to 6-year follow-up of 67 children who remained on the ketogenic diet less than one year. *Epilepsia, 47*(2), 425–430.

Martino, S., di Girolamo, I., Orlacchio, A., Datti, A., & Orlacchio, A. (2009). MicroRNA implications across neurodevelopment and neuropathology. *Journal of Biomedicine & Biotechnology, 2009,* 654346.

Mason, C., & Manzotti, E. (2010). Defeating stem cell tourism. Foreword. *Regenerative Medicine, 5*(5), 681–686.

Mattis, V. B., & Svendsen, C. N. (2011). Induced pluripotent stem cells: A new revolution for clinical neurology? Lancet Neurology, 10(4), 383–394.

Michalon, A., Sidorov, M., Ballard, T. M., Ozmen, L., Spooren, W., Wettstein, J. G., Jaeschke, G., et al. (2012). Chronic pharmacological mGlu5 inhibition corrects fragile X in adult mice. *Neuron*, *74*(1), 49–56.

Miller, B. H., Zeier, Z., Xi, L., Lanz, T. A., Deng, S., Strathmann, J., Willoughby, D., et al. (2012). MicroRNA-132 dysregulation in schizophrenia has implications for both neurodevelopment and adult brain function. *Proceedings of the National Academy of Science, USA*, *109*(8), 3125–3130.

Nudelman, I., Rebibo-Sabbah, A., Cherniavsky, M., Belakhov, V., Hainrichson, M., Chen, F., Schacht, J., et al. (2009). Development of novel aminoglycoside (NB54) with reduced toxicity and enhanced suppression of disease-causing premature stop mutations. *Journal of Medicinal Chemistry*, *52*(9), 2836–2845.

Olson, S. D., Pollock, K., Kambal, A., Cary, W., Mitchell, G. M., Tempkin, J., Stewart, H., et al. (2012). Genetically engineered mesenchymal stem cells as a proposed therapeutic for Huntington's disease. *Molecular Neurobiology*, *45*(1), 87–98.

Osterweil, E. K., Chuang, S. C., Chubykin, A. A., Sidorov, M., Bianchi, R., Wong, R. K., & Bear, M. F. (2013). Lovastatin corrects excess protein synthesis and prevents epileptogenesis in a mouse model of fragile X syndrome. *Neuron*, *77*(2), 243–250.

Plowman, L., & McPake, J. (2013). Seven myths about young children and technology. *Childhood Education*, *89*(1), 27–33.

Plowman, L., Stevenson O., Stephen C., & McPake J (2012). Preschool children's learning with technology at home. *Computers & Education*, *59*(1), 30–37.

Qureshi, I. A., Mattick, J. S., & Mehler, M. F. (2010). Long non-coding RNAs in nervous system function and disease. *Brain Research*, 1338, 20–35.

Ramaswamy, S., Soderstrom, K. E., & Kordower, J. H. (2009). Trophic factors therapy in Parkinson's disease. *Progress in Brain Research*, *175*, 201–216.

Rogers, S. J., Estes, A., Lord, C., Vismara, L., Winter, J., Fitzpatrick, A., Guo, M., & Dawson, G. (2012). Effects of a brief Early Start Denver model (ESDM)–based parent intervention on toddlers at risk for autism spectrum disorders: A randomized controlled trial. *Journal of the American Academy of Child & Adolescent Psychiatry*, *51*(10), 1052–1065.

Romero-Zerbo, Y., Decara, J., el Bekay, R., Sanchez-Salido, L., Del Arco-Herrera, I., de Fonseca, F. R., & de Diego-Otero, Y. (2009). Protective effects of melatonin against oxidative stress in Fmr1 knockout mice: A therapeutic research model for the fragile X syndrome. *Journal of Pineal Research*, *46*(2), 224–234.

Rosser, A. E., Barker, R. A., Harrower, T., Watts, C., Farrington, M., Ho, A. K., Burnstein, R. M., et al. (2002). Unilateral transplantation of human primary fetal tissue in four patients with Huntington's disease: NEST-UK safety report ISRCTN no. 36485475. *Journal of Neurology, Neurosurgery, & Psychiatry*, *73*(6), 678–685.

Rossignol, D. A., & Frye, R. E. (2012). A review of research trends in physiological abnormalities in autism spectrum disorders: Immune dysregulation, inflammation, oxidative stress, mitochondrial dysfunction and environmental toxicant exposures. *Molecular Psychiatry*, *17*(4), 389–401.

Sadan, O., Shemesh, N., Cohen, Y., Melamed, E., & Offen, D. (2009). Adult neurotrophic factor-secreting stem cells: A potential novel therapy for neurodegenerative diseases. *Israel Medical Association Journal*, *11*(4), 201–204.

Schumann, G., Johann, M., Frank, J., Preuss, U., Dahmen, N., Laucht, M., Rietschel, M., et al. (2008). Systematic analysis of glutamatergic neurotransmission genes in alcohol dependence and adolescent risky drinking behavior. *Archives of General Psychiatry*, *65*(7), 826.

Shen, L., Zhang, S., & Zhu, Y. (2012). Research on the design of optimizing the selection of iPad educational resources. *System of Systems Engineering* (Genoa, Italy) 789–792.

Siniscalco, D., Sapone, A., Cirillo, A., Giordano, C., Maione, S., & Antonucci, N. (2012). Autism spectrum disorders: Is mesenchymal stem cell personalized therapy the future? Journal of Biomedicine & Biotechnology, 2012, 480289.

Sleeboom-Faulkner, M. (2013). Experimental treatments: Regulating stem-cell therapies worldwide. *Nature*, *495*(7439), 47.

Suzuki, M., McHugh, J., Tork, C., Shelley, B., Klein, S. M., Aebischer, P., & Svendsen, C. N. (2007). GDNF secreting human neural progenitor cells protect dying motor neurons, but not their projection to muscle, in a rat model of familial ALS. *PLoS One*, *2*(1), e689.

Tal, T. L., & Tanguay, R. L. (2012). Non-coding RNAs—novel targets in neurotoxicity. *Neurotoxicology*, *33*(3), 530–544.

Utari, A., Adams, E., Berry-Kravis, E., Chavez, A., Scaggs, F., Ngotran, L., Boyd, A., et al. (2010). Aging in fragile X syndrome. *Journal of Neurodevelopmental Disorders*, *2*(2), 70–76.

Vaishnavi, V., Manikandan, M., Tiwary, B. K., & Munirajan, A. K. (2013). Insights on the functional impact of microRNAs present in autism-associated copy number variants. *PLoS One*, *8*(2), e56781.

van Eeghen, A. M., Pulsifer, M. B., Merker, V. L., Neumeyer, A. M., van Eeghen, E. E. Thibert, R. L., Cole, A. J., et al. (2013). Understanding relationships between autism, intelligence, and epilepsy: A cross-disorder approach. *Developmental Medicine & Child Neurology*, *55*(2), 146–153.

Wang, J. Y., Hessl, D., Iwahashi, C., Cheung, K., Schneider, A., Hagerman, R. J., Hagerman, P. J., et al. (2013). Influence of the fragile X mental retardation (FMR1) gene on the brain and working memory in men with normal FMR1 alleles. *Neuroimage*, *65*, 288–298.

Weiqin, C. (2012). Multitouch tabletop technology for people with autism spectrum disorder: A review of the literature. *Procedia Computer Science*, *14*, 198–207.

Westmark, C. (2014). Soy Infant formula and seizures in children with autism: A retrospective study. *PLoS One*, *9*(3), e80488.

Wilczynski, G. M., Konopacki, F. A., Wilczek, E., Lasiecka, Z., Gorlewicz, A., Michaluk, P., et al. (2008). Important role of matrix metalloproteinase 9 in epileptogenesis. *The Journal of Cell Biology*, *180*(5), 1021–1035.

Winarni, T. I., Schneider, A., Borodyanskara, M., & Hagerman, R. J. (2012). Early intervention combined with targeted treatment promotes cognitive and behavioral improvements in young children with fragile X syndrome. *Case Reports in Genetics*, *2012*, 280813.

Wirojanan, J., Jacquemont, S., Diaz, R., Bacalman, S., Anders, T. F., Hagerman, R. J., & Goodlin-Jones, B. L. (2009). The efficacy of melatonin for sleep problems in children with autism, fragile X syndrome, or autism and fragile X syndrome. *Journal of Clinical Sleep Medicine*, *5*(2), 145–150.

INDEX

fig denotes figure; *t* denotes table; **bold** denotes photo

monoamine oxidase–inhibiting (MAO-I) effects, 80
monoamines, 76, 80, 117, 134, 146–147
Morrison, A. P., 60
Morris Water Maze (MWM), 269
moving treatment targets, 13*fig*
Mowat Wilson syndrome, 243
mRNA, splicing of, 313*fig*
MR spectroscopy (MRS), 16
MSCs (mesenchymal stem cells/marrow stromal cells), 347–349
MTHFR, 76
mTOR (mammalian Target of Rapamycin), 178, 187–188, 192, 198, 335
mTORC1, 188
mTORC2, 188
mTOR inhibitors, 178, 194, 195, 204, 205, 206–207, 208
mTOR overactivation syndromes, 178, 188, 192–193, 198, 201
Multimodal Treatment of ADHD (MTA) study, 107, 116
muscular dystrophies
    asymmetrical scapular winging, **318**
    BMD. *See* Becker muscular dystrophy (BMD)
    DGC, 310*fig*
    diagnostic testing, 307–309
    DMD. *See* Duchenne muscular dystrophy (DMD)
    dystrophin gene, 312*fig*
    dystrophinopathies, 305–307
    facioscapulohumeral dystrophy, 317–320
    Gower's sign, **308**
    introduction, 305
    limb-girdlemuscular dystrophy, 321–327
    myotonic muscular dystrophy, types 1 and 2, 314–317
    percussion myotonia, **315**
    photos, **307**
    splicing of mRNA, 313*fig*
    summary of autosomal dominant and autosomal recessive subtypes of limb-girdlemuscular dystrophies, 322*t*–325*t*

summary of selected findings in Duchenne and Becker muscular dystrophy, 309*t*
translations (normal, incomplete, PTC-124-facilitated), 314*fig*
treatment, 309–314
MWM (Morris Water Maze), 269
myelin, 3, 295
myelination, 3, 55, 78, 162, 188, 276
myostatin inhibitors, 311, 320
myotonic dystrophy, 314–317, 320, 326
myotonic muscular dystrophy type 1 (DM1), 314–316, 320
myotonic muscular dystrophy type 2 (DM2), 316, 320

N-acetylcysteine (NAC), 33, 34, 92, 232, 339
NAChR (nicotinic acetylcholine receptor) agonists, 59
naltrexone, 32, 144, 151
NAP + SAL treatment, 276
NAPVSIPQ (NAP), 276
National Institute for Health and Clinical Excellence (NICE), 107
National Institute of Mental Health (NIMH), 14, 63
NE (norepinephrine). *See* norepinephrine (NE)
negative symptoms
    of psychosis, 49
    of schizophrenia, 44
nerve growth factor (NGF), 147, 279
Neul, J. L., 137
neuroanatomical and neurophysiological features, in MDD, 74–75
neurodegenerative disorders, commonalities with neurodevelopmental disorders, 335–337
neurodevelopment
    in DS, 275–276
    key elements in, 2–4
neurodevelopmental disorders, commonalities with neurodegenerative disorders, 335–337
neurodevelopmental perturbations in serotonin and dopamine neurotransmission, as epigenetic process, 11

peripheral blood mononuclear cells
(PBMCs), 88
pervasive developmental disorders
(PDD) category, 22–23
pesticides, 27, 340–341
Peters, S. U., 253
Peutz-Jeghers syndrome, 193
pharmacological treatments
for ADHD, currently, 116–120
for ADHD, future, 120–121
for MD, 317
Phelan-McDermid syndrome, 24
phenobarbital, 244
phenylalanine (Phe), 296, 297, 298, 299
phenylalanine ammonia lyase treatment,
301
phenylalanine hydroxylase (PAH), 294,
296, 297, 298, 299, 300, 301
phenylalanine hydroxylase deficiency
(PKU)
classification of, 297–298
clinical features of, 295
diagnosis and testing of, 296–297
GABA abnormalities, 334
introduction, 294
investigations/clinical trials under
way, 301–302
LNAA transporters, 299
molecular genetic testing, 297
phenylalanine ammonia lyase
treatment, 301
sapropterin treatment, 299–301
schematic role of sapropterin in
activation of phenylalanine
hydroxylase, 296fig
targeted treatments in, 298–302
traditional management of, 298
phenylketonuria
biology of, 296
clinical features of, 295
introduction, 294
PI3K inhibitors, 232
picrotoxin (PTX), 268
PiktoPlus, 343
Pitt Hopkins syndrome, 243
PKU diet, 300, 301
PKU/hyperphenylalaninemia, clinical
features of, 295
platinum chemotherapeutics, 340
PMDD, 84

POG2, 29
polybrominated diphenyl ethers
(PBDEs), 27
polyethylene glycol powder, 133
polymerase chain reaction (PCR), 220,
247
Pompe disease, 312
positive symptoms
of psychosis, 47–48, 48t
of schizophrenia, 44, 45
PositScience, 59
post-transcriptional regulation, 145
Povey, Sue, 186
Prader-Willi syndrome, 243, 245
primary ovarian insufficiency (FXPOI),
215, 219, 222
Premutation, 4,7,8,9,15,28,215,332,334,
336,341,342,349
Pringle, J. J., 177
PRKAG2, 192
Procentra, 117
prodromal syndromes, clinical high-
risk criteria from the structured
interview for, 51t
Proloquo2Go, 343
propranolol, 32
proximal myotonic myopathy (PROMM),
316
psychiatric and physical illness, model
of multiple pathways leading to,
83fig
psychosis
definition, 44, 54
early intervention programs and
cognitive therapy for, 59–60
PTC 124, 311
PTEN, 16, 24, 25, 28, 29, 193, 201
PTX (picrotoxin), 268
putative depressogenic circuits/tracts, 75

quetiapine, 57, 58
Quillivant XR, 117

R106W mutation, 135, 138
R133C mutation, 135, 137, 138, 145
R168X mutation, 137, 138
R255X mutation, 138
R270X mutation, 138
R294X mutation, 131, 137, 138
R306C mutation, 131, 138

Rogers, Sally, 222
"Rolando" variant of RTT, 132
ROS (reactive oxygen species), 8, 276, 277, 278, 336
Rosser, A. E., 347
RTK (receptor tyrosine kinases), 164
RTT (Rett syndrome). *See* Rett syndrome (RTT)

SALLRSIPA (SAL), 276
Sam 68, 9
Sampson, J. R., 203
Sapolsky, R. M., 82
sapropterin, 296*fig*, 299–301
sapropterin hydrochloride, 301
Sato, A., 202
scapulo-peroneal muscular dystrophy syndromes, 320
schizophrenia
    as "cancer of the mind," 46
    "common disease, common variant" hypothesis, 52
    "common disease, rare variant" hypothesis, 52
    computerized cognitive training for impaired neural system functioning, 61–63
    core clinical features of, 47–50, 48*t*
    definition, 44
    development of targeted treatments for, 56–63
    early detection of, 46–51
    early intervention programs and cognitive therapy for, 59–60
    environmental risk factors, 53–54
    epidemiological features of, 46–47
    essential features of, 46–51
    etiology and pathophysiology of, 51–56
    future directions for study of, 63
    GABA abnormalities, 334
    genetic risk factors, 51–53
    introduction, 44–46
    models of pathophysiology in, 55–56
    as neurocognitive disorder, 45
    as neurodevelopmental disorder, 45
    neurodevelopmental model of, 54*fig*
    onset and course of, 50–51
    pharmacological treatment landscape for, 57–59

shared polygenic variation between bipolar disorder and, 52
    stress-vulnerability model of, 55
scoliosis, 131, 132, 133, 161, 168, 241, 306, 309
Seaside Therapeutics, 33, 223, 224
SEGAs (subependymal giant cell astrocytomas), 178, 179, 190, 191, 194, 199, 203–205
seizures
    in AS, 242, 244, 332
    in ASD, 30, 332
    in CFC, 168
    as commonality across disorders, 332–333
    in FXS, 332
    in RTT, 133, 322
    in TSC, 189, 191, 194–195, 200, 332
sensory processing abnormalities, in schizophrenia, 49
Sequenced Treatment Alternatives to Relieve Depression (STAR*D), 81
serine/threonine kinase mammalian target of rapamycin (Akt-mTOR) pathway, 25, 29
serotonin, 11, 57, 76, 77, 79, 80, 81, 109, 119, 135, 146, 147, 149, 295, 336
serotonin-norepinephrine reuptake inhibitors (SNRIs), 91
serotonin reuptake inhibitors (SSRIs), 31, 84, 87, 91, 133, 197, 222, 272, 273, 342
sertraline, 222
serum brain-derived neurotrophic (BDNF), 62
serum creatine kinase, 307, 309, 316, 319, 326
SGS -111, 277
SHANK2, 24, 28
SHANK3, 24, 25
Sibutramine, 121
Silverman, J. L., 32
single nucleotide variations/mutations (SNVs), 15
SIRT1, 141
60 Minutes, 349
SLC6A4, 76
sleep, 242, 244, 339
    See also melatonin
"sleep clock," 34

TSAlliance (US), 198
TSC (tuberous sclerosis complex). *See*
    tuberous sclerosis complex (TSC)
TSC1, 24, 25, 178, 179, 180, 186, 187,
    188, 189, 203, 332
TSC1-TSC2 complex, as molecular
    switchboard, 187, 199
TSC2, 178, 179, 180, 186, 187, 188, 189,
    192, 193, 203, 332
TSC-Associated Neuropsychiatric
    Disorders Checklist (TAND
    Checklist), 191
TSCi (Tuberous Sclerosis Complex
    International), 198
tuberin, 178, 186
Tuberous Sclerosis Association (UK), 198
tuberous sclerosis complex (TSC)
    animal models of ASD in, 201
    animal models of epilepsy in, 200–202
    animal models of neurocognition in,
        199–200
    animal models of renal and skin
        manifestations, 199
    animal models of targeted treatments
        in, 198–202
    behavioral manifestations of, 180–183
    clinical diagnostic criteria, 189–190
    clinical features of, 179–186
    clinical trials in, 203–206
    clinical trials of neuropsychiatric
        manifestations and epilepsy,
        205–206
    clinical trials of SEGA, AML, and facial
        angiofibromata, 203–205
    clinical utility of mTOR inhibitors in,
        206–207
    current management of, 193–198
    diagnosis of, 189–191
    as disorder with variable expression,
        179
    future prospects for targeted
        treatments in, 207–208
    as having age-related expression of
        features, 179
    initial workup of newly diagnosed
        individuals, 190
    intellectual ability/disability, 184–185
    introduction, 177–178
    management of neuropsychiatric
        manifestations in, 195–196

    management of physical
        manifestations of, 194–195
    molecular mechanisms of, 186–189
    neuropsychiatric manifestations of,
        180
    neuropsychological profiles, 185–186
    physical characteristics of, 181*t*–182*t*
    physical manifestations of, 179–180
    psychiatric manifestations of,
        183–184
    related disorders, 191–193
    scholastic/academic disorders, 185
    seizures, 189, 191, 194–195, 200, 332
    signaling pathway, 187*fig*
    surveillance guidelines, 190–191
    targeted treatments in, 198–207
    upregulation of mTOR system, 335
Tuberous Sclerosis Complex
    International (TSCi), 198
TuberOus SClerosis registry to increase
    disease Awareness (TOSCA), 180
"21st Century Snakeoil," 349
tyrosine, 144, 146, 166, 296, 298, 299
tyrosine hydroxylase (TH), 146
tyrosine-related kinase B (TrkB),
    149–150

U0126 MEK1/2 inhibitor, 169
ube3a, 255
Ube3a, 248–249, 250
UBE3A deletion, 245
UBE3A gene, 24, 25, 245, 247, 248, 253,
    256
UBE3A mutation, 242, 246
Ubiquinol (ubiquinone), 340
uniparental disomy (UPD), 242,
    245–246, 247, 256
U.S. Food and Drug Administration
    (FDA), 120, 159, 178, 198, 199,
    204, 205, 206, 227, 230, 248, 249,
    310, 340
Utari, A., 229
utrophin upregulators, 311

vagal nerve stimulation (VNS), 195
valproate, 4, 133, 333
valproic acid, 4, 25, 244, 340
VAS (Visual Analog Scale), 226, 229, 231
vascular endothelial growth factor
    (VEGF), 335